Oncology
Lecture Notes

This title is also available as an e-book.
For more details, please see
www.wiley.com/buy/9781118842096
or scan this QR code:

Oncology
Lecture Notes

Mark Bower

Professor of Oncology
Chelsea and Westminster Hospital and
Imperial College School of Medicine
London, UK

Jonathan Waxman

Professor of Oncology
Hammersmith Hospital
Imperial College School of Medicine
London, UK

Third Edition

WILEY Blackwell

Registered office: John Wiley & Sons, Ltd, The Atrium, Southern Gate, Chichester, West Sussex,
PO19 8SQ, UK

Editorial offices: 9600 Garsington Road, Oxford, OX4 2DQ, UK
The Atrium, Southern Gate, Chichester, West Sussex, PO19 8SQ, UK
111 River Street, Hoboken, NJ 07030-5774, USA

For details of our global editorial offices, for customer services and for information about how to
apply for permission to reuse the copyright material in this book please see our website at
www.wiley.com/wiley-blackwell

Library of Congress Cataloging-in-Publication Data

Bower, Mark, author.
Lecture notes. Oncology / Mark Bower, Jonathan Waxman. – Third edition.
p. ; cm.
Oncology
Oncology lecture notes
Includes bibliographical references and index.
ISBN 978-1-118-84209-6 (pbk.)
I. Waxman, Jonathan, author.   II. Title.   III. Title: Oncology.   IV. Title: Oncology lecture notes.
[DNLM: 1. Neoplasms. QZ 200]
RC254.5
616.99′4–dc23

                            2015004427

A catalogue record for this book is available from the British Library.

Wiley also publishes its books in a variety of electronic formats. Some content that appears in print
may not be available in electronic books.

Cover image: Stockphoto@royalsrockphoto

Set in 8.5/11pt Utopia by Aptara Inc., New Delhi, India

1 2015

Contents

Preface, vi
About the companion website, vii

Part 1 Introduction to oncology

1 What is cancer?, 3

2 The scientific basis of cancer, 22

3 The principles of cancer treatment, 52

4 Cancer and people, 96

Part 2 Types of cancer

5 Breast cancer, 107

6 Central nervous system cancers, 116

7 Oesophageal cancer, 124

8 Gastric cancer, 128

9 Hepatobiliary cancer, 132

10 Pancreatic cancer, 137

11 Colorectal cancer, 143

12 Kidney cancer, 151

13 Bladder cancer, 156

14 Prostate cancer, 161

15 Testis cancer, 169

16 Gestational trophoblastic disease, 175

17 Cervical cancer, 178

18 Endometrial cancer, 183

19 Ovarian cancer, 186

20 Head and neck cancers, 193

21 Thyroid cancer, 200

22 Adrenal cancers, 203

23 Carcinoid tumours, 206

24 Pituitary tumours, 210

25 Parathyroid cancers, 212

26 Lung cancer, 214

27 Mesothelioma, 224

28 The leukaemias, 227

29 Hodgkin's lymphoma, 238

30 Non-Hodgkin's lymphoma, 244

31 Myeloma, 252

32 Non-melanoma skin tumours, 258

33 Melanoma, 264

34 Paediatric solid tumours, 271

35 Cancers in teenagers and young adults, 279

36 Bone and soft tissue sarcomas, 281

37 Cancer of unknown primary, 289

38 Immunodeficiency-related cancers, 295

Part 3 The practice of oncology

39 Paraneoplastic complications of cancer, 303

40 Oncological emergencies, 314

41 End of life care, 334

42 Cancer survivorship, 339

Index, 341

Preface

Cancer is fabulous, and without a doubt, the most interesting and exciting of all the medical specialities. So you were right to buy this book.

When the authors of *Lecture Notes in Oncology* entered specialty training, we were told by our learned professors and mentors that we had made great career choices because oncology was at the forefront of the scientific advances in medicine.

At that time we were also told by these formidable men, and they were all men because there were no female oncology consultants in that era, that as a result of these advances incurable diseases were now curable. Four cancers were enumerated to encourage our interest in cancer; we were told that lymphoma, testicular cancer, choriocarcinoma and childhood leukaemia were curable. The number of patients cured was, of course, small but this at least was a start.

It is with joy that we admit that our teachers were right. It was a start that has led on to a galaxy of incredible treatments that have transformed the lives of patients. Cancer is indeed at the vanguard of modern medicine and changes in our understanding of how cancer cells work at the molecular level have been translated into a plethora of therapies that target these unique defects in cancer cells.

But it is not only these sparkling new treatments that are important in reducing cancer mortality. Screening strategies that detect and eliminate early cancers or their precursors have been developed and prophylactic vaccines that protect us from acquiring cancer-causing infections are available. As a consequence, death rates have fallen in many common cancers and the stigma of a cancer diagnosis has diminished.

Cancer has, of course, become politicized, as the reader of this preface might have noticed. We have the drugs, but in the United Kingdom at least dubious cost–benefit calculations mean that many of the drugs that would help our patients are branded as apparently unaffordable. We would urge the readers of this book to become involved politically and campaign for the right of patients to receive the treatment they need.

Mark Bower
Jonathan Waxman

About the companion website

Don't forget to visit the companion website for this book:

 www.lecturenoteseries.com/oncology

There you will find valuable material designed to enhance your learning, including:

- Interactive multiple choice questions
- Case studies

Scan this QR code to visit the companion website

Part 1

Introduction to oncology

What is cancer?

Cancer is not a single illness but a collection of many diseases that share common features. Cancer is widely viewed as a disease of genetic origin. It is caused by mutations of DNA and epigenetic changes that alter gene expression, which make a cell multiply uncontrollably. However, the description and definitions of cancer vary depending on the perspective as described below.

Epidemiological perspective

Cancer is a major cause of ill health. In 2011, in the United Kingdom, there were:

- 434,115 new cases of cancer
- 159,178 deaths from cancer

There are more than 200 different types of cancer, but four of them (breast, lung, colorectal and prostate) account for over half of all new cases (Table 1.1). Overall, it is estimated that one in three people will develop some form of cancer during their lifetime. In the period 1976–2009, the age-standardized incidence of cancer increased by 22% in men and 42% in women but have remained fairly constant over the last decade (Figures 1.1 and 1.2).

Cancer incidence refers to the number of new cancer cases arising in a specified period of time. Prevalence refers to the number of people who have received a diagnosis of cancer who are alive at any given time, some of whom will be cured and others will not. Therefore, prevalence reflects both the incidence of cancer and its associated survival pattern (Box 1.1). In 2010, approximately 3% of the population of the United Kingdom (around 2 million people) are alive having received a diagnosis of cancer. Over a million Britons are cancer survivors having lived more than 10 years since being diagnosed with cancer.

The epidemiology of cancer is littered with jargon, and some of the key terms are defined in Box 1.1.

Box 1.1 Understand the Geek-speak of epidemiology

Cancer incidence is the number of new cancer cases arising in a specified period of time.

Cancer prevalence is the number of people who have received a diagnosis of cancer who are alive at any given time, some of whom will be cured and others will not.

Cancer mortality is the number of deaths due to cancer in a specific time period and defined population.

Age-specific rates. To overcome problems of different population age structures, age-specific rates for an age range (usually 5–10 years) are published. For example, age-specific incidence rates of breast cancer in women aged 50–54 years.

Standardization is used to remove the effect of a variable that you are not interested in studying (often age or gender).

Oncology: Lecture Notes, Third Edition. Mark Bower and Jonathan Waxman.
© 2015 by John Wiley & Sons, Ltd. Published 2015 by John Wiley & Sons, Ltd.
Companion Website: www.lecturenoteseries.com/oncology

Table 1.1 Most frequent cancers according to age and gender

Age	0–14 yr	15–24 yr	25–49 yr	50–74 yr	>74 yr
Male	Leukaemia	Testis	Testis	Prostate	Prostate
	Brain tumour	Hodgkin lymphoma	Melanoma	Lung	Lung
	Lymphoma	Leukaemia	Bowel	Bowel	Bowel
Female	Leukaemia	Hodgkin lymphoma	Breast	Breast	Breast
	Brain tumour	Melanoma	Melanoma	Lung	Bowel
	Lymphoma	Ovary	Cervix	Bowel	Lung

Age standardized rates. This corrects the crude rates to a "standardized population". The same "standard population" is used for all rates to allow comparisons.

Standardized ratios. Standardized incidence ratio (SIR) and mortality ratio (SMR) compare the age-specific rate in the study population with those of a control population.

Relative risk (also known as risk ratio) is the ratio of the risk of disease (e.g. lung cancer) amongst people exposed to a risk factor (e.g. smoking) to the risk amongst unexposed people (e.g. non-smokers). Data are calculated from cohort studies from which the incidence can be calculated.

Odds (as every gambler knows) is the ratio of the occurrence of an event to that of non-occurrence. If 20 out of every 100 smokers develop lung cancer, the odds are 20:80 or 1 in 4 (whilst the probability of developing lung cancer is 20/100 or 0.2).

Odds ratio compares the odds of an event in two different populations.

Sociological perspective

People living with cancer adopt a medically sanctioned form of deviant behaviour described in the 1950s by Talcott Parsons as "the sick role". In order to be excused from their usual duties and not to be considered responsible for their illness, patients are expected to seek professional advice and to adhere to treatments in order to get well. Medical practitioners are empowered to sanction their temporary absence from the workforce and family duties as well as to absolve them of blame. This behavioural model minimizes the impact of illness on the society and reduces the secondary gain that the patient benefits from as a consequence of their illness. However, as Ivan Illich pointed out, it also sets up physicians as agents of social control by medicalizing health and contributing to iatrogenic illness – "a medical nemesis". Of all the common medical diagnoses, cancer probably carries the greatest stigma and is associated with the most fear. The many different ways in which cancer affects people has been explored in literature (Table 1.2).

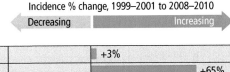

Incidence % change, 1999–2001 to 2008–2010

	Decreasing	Increasing
All cancers excl. NMSC		+3%
Malignant melanoma		+65%
Liver		+44%
Kidney		+26%
Oral		+26%
Prostate		+22%
Lung	−15%	
Larynx	−15%	
Bladder	−23%	
Stomach	−32%	

Figure 1.1 Fastest changing cancer incidences in men in the United Kingdom over the last decade. NMSC, non-melanoma skin cancer.

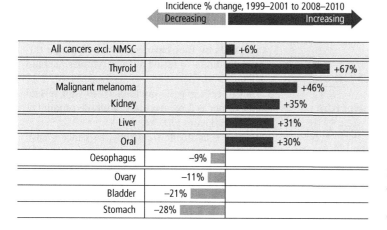

Incidence % change, 1999–2001 to 2008–2010

	Decreasing	Increasing
All cancers excl. NMSC		+6%
Thyroid		+67%
Malignant melanoma		+46%
Kidney		+35%
Liver		+31%
Oral		+30%
Oesophagus	–9%	
Ovary	–11%	
Bladder	–21%	
Stomach	–28%	

Figure 1.2 Fastest changing cancer incidences in women in the United Kingdom over the last decade.

Experimental perspective

In the laboratory, a number of characteristics define a cancer cell growing in culture. The four features listed below are used by scientists experimentally to confirm the malignant phenotype of cancer cells:

1. Cancer cells are clonal, having all derived from a single parent cell.
2. Cancer cells grow on soft agar in the absence of growth factors.
3. Cancer cells cross artificial membranes in culture systems.

Table 1.2 Tip top cancer books

	Title	Author
1	Cancer Ward	Alexander Solzhenitsyn
2	A Very Easy Death	Simone de Beauvoir
3	Age of Iron	J. M. Coetzee
4	Cancer Vixen	Marisa Acocella Marchetto
5	One in Three	Adam Wishart
6	C: Because Cowards Get Cancer, Too	John Diamond
7	Before I Say Goodbye	Ruth Picardie
8	Illness as Metaphor	Susan Sontag
9	The Black Swan	Thomas Mann
10	Mom's Cancer	Brian Fies
11	Coda	Simon Gray
12	Cancer Tales	Nell Dunn
13	A Grief Observed	C. S. Lewis

4. Cancer cells form tumours if injected into immunodeficient strains of mice (Box 1.2).

Box 1.2 Onco-mice

Mice have been used as a laboratory model in cancer research for a century. In the 1930s, Sir Ernest Kennaway showed that polycyclic aromatic hydrocarbons were carcinogenic by inducing skin cancers in mice. In 1969m the first inbred mice were developed that were essentially genetically identical except for gender. These strains allowed the transfer of cells and tissues between mice without rejection, as they are syngeneic (genetically identical). This has allowed the effects of experimental treatments on murine cancers to be evaluated in laboratory mice. Some inbred strains also spontaneously develop cancers (e.g. BALB/c mice frequently develop lung tumours), so the effects of cancer prevention strategies can be studied. The development of immunodeficient mice allowed the transfer and study of human cancer cells in mice without the mice rejecting the xenograft (graft between different species). The first immunodeficient mice were "nude mice", an inbred strain that lacks a thymus gland and T lymphocytes; they are hairless because of a mutation in a linked genetic locus. Subsequently, in 1983, even more immunodeficient severe combined immunodeficiency (SCID) mice were developed that lack both T and B cells. Genetically modified transgenic mice have been manufactured by knocking out specific genes ("knockout mice") or adding extra trans-genes, usually from different species ("transgenic mice"), to embryonic stem cells. These mice are used to elucidate the influence of individual genes on the phenotype. Finally, mice were the original source of monoclonal antibodies produced by immunizing inbred mice with the desired antigen and fusing spleen cells from the mouse with myeloma cells to yield hybridoma cells that produce monoclonal antibodies.

Histopathological perspective

Cancer is usually defined by various histopathological features, most notably invasion and metastasis, that are observed by gross pathological and microscopic examinations. Laminin staining of the basement membrane may assist the histopathologist in identifying local invasion by tumours that breach the basement membrane. In addition, a number of microscopic features point to the diagnosis of cancer:

1. The arrangement of tumour cells (their "architecture") is less organized than that of their parent tissues, with heterogeneous cells of varying sizes and orientation with respect to one another despite their clonal origin (Figure 1.3).

2. Cancer cells have more nuclear DNA than normal cells, so they have comparatively larger nuclei, leading to a raised nuclear:cytoplasmic ratio (Figure 1.4).

3. Cancer cells may be multinucleated with several nuclei per cell or may have multiple prominent nucleoli (Figure 1.5).

4. Cancer cells divide frequently, so cancers have many mitotic figures (Figure 1.6).

5. Cancer cells will commonly have densely coloured or hyperchromatic nuclei with wrinkled nuclear edges (Figure 1.7).

Molecular perspective

At a molecular level, six basic steps or "hallmarks" that turn a cell into a cancer were described in 2000 by Douglas Hanahan and Robert Weinberg. In 2011,

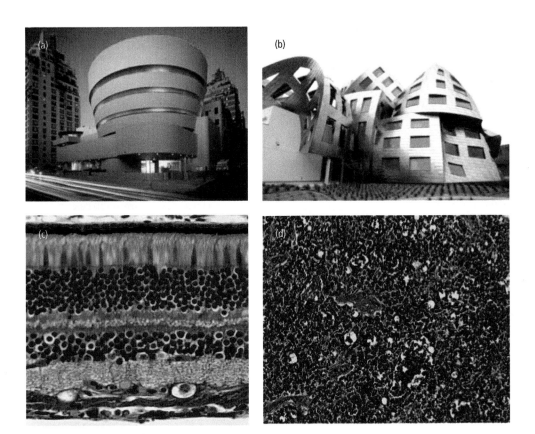

Figure 1.3 The Frank architecture of cancer. Normal tissue architecture is ordered, structured and controlled like a Frank Lloyd Wright building. Cancer tissues are higgledy-piggledy heaped on top of each other without any apparent planning like some of the buildings of Frank Gehry. (a) Frank Lloyd Wright designed the Guggenheim museum in New York. (b) Frank Gehry designed the Lou Ruvo centre for brain health in Las Vegas. (c) Normal retina histology. (d) Retinoblastoma histology.

High nuclear:cytoplasmic ratio

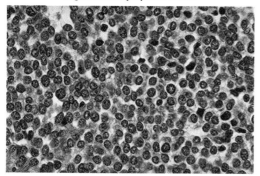

Figure 1.4 Ewing's sarcoma cells with large prominent purple nuclei surrounded by a thin pink rim of cytoplasm, demonstrating the high nuclear:cytoplasmic ratio of cancer cells.

Mitotic figure

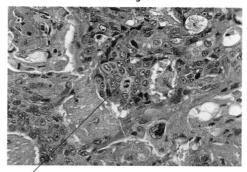

A mitotic figure is seen, surrounded by a poorly differentiated squamous cell cancer of the lung

Figure 1.6 Poorly differentiated squamous cell lung cancer with a prominent mitotic figure.

a further two "enabling hallmarks" were added that contribute to the ability of cells to acquire the six hallmarks and a further two "emerging hallmarks" required for cancer cells to continue to survive as tumours. Molecular features that identify a cancer and make it behave differently from a normal cell are described in Chapter 2. The six original properties are:

1. Grow without a trigger (self-sufficiency in growth stimuli).
2. Do not stop growing (insensitivity to inhibitory stimuli).
3. Do not die (evasion of apoptosis).
4. Do not age (immortalization).
5. Feed themselves (neoangiogenesis).
6. Spread (invasion and metastasis).

How to read a histology report

The diagnosis of cancer is most commonly established following a histopathological examination of a biopsy or tumour resection (Figure 1.8). A histopathological report should include both gross pathological features (tumour size and number and size of lymph nodes examined) and microscopic findings (tumour grade, architecture, mitotic rate, margin involvement and lymphovascular invasion). The grade and stage of a cancer are important prognostic factors that may influence therapy options (Box 1.3).

Hyperchromatic nuclei

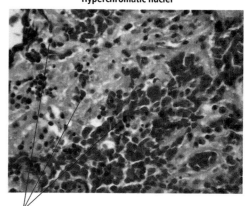

Dark staining, hyperchromatic nuclei in small cell lung cancer specimen

Figure 1.7 Small cell lung cancer containing several darkly stained hyperchromatic nuclei.

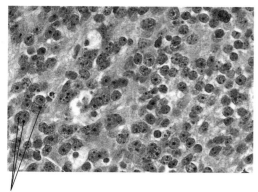

Prominent nucleoli

Figure 1.5 Many large dark nucleoi are seen here within the nuclei of cancer cells in this prostate adenocarcinoma.

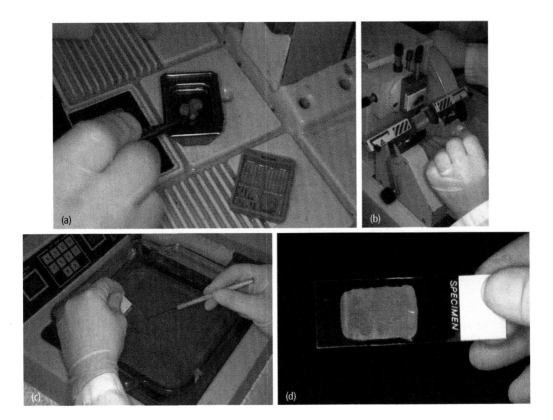

Figure 1.8 Preparing a histology slide. (a) Tissue is embedded in paraffin wax. (b) Thin sections of the tissue are sliced by a microtome. (c) Tissue sections are floated onto a glass slide. (d) The tissue sections on the glass slide are then stained.

Box 1.3 Histopathology definitions

Quantitative changes: too small

Atrophy

Acquired shrinkage due to a decrease in the *size or number* of cells of a tissue, for example, decrease in size of the ovaries after the menopause.

Quantitative changes: too big

Hypertrophy

Increase in the size of an organ or tissue due to an increase in the *size* of individual cells, for example, pregnant uterus.

Hyperplasia

Increase in the *size* of an organ due to an increase in the *number* of cells, for example, lactating breast.

Qualitative changes

Metaplasia

Replacement of one cell type in an organ by another. This implies changes in the differentiation programme and is usually a response to persistent injury. It is reversible so that removal of the source of injury results in reversion to the original cell type; for example, squamous metaplasia of laryngeal respiratory epithelium in a smoker. Chronic irritation from smoking causes the normal columnar respiratory epithelium to be replaced by the more resilient squamous epithelium.

Dysplasia

Dysplastic changes are changes in cell type, as for metaplasia, that do not revert to normal once the injury is removed; for example, cervical dysplasia initiated by human papillomavirus infection persists after eradication of the virus. Dysplasia is usually considered to be part of the spectrum of changes leading to neoplasia.

Invasion

The capacity to infiltrate the surrounding tissues and organs is a characteristic of cancer.

Metastasis

The ability to proliferate in distant parts of the body after tumour cells have been transported by lymph or blood or along body spaces.

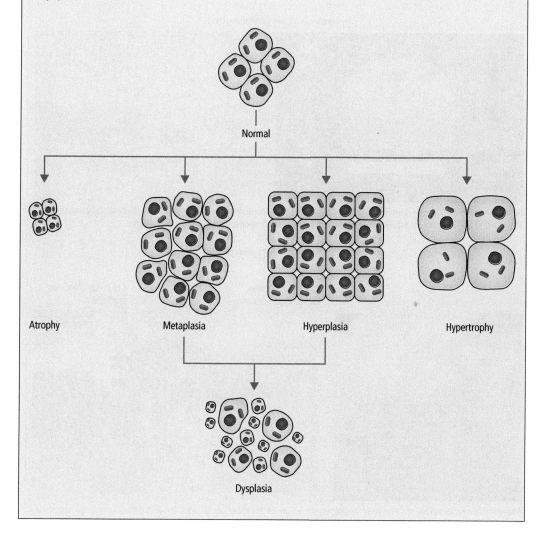

Atrophy of testes

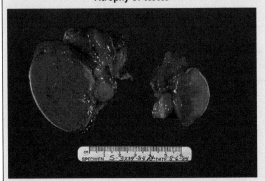

Testicular atrophy is a reduction in the size and function of the testes and may be caused by anabolic steroid use.

Hypertrophic cardiomyopathy (HCM)

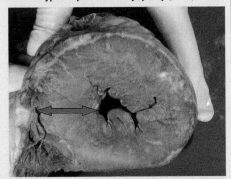

Concentric thickening of the heart muscle caused by an increase in the size of the heart muscle cells (myocytes)

Hyperplasia of the prostate gland

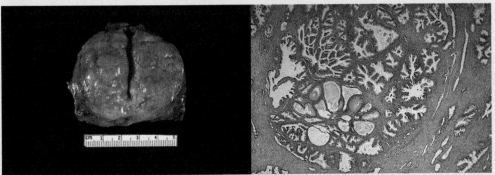

Benign prostatic hyperplasia is an increase in the number of cells. The normal prostate is 3–4 cm in diameter, by comparison. The prostate is filled with enlarged crowded glands, but there is still stroma between adjacent glands.

Metaplasia in Barrett's oesophagus

Normal squamous oesophageal mucosa

Columnar glandular epithelium

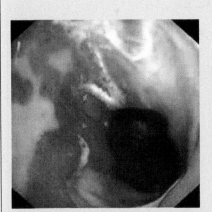

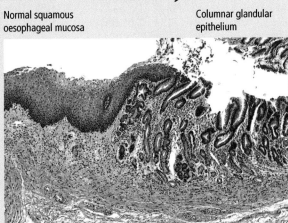

The reversible replacement of the normal squamous epithelium of the lower oesophagus (on left) with columnar glandular mucosa similar to that found in the stomach (on right)

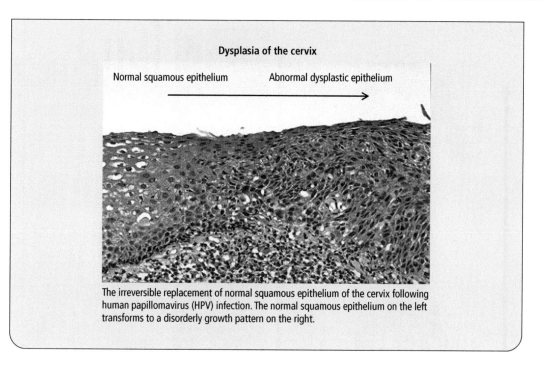

Dysplasia of the cervix

Normal squamous epithelium   Abnormal dysplastic epithelium

The irreversible replacement of normal squamous epithelium of the cervix following human papillomavirus (HPV) infection. The normal squamous epithelium on the left transforms to a disorderly growth pattern on the right.

A histopathological definition of cancer: is it malignant or benign?

Malignancy is usually characterized by various behavioural features, most notably invasion and metastasis. However, the histopathologist may have to identify a cancer without this information. Cancers are composed of clonal cells (all are the progeny of a single cell) and have lost control of their tissue organization and architecture. In addition to the natural history, a number of physical properties help to distinguish between benign and malignant tumours (Table 1.3). However, there is no single histological feature that defines a cancer nor indeed that separates benign from malignant tumours. In general, benign tumours are rarely life-threatening but may cause health problems on account of their location (by pressure or obstruction of adjacent organs) or by overproduction of hormones. In contrast, malignant tumours usually follow a progressive course and unless successfully treated are frequently fatal.

Is it *in situ* or invasive?

Invasive cancers extend into the surrounding stroma (Figure 1.9). However, tumours that exhibit all the microscopic features of cancers but do not breach the original basement membrane are termed *in situ* (non-invasive) cancers. Examples include *in situ* breast cancer confined to the mammary ducts (ductal carcinoma *in situ* (DCIS)) or lobules (lobular carcinoma *in situ* (LCIS)) (Figure 1.9). Similar pre-invasive *in situ* cancers have been found in many organs (e.g. cervix, anus, prostate, bronchus) and are believed to represent a stage in the progression from dysplasia to cancer (Figure 1.10).

Table 1.3 Histological features of benign and malignant tumours

Features of malignancy	Features of benign tumours
Macroscopic features	
Invade and metastasize	Do not invade or metastasize
Rapid growth	Slow growing
Not clearly demarcated	Clearly demarcated from surrounding tissue
Surface often ulcerated and necrotic	Surface smooth
Cut surface heterogenous	Cut surface homogenous
Microscopic features	
Often high mitotic rate	Low mitotic rate
Nuclei pleomorphic and hyperchromatic	Nuclear morphology often normal
Abnormal mitoses	Mitotic figures normal

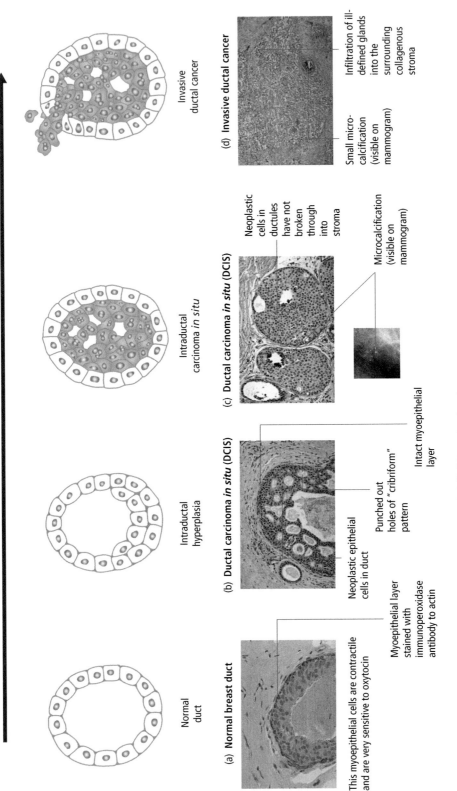

Figure 1.9 (a) Normal breast duct. (b)+(c) Ductal carcinoma *in situ* (DCIS). (d) Invasive ductal cancer.

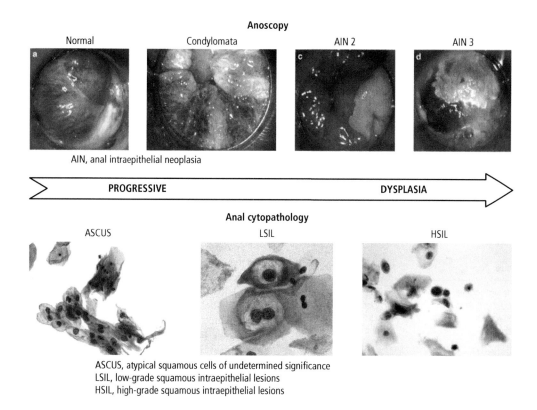

Figure 1.10 Progression of pre-invasive anal cancer with associated cytopathology changes.

Histopathologist's nomenclature: name that cancer

The histopathologists' lexicon often can be a tool for obfuscation, but follow a few simple rules and you can translate their lingo. The suffix -oma usually denotes a benign tumour (although it simply means "swelling" and some -omas are not tumours, e.g. xanthoma). If a tumour is malignant, the suffix -carcinoma (Greek for crab) is used for epithelial cancers or -sarcoma (Greek for flesh) for connective tissue cancers. The prefix is determined by the cells of origin of the tumour (e.g. adeno- for glandular epithelium), qualified by the tissue of origin (e.g. prostatic adenocarcinoma). There are numerous exceptions to this systematic nomenclature; for example, leukaemias and lymphomas are malignant tumours of the bone marrow and lymphoid tissue, respectively. As a general rule, neoplasms are classified according to the type of normal tissue they most closely resemble. The four major categories are: epithelial, connective tissue, lymphoid and haemopoietic tissue, and germ cells (Tables 1.4, 1.5, 1.6 and 1.7). The latter arises in totipotential cells and can develop into any cell type. Germ cell tumours

Table 1.4 Nomenclature of epithelial tumours

Epithelium	Benign tumour	Malignant tumour
Squamous	Squamous papilloma	Squamous carcinoma
Glandular	Adenoma	Adenocarcinoma
Transitional	Transitional papilloma	Transitional carcinoma
Liver	Hepatic adenoma	Hepatocellular carcinoma
Skin	Papilloma	Squamous cell carcinoma
		Basal cell carcinoma
Skin melanocyte	Naevus	Malignant melanoma

Table 1.5 Nomenclature of connective tissue tumours

Tissue	Benign tumour	Malignant tumour
Bone	Osteoma	Osteosarcoma
Cartilage	Chondroma	Chondrosarcoma
Fat	Lipoma	Liposarcoma
Smooth muscle	Leiomyoma	Leiomyosarcoma
Striated muscle	Rhabdomyoma	Rhabdomyosarcoma
Blood vessel	Angioma	Angiosarcoma
Fibrous tissue	Fibroma	Fibrosarcoma

Table 1.6 Nomenclature of haematological tumours

Tissue	Malignant tumour
Node lymphocyte	Lymphoma
Marrow lymphocyte	Lymphocytic leukaemia
Granulocyte	Myeloid leukaemia
Plasma cell	Myeloma

contain a variety of different mature and/or immature tissues from different embryonic germ layers and these are given names with the root terato- (Greek for monster). In addition, as with most fields of medicine where physicians try to leave their mark, there are a number of eponymous names (e.g. Hodgkin's disease). In 1832, Thomas Hodgkin (of Guy's Hospital) described seven cases of the tumour that bears his name, but re-examination in 1926 revealed that the diagnosis was inaccurate in four of the seven cases.

Tumour grading

Tumours are graded according to the degree of tissue differentiation (Box 1.4). Cancers that closely resemble their tissue of origin are graded as well-differentiated cancers. Cancers that look nothing like the original tissue and have histological features of aggressive growth with high mitotic rates are graded as poorly differentiated cancers. The grade of a tumour is of prognostic significance (Figure 1.11).

In addition, pathologists may identify other features that relate to the natural behaviour of a tumour, such as lymphovascular invasion and perineural invasion, which usually denotes a worse prognosis (Figure 1.14). The molecular properties of a cancer can also influence the biology, prognosis and treatment of a tumour. For example, the gene expression profile of a breast cancer may be determined by gene expression microarray chip technology, and the results assist clinicians in optimizing adjuvant therapy (Figure 1.12).

Unknown primary identification (standard histological techniques)

Occasionally patients present with metastatic cancer without an obvious primary tumour site and, in addition to a careful clinical and radiological examination, the pathologist may provide a clue to the origins of the cancer. Most unknown primary cancers are adenocarcinoma (60%) and the remainder are poorly differentiated carcinomas (30%) and squamous cell carcinomas (5%). Light microscopy may provide pointers; for example, the presence of melanin pigment favours melanoma, whilst the presence of mucins, which are gel-forming lubricating proteins, is common in gastrointestinal, breast and lung cancers but less

Table 1.7 Nomenclature of germ cell tumours

Tissue	Benign tumour	Malignant tumour (male)	Malignant tumour (female)
Germ cell	Mature teratoma/ dermoid cyst	Non-seminomatous germ cell tumour/ malignant teratoma	Immature teratoma/embryonal carcinoma
	–	Seminoma	Dysgerminoma

Box 1.4 Grading breast cancer (Scarff–Bloom–Richardson system)

1 Frequency of cell mitosis (score 1–3)

2 Tubule formation (score 1–3)

3 Nuclear pleomorphism (score 1–3)

Total score: 3–5 = Grade 1 tumour (well differentiated), 6–7 = Grade 2 (moderately differentiated), 8–9 = Grade 3 (poorly differentiated). The 5-year overall survival for grades 1, 2 and 3 are 95%, 75% and 50%, respectively.

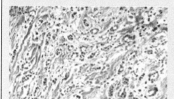 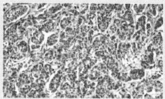 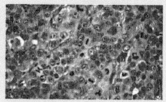

Grade 1
Well
differentiated
(bad)

Grade 2
Moderately
differentiated
(worse)

Grade 3
Poorly
differentiated
(worst)

Figure 1.11 Grading breast cancer.

---

common in ovarian cancers and is rare in renal and thyroid cancers. Immunocytochemical staining of tissue samples uses antibodies to specific proteins to aid the pathologist in tissue identification. For example, the presence of oestrogen and progesterone receptors favours a diagnosis of breast cancer (Figure 1.13), whilst prostate-specific antigen and prostatic acid phosphatase staining points to prostatic adenocarcinoma. Similarly, cytokeratin expression patterns may provide helpful hints about the origin of metastatic cancers (Box 1.5). Cell surface immunophenotyping is a sophistication of immunocytochemistry that is frequently applied to haematological malignancies. The pattern of immunoglobulin, T-cell receptor and cluster designation (CD) antigen expression on the surface of lymphomas is helpful in their diagnosis and classification. Immunophenotyping can be achieved by immunohistochemical staining, immunofluorescent staining or flow cytometry.

Unknown primary identification (special histological techniques)

The study of intracellular organelles by electron microscopy may identify the cellular origin of a tumour; for example, the presence of melanosomes in melanomas and dense core neurosecretory granules in neuroendocrine tumours. Further laboratory techniques to aid diagnosis include molecular studies of

DNA rearrangements that characterize malignancies. Monoclonal immunoglobulin gene rearrangements are present in B-cell malignancies and rearrangements of T-cell receptor genes occur in T-cell tumours. In addition, a number of chromosomal translocations involving the immunoglobulin genes (heavy chain on chromosome 14q32, light chains on 2p12 and 22q11) and T-cell receptor genes (TCRα on 14q11, TCRβ on 7q35, TCRγ on 7p15, TCRδ on 14q11) occur in malignancies arising from these cell types. For instance, low-grade follicular lymphomas rearrange the Bcl-2 gene on 18q21 (e.g. t(14;18)(q32;q21)), most Burkitt lymphomas rearrange the Myc oncogene on 8q24 (e.g. t(8;14)(q24;q32)) and most mantle cell lymphomas rearrange Bcl-1 on 11q13 (e.g. t(11;14)(q13;q32)). These rearrangements may be detected by karyotype analysis of mitotic chromosome preparations or by molecular techniques including Southern blotting and polymerase chain reaction (Box 1.6 and Table 1.8). Less commonly, these same methods may assist the diagnosis of solid tumours that are associated with specific chromosomal abnormalities such as the i(12p) isochromosome found in germ cell tumours and the t(11;22)(q24;q12) translocation seen in Ewing's sarcoma and peripheral neuroectodermal tumours. In addition to translocations, gene amplification may be detected and may have prognostic significance; for example, the amplification of the n-Myc oncogene in neuroblastoma is an adverse prognostic variable.

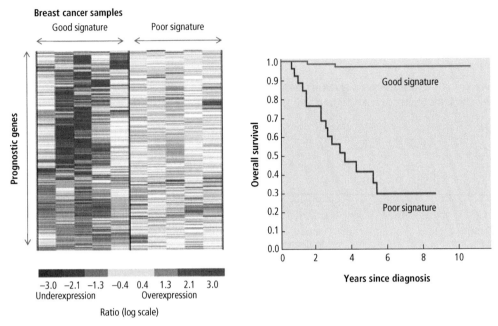

Gene expression array

Figure 1.12 Gene expression profiles for breast cancer samples differentiate tumours into good- and poor-prognosis signatures that predict survival.

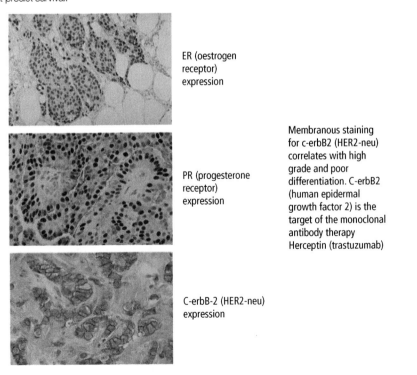

ER (oestrogen receptor) expression

PR (progesterone receptor) expression

Membranous staining for c-erbB2 (HER2-neu) correlates with high grade and poor differentiation. C-erbB2 (human epidermal growth factor 2) is the target of the monoclonal antibody therapy Herceptin (trastuzumab)

C-erbB-2 (HER2-neu) expression

Figure 1.13 Immunocytochemical staining in breast cancer.

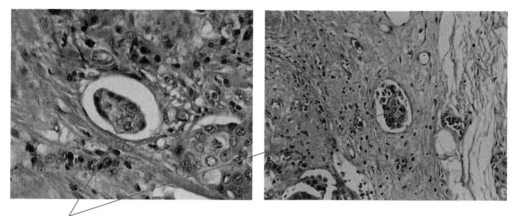

Invasive transitional cell cancer of the bladder with cancer cells present in lymphatic channels

(a)

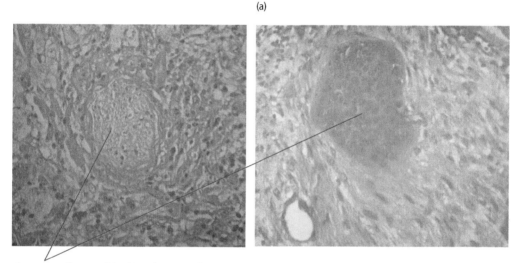

Squamous cell cancer of the skin with cancer cells present within nerve sheaths that are delineated by a concentric layer of perineural epithelial cells

(b)

Figure 1.14 (a) Lymphatic invasion and (b) perineural invasion.

Cancer epidemiology

Epidemiology in the United Kingdom

Cancer is now the most common cause of death in the United Kingdom (if cardiovascular and cerebrovascular diseases are classed separately).

- One in three people in the United Kingdom will de-velop a cancer (434,115 in 2011).
- One in four die of cancer (159,178 in 2011).

Global epidemiology

The current world population is 6 billion with 10 million new cancer cases and 6 million cancer deaths annually. Projections for 2020 are a global population of 8 billion; 20 million new cancer cases and 12 million deaths annually. Tobacco contributes to 3 million cases (chiefly lung, head, neck and bladder cancers), diet to an estimated 3 million cases (upper gastrointestinal, colorectal) and infection to a further 1.5 million cases (cervical, stomach, liver, bladder and lymphomas) globally. The incidence of different types of cancer varies geographically

Box 1.5 **Cytokeratins**

Cytokeratins are intermediate filament proteins that form the cytoskeleton within a cell. They are expressed in pairs comprising a type I (cytokeratins 9–20) and a type II (cytokeratins 1–8) cytokeratin. Different tissues express different pairs and immunocytochemical staining for cytokeratins can help identify the likely tissue origins of cancers cells. For example, in disseminated peritoneal metastases, CK7 expression favours an ovarian origin, whilst lack of CK7 is more common in colorectal cancer (Figure 1.3).

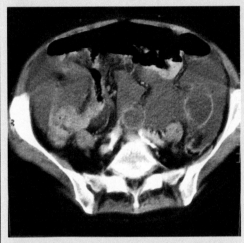

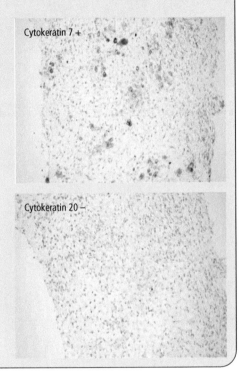

Cytokeratin 7 +

Cytokeratin 20 –

A 78-year-old woman presents with bowel obstruction and ascites. The CT scan shows extensive ascites and omental thickening. CT-guided biopsy of peritoneal deposits demonstrates adenocarcinoma, immunocytochemistry for cytokeratins (CK7+ and CK20–) suggests an ovarian rather than colonic primary

according to the risk factors and demographics of the local population (Figure 1.15) However, there is a general correlation between increasing wealth and increasing cancer incidence. This is attributable to tobacco use, diet and increased longevity in wealthy populations. There are intriguing exceptions; for example, the Gulf States of Kuwait, Qatar, Bahrain, United Arab Emirates and Saudi Arabia have lower cancer incidences than would be predicted from their per capita gross national product. Consideration also has to be given to the variable standard of reporting of cancer statistics in different countries.

Table 1.8 Examples of chromosomal abnormalities in cancers

Chromosome defect	Karyotype	Tumour	Candidate gene
Monosomy	45,XY −22	Meningioma	NF2
Trisomy	47,XX +7	Papillary renal carcinoma	MET
Deletion	46,XY del(11)(p13)	Wilms' tumour	WT1
Duplication	46,XX dup(2)(p23-24)	Neuroblastoma	n-Myc
Inversion	46,XY inv(16)(p13q22)	Acute myeloid leukaemia (M4Eo)	MYH11/core-binding factor b
Isochromosome	47,XX i(12p)	Testicular germ cell tumour	
Translocation	46,XX t(9;22)(q34;q11)	Chronic myeloid leukaemia	bcr/abl

Box 1.6 The language of chromosomes – karyotype nomenclature

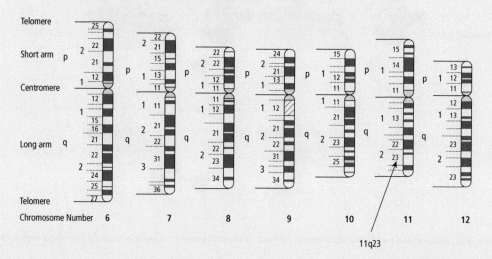

Each arm of a chromosome is divided into one to four major regions, depending on the chromosomal length; each band, positively or negatively stained, is given a number that rises as the distance from the centromere increases. The normal male is designated as 46,XY and the normal female as 46,XX.

For example, 11q23 designates the chromosome (11), the long arm (q), the second region distal to the centromere (2) and the third band (3) in that region.

Polyploid

A cell with more than one complete chromosome set or with multiples of the basic number of chromosomes characteristic of the species; in humans this would be 69,92, etc.

Aneuploid

Individual with one or more chromosomes in addition or missing from the complete chromosome set; for example, trisomy 21 (47,XX +21).

Deletion

The loss of a chromosome segment from a normal chromosome.

Duplication

An extra piece of chromosome segment which may be attached to the same homologous chromosome or transposed to another chromosome in the genome.

Inversion

A change in the linear sequence of the genes in a chromosome that results in the reverse order of genes in a chromosome segment. Inversions may be pericentric (two breaks on either side of the centromere) or paracentric (both breaks on the same arm).

Isochromosome

Breaks in one arm of a chromosome followed by duplication of the other arm of the chromosome to produce a chromosome with two arms that are both short (p) or both long (q) arms.

Translocations

Translocations are the result of the reciprocal exchange of terminal segments of non-homologous chromosomes.

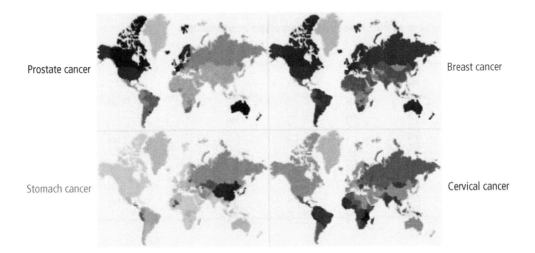

Prostate cancer

Breast cancer

Stomach cancer

Cervical cancer

Figure 1.15 Global incidences for prostate, breast, stomach and cervical cancers. Darker colours denote higher incidence.

Cancer charities

Cancer charities

The United Kingdom has 640 cancer charities to counter the disease. Their expenditure increases awareness of cancer, improves diagnosis and treatment capability and provides care for patients with the disease. The total income generated by the top 20 UK cancer charities in 2004 was £758 million, and the average charitable efficiency was 64% providing £488 million for spending on patients' care and research. The two largest UK cancer charities, the Imperial Cancer Research Fund (ICRF) and the Cancer Research Campaign (CRC) merged to form Cancer Research UK (CRUK) in 2002. CRUK is the largest volunteer-supported cancer research organization in the world, with 3000 scientists and an annual scientific spend of more than £460 million – raised almost entirely through public donations.

Cancer hospitals

Philanthropists and social reformers during the 19th century tried to provide free medical care for the poor. William Marsden, a young surgeon opened a dispensary for advice and medicines in 1828. His grandly named London General Institution for the Gratuitous Cure of Malignant Diseases – a simple four-storey house in one of the poorest parts of the city – was conceived as a hospital to which the only passport should be poverty and disease and where treatment was provided free of charge. The demand for Marsden's free services was overwhelming, and by 1844 his dispensary, now called the Royal Free Hospital, was treating 30,000 patients a year. In 1846 when his wife died of cancer, Marsden opened a small house in Cannon Row, Westminster, for patients suffering from cancer. Within 10 years, the institution moved to Fulham Road and became known as the Cancer Hospital, of which Marsden was the senior surgeon. The hospital was incorporated into the National Health Service in 1948 and renamed the Royal Marsden Hospital in 1954. Although other cancer hospitals have been established in Manchester (the Christie Hospital) and Glasgow (the Beatson Hospital), the Royal Marsden Hospital remains the most renown. With the recent emphasis on multidisciplinary approaches to cancer, single specialty hospitals are less in vogue and the majority of cancer departments are within large teaching hospitals.

Cancer celebrities

Celebrities influence public perceptions and behaviour inordinately and this is as true in oncology as elsewhere. Celebrities with cancer have contributed in three main ways: personal accounts bring patients' experiences into the limelight, reports of celebrity patients increase public awareness and may encourage health-seeking behaviour such as stopping smoking and celebrity patients may support cancer charities and encourage donations. Prominent examples of

Table 1.9 Rock star cancer deaths

	Year of death	Age	Cause of death
Donna Summer	2012	63	Lung cancer
Poly Styrene (XRay Spex)	2011	53	Breast cancer
Malcolm McLaren (Sex Pistols' manager)	2010	64	Mesothelioma
Ari Up (The Slits)	2010	48	Breast cancer
Richard Wright (Pink Floyd)	2008	65	Cancer (type undisclosed)
Syd Barrett (Pink Floyd)	2006	60	Pancreas cancer
Johnny Ramone (The Ramones)	2004	55	Prostate cancer
Joey Ramone (The Ramones)	2001	49	Non-Hodgkin's lymphoma
George Harrison (The Beatles)	2001	58	Non-small cell lung cancer
Ian Dury (Ian Dury & The Blockheads)	2000	58	Colorectal cancer
Dusty Springfield	1999	60	Breast cancer
Carl Wilson (The Beach Boys)	1998	52	Lung cancer
Eva Cassidy	1996	33	Melanoma
Frank Zappa	1993	53	Prostate cancer
Freddy Mercury	1991	45	Kaposi's sarcoma
Bob Marley	1981	36	Melanoma

patient's perspectives include John Diamond's account in *C: Because Cowards Get Cancer, Too* and Ruth Picardie's *Before I Say Goodbye*, both moving accounts by accomplished journalists. Celebrity patients can influence the treatment choices that the public make. Following Nancy Reagan's mastectomy for localized breast cancer in 1987, there was a 25% decline in American women choosing breast-conserving surgery over mastectomy. Her husband's successful surgery for Dukes' B colon cancer whilst president in 1984 increased awareness and propelled the warning signs of colon cancer into the media. Similarly, the diagnosis and death from cervical cancer in 2009 of Jade Goody, a *Big Brother* celebrity, led to an increased uptake of cervical cancer screening, especially amongst young women in the United Kingdom. Successful cancer treatment is often most widely publicized and no article describing Lance Armstrong's seven consecutive Tour de France cycling victories is complete without a mention of his treatment for metastatic non-seminomatous germ cell tumour, which involved bilateral thoracotomies and neurosurgery, and his two children conceived with stored sperm banked prior to chemotherapy. Other celebrity patients have used their wealth and fame to establish and support charitable projects to support cancer research and treatment including Bob Champion, the steeple chase jockey treated for testicular cancer in the 1979, and Roy Castle, a lifelong non-smoker who was diagnosed with lung cancer in 1992. Of course, no one is immune to cancer; even rock stars whose deaths are more traditionally associated with suicide and substance abuse (Table 1.9).

 KEY POINTS

- One in three people in the United Kingdom develop cancer, and one in four die of cancer
- Breast, colorectal, lung and prostate cancers account for over half of all cancers in the United Kingdom
- The histopathologist diagnoses cancer on the basis of microscopic features and characterizes the tumour as benign or malignant, *in situ* or invasive, as well as identifying the likely tissue of origin and grading
- In the case of cancer of unknown primary, specialist immunohistochemical stains, chromosomal and molecular analyses may identify the origin of the cancer

2

The scientific basis of cancer

Learning objectives

✓ List the six hallmarks of cancer with examples

✓ Describe the enabling and emerging characteristics of cancers

✓ Classify the epigenetic changes that contribute to cancers

✓ Explain the hereditary and environmental causes of cancers with examples

The hallmarks of cancer

At a molecular level, six basic steps or "hallmarks" that turn a cell into a cancer were described in 2000. In 2011, a further two "enabling hallmarks" were added that contribute to the ability of cells to acquire the six hallmarks and a further two "emerging hallmarks" required for cancer cells to continue to survive as tumours.

The original six hallmarks of cancer are:

1. Cancer cells grow by themselves, with no need for external growth stimuli.
2. Once started, cancer cells continue to grow and will ignore any external signals telling them to stop.
3. Cancer cells bypass the normal cell mechanisms for planned cell death, known as apoptosis.
4. Cancer cells remain forever young by replenishing their own stocks of telomeres. As normal cells age they lose telomeres, leading eventually to an inability to divide.
5. Cancer cells can feed their own tumours through neoangiogenesis.
6. Cancer cells can spread to distant organs via metastases.

It is probable that all six are necessary to a greater or lesser extent. Some molecular changes may contribute to more than one of the six capabilities (e.g. a mutation on the p53 gene may contribute to both avoidance of apoptosis and insensitivity to inhibitory stimuli).

A number of mechanisms may contribute to the acquisition of these six properties, including genomic instability as a consequence of deficient DNA repair (lack of caretaking) or loss of cell cycle arrest/death in response to DNA damage (lack of gatekeeping). Many new treatment strategies for cancer aim to interrupt these steps.

The two enabling hallmarks of cancer are:

7. Cancer cells are prone to mutations due to genome instability.
8. Inflammation promotes the growth of cancers.

The two emerging hallmarks of cancer are:

9. Cancers avoid destruction by the host immune system.
10. Cancer cells deregulate cellular metabolism.

Oncology: Lecture Notes, Third Edition. Mark Bower and Jonathan Waxman.
© 2015 by John Wiley & Sons, Ltd. Published 2015 by John Wiley & Sons, Ltd.
Companion Website: www.lecturenoteseries.com/oncology

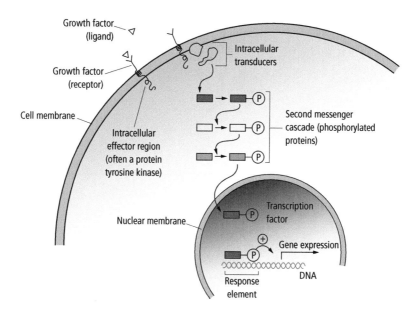

Figure 2.1 Signal transduction pathway.

1. Sustaining proliferative signalling (growing by themselves)

The instructions to cells to grow and start dividing are transmitted to cells by extracellular growth factor ligands that bind cell surface receptors. This results in the reversible phosphorylation of tyrosine, threonine or serine residues. The transfer of these molecular switches from activated receptors to downstream nuclear transcription activators is known as signal transduction (Figure 2.1). This cascade results in amplification of the initial stimulus.

Cancers achieve self-sufficiency in growth factors and are not dependent on extracellular concentrations of growth factors for continued growth. The majority of dominant oncogenes act on this mechanism by one of the following mechanisms:

- Overproducing growth factors, for example, glioblastomas produce platelet-derived growth factor (PDGF)
- Overproducing growth factor receptors, for example, epidermal growth factor receptor (EGFR/erbB) overexpression in breast cancers
- Mutations of the receptor or components of the signalling cascade, which are constitutively active, for example, mutations of Ras in lung and colonic cancers

2. Evading growth suppressors

Many normal cells grow throughout their lifespan and the co-ordination of their growth, differentiation, senescence and death is controlled by the cell cycle. Antiproliferative signals may be received by cells as soluble growth inhibitors or fixed inhibitors in the extracellular matrix. They act on the cell cycle clock (Box 2.1 and Figure 2.3), most frequently arresting transit through G1 into the S phase. Cancer cells ignore these "STOP" signals.

The co-ordination of the cell cycle and its arrest at checkpoints in response to DNA damage is achieved by sequential activation of kinase enzymes that ultimately phosphorylate and dephosphorylate the retinoblastoma protein (Rb). Periodic activation of these cyclin–cyclin-dependent kinase (CDK) complexes drives the cell cycle forward (Figure 2.2). Phosphorylation of Rb releases E2F, a transcription factor, which is then able to promote the expression of a number of target genes resulting in cell proliferation. The brakes that balance this system are CDK inhibitors (CKIs). Interference in elements of the cell cycle regulatory process is a common theme in malignancy (Table 2.1).

Examples of independence of cell cycle checkpoints:

- Cancer cells may overproduce cyclins (e.g. cyclins D and E) and CDKs (e.g. Cdk2 and Cdk4).

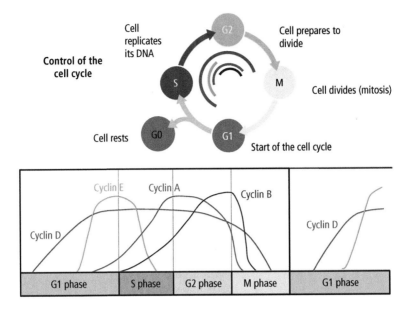

Figure 2.2 Oscillating levels of cyclins through the phases of the cell cycle.

- Cancer cells under-express or have mutations of CKIs (e.g. p16).
- Cancers have germline or somatic mutations of tumour suppressor genes (p53 and Rb).
- Human papillomavirus (HPV) oncoproteins inactivate Rb and p53.

G1/S checkpoint

An important checkpoint or restriction point in the cell cycle occurs in G1 to ensure that errors in DNA are not replicated, but instead are either repaired or that the cell dies by apoptosis. This is initiated by

Table 2.1 Examples of the six features and their molecular basis in cancers

Feature	Colorectal cancer	Glioma	Head and neck squamous cancer
1. Growth factor independence	KRAS mutation	EGFR amplification or mutation NF1 loss	EGFR mutation
2. Over-riding inhibitory signals	SMAD2/SMAD4 mutation	CDK4/p16 mutation	Cyclin D amplification p16 and p21 mutation
3. Evasion of apoptosis	p53 mutation	p53 mutation/MDM2 overexpression	p53 mutation
4. Immortalization	hTERT re-expression	hTERT re-expression	hTERT re-expression
5. Angiogenesis	VEGF expression	PDGF/PDGFR overexpression	Nitric oxide pathway activation of VEGF
6. Invasion and metastasis	APC, inactivate E-cadherin	Cathepsin D, MMP-2 and -9 and UPA overexpression	Cathepsin D, MMP-1, -2 and -9 overexpression

APC, adenomatous polyposis coli gene; EGFR, endothelial growth factor receptor; hTERT, human telomerase reverse transcriptase; MMP, matrix metalloproteinase; PDGF, platelet-derived growth factor; PDGFR, platelet-derived growth factor receptor; VEGF, vascular endothelial growth factor; UPA, urokinase-type plasminogen activator; SMAD, small mothers against decapentaplegic; CDK, cyclin-dependent kinase; KRAS, Kirsten rat sarcoma viral oncogene.

damaged DNA and is co-ordinated by p53, the gene that is probably most commonly mutated in cancers overall. Additional checkpoints are present in the S and G2 phases to allow cells to repair errors that occur during DNA duplication and thus prevent the propagation of these errors to daughter cells.

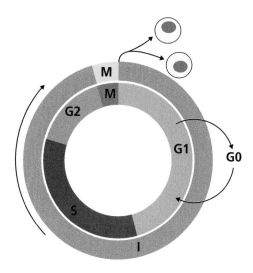

Figure 2.3 The cell cycle.

Box 2.1 The cell cycle (Figure 2.3)

There are five cell cycle phases:

Quiescent phase (G0)
Normal cells grown in culture will stop proliferating once they become confluent or are deprived of growth factors and enter a quiescent state called G0. Most cells in the normal tissue of adults are in a G0 state. Once the cell leaves G0, it starts the cell cycle:

First gap phase (G1) (duration 10–14 hours)
This occurs prior to DNA synthesis. Cells in G0 and G1 are receptive to growth signals, but once they have passed a restriction point are committed to DNA synthesis (S phase).

Synthesis phase (S) (duration 3–6 hours)
During this phase DNA replication occurs and the cell becomes diploid.

Second gap phase (G2) (duration 2–4 hours)
This occurs after DNA synthesis and before mitosis (M) and completion of the cell cycle. There is an important checkpoint at this stage to ensure there have been no duplication mistakes before mitosis and cell division.

Mitosis (M) (duration 1 hour)
Cell division completes the cell cycle.

---

3. Resisting cell death

Apoptosis is a pre-programmed sequence of cell suicide that occurs over 30–120 minutes. Apoptosis commences with condensation of cellular organelles and swelling of the endoplasmic reticulum. The plasma membrane remains intact, but the cell breaks up into several membrane-bound apoptotic bodies, which are phagocytosed. Confining the process within the cell membrane reduces activation of both inflammatory and immune responses, so that programmed cell death does not cause autoimmune disease or inflammation. Amongst the molecules that control apoptosis are the Bcl-2 family that confusingly includes both pro-apoptosis members (e.g. Bax) and anti-apoptosis members (e.g. Bcl-2).

In mammalian cells two pathways initiate apoptosis (Figure 2.4):

1. **Intracellular triggers:** DNA damage leads via p53 to activation of pro-apoptotic members of the Bcl-2 family. This causes release of cytochrome c from mitochondria, which in turn activates the caspase (**c**leaves after **asp**artate prote**ase**) cascade.
2. **Extracellular triggers:** Binding of extracellular ligands to the cell surface death receptor super-family (including CD95/Fas and tumour necrosis factor (TNF) receptors) leads to a death-inducing cytoplasmic signalling complex that activates the caspase cascade.

Ultimately both pathways activate the caspase cascade, a series of protease enzymes that result in cell apoptosis. Evasion of this pathway is a prerequisite for malignant cell proliferation and a number of strategies to this end have been identified (Table 2.1).

4. Enabling replicative immortality

In culture, cells can divide a limited number of times, up to the "Hayflick limit" (60–70 doublings in the case of human cells in culture), before the cell population enters crisis and dies off. This senescence is attributed to progressive telomere loss, which acts as a mitotic clock (Figure 2.5). Telomeres are the end segments of chromosomes and are made up of thousands of copies of a short six-base pair sequence (TTAGGG).

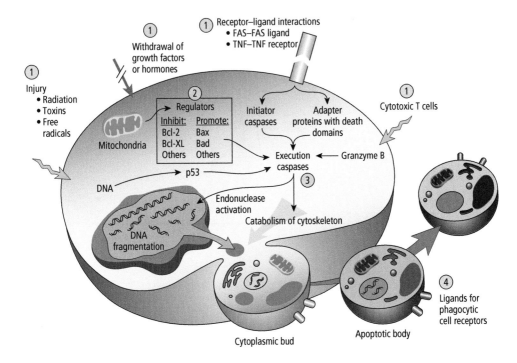

Figure 2.4 The apoptotic pathway.

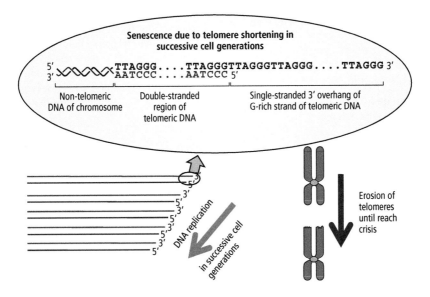

Figure 2.5 Telomerase, telomere length, senescence and immortalization.

DNA replication always follows a 5′ to 3′ direction so that manufacturing the 3′ ends of the chromosomes cannot be achieved by DNA polymerases and each time a cell replicates its DNA ready for cell division, 50–100 base pairs are lost from the ends of chromosomes. Eventually the protective ends of chromosomes are eroded and end-to-end chromosomal fusions occur with karyotypic abnormalities and death of the affected cell.

Normal germ cells and cancer cells avoid this senescence, acquiring immortality in culture usually by upregulating the expression of human telomerase reverse transcriptase (hTERT) enzyme that uses an RNA template and RNA-dependent DNA polymerase to add the six-base pair sequence back onto the ends of chromosomes to compensate for the bases lost during DNA replication (Table 2.1). Dyskeratosis congenita is an inherited condition, characterized by many abnormalities, including premature ageing and an increased risk of skin and gut cancers. It is due to mutations of components of the telomerase complex including the telomerase RNA and dyskerin.

5. Angiogenesis

All tissues including cancers require a supply of oxygen and nutrients. For cancers to grow larger than about 0.4 mm in diameter, a new blood supply is needed to deliver these. The growth of new blood vessels from pre-existing vasculature is termed angiogenesis. The "angiogenic switch" denotes the ability of tumours to recruit new blood vessels by producing growth factors and is necessary for tumour growth and metastasis. Angiogenesis is determined by the balance of angiogenesis promoters and inhibitors (Figure 2.6).

Vascular endothelial growth factors (VEGF-A to -E) are a family of growth factor homodimers that act via one of three plasma membrane receptors (VEGFR-1 to -3) on endothelial cells. Overproduction of VEGF and/or FGF (fibroblast growth factor) is a common theme in many tumours (Table 2.1). Angiogenesis may be measured microscopically as microvessel density in an area of tumour or by assays of angiogenic factors. These measures are of prognostic significance in several human tumours. Angiogenesis

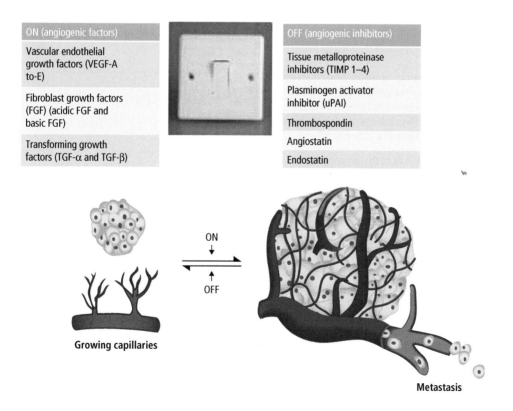

ON (angiogenic factors)	OFF (angiogenic inhibitors)
Vascular endothelial growth factors (VEGF-A to-E)	Tissue metalloproteinase inhibitors (TIMP 1–4)
Fibroblast growth factors (FGF) (acidic FGF and basic FGF)	Plasminogen activator inhibitor (uPAI)
	Thrombospondin
Transforming growth factors (TGF-α and TGF-β)	Angiostatin
	Endostatin

ON
↓
↑
OFF

Growing capillaries

Metastasis

Figure 2.6 The angiogenic switch.

is becoming a major focus of anticancer drug development. It is an attractive target for several reasons. Angiogenesis is a normal process in growth and development but is quiescent in adult life except during wound healing and menstruation, so side effects are predicted to be minimal. As the target will be normal endothelial cells without any genetic instability, there should be little capacity to acquire resistance. Each capillary supplies a large number of tumour cells, so the effects should be magnified in terms of tumour cell kill. Anti-angiogenic agents should have easy access to their target through the blood stream. In combination, these elements make anti-angiogenic therapies attractive, and several pharmaceutical companies have invested heavily in attempts to develop these agents. Bevacizumab is a monoclonal antibody that binds to VEGF; it was originally licensed for use in colon cancer and is also a valuable treatment for age-related macular degeneration, which is caused by retinal vessel proliferation.

Examples of neoangiogenesis in cancers:

- Colorectal cancer cells may produce VEGF.
- Glioma cells overexpress PDGF and PDGF receptor (PDGFR).
- Head and neck cancers activate VEGF via the nitric oxide pathway.

6. Invasion and metastasis

The properties of tissue invasion and metastatic spread are the histopathological hallmarks of malignant cancers that discriminate them from benign. A number of sequential steps have been identified in the process of metastatic spread of cancers:

1. Motility and invasion from the primary site.
2. Embolism and circulation in lymph or blood.
3. Arrest in a distant vascular or lymphatic capillary and adherence to the endothelium.
4. Extravasation into the target organ parenchyma.

Central to many of these steps is the role of cell–cell adhesion that controls the contact between cells and cell–extracellular matrix connections that influence the relationship between a cell and its environment. These interactions are regulated by cell adhesion molecules. Members of the cadherin and immunoglobulin superfamilies modulate cell–cell interactions whilst integrins control cell–extracellular matrix interactions. Alterations of cadherin, adhesion molecule and integrin expression are a common feature of metastatic cancer cells (Table 2.1).

Tumours may migrate as single cells or as collections of cells. The former strategy is used by lymphoma

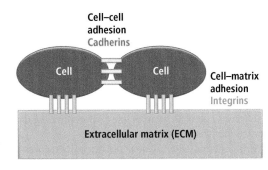

Figure 2.7 Cell–cell and cell–matrix interactions.

and small-cell lung cancer cells. It requires changes in integrins that mediate the cell–extracellular matrix interaction and matrix-degrading proteases. Metastatic migration as clumps of cancer cells is common for most epithelial tumours. In addition, this needs changes in cell–cell adhesion through cadherins and other adhesion receptors, as well as cell–cell communication via gap junctions (Figure 2.7).

Examples of invasion in cancers

- Colorectal cancer cells inactivate E-cadherin via APC and have altered expression of integrins.
- Melanoma cells overexpress MMP-2 and -9.

How to acquire the six capabilities (enabling hallmarks)

7. Cancer cells are prone to mutations due to genome instability

Cancer is really a genetic disease caused by mutations of cellular DNA that do not occur in the germ cells (oocytes and sperm). One of our lines of defense against cancer is to repair errors in DNA or to eradicate cells that have accumulated extensive DNA damage. However, DNA mutations tend to go uncorrected in cancer cells because their DNA replication is error-prone, their DNA repair mechanisms are deficient and their DNA damage cell cycle arrest and apoptosis responses are uncoupled. Altogether cancer cells are said to have genetic instability and this enables them to acquire the six hallmarks of a cancer cell. Sometimes these mutations develop in a stepwise fashion as the cell phenotype becomes more abnormal.

Box 2.2 How cancers metastasize: routes and destinations

Routes of metastasis

Breast cancer cells that leave a primary tumour in blood vessels will be carried in the blood first through the heart and then to the capillary beds of the lungs. Some cancer cells might form metastases in the lung (Figure a), whilst others pass through the lung to enter the systemic arterial system, where they are transported to remote organs, such as bones (Figure b) or skin (Figure e). By contrast, colon cancer cells will be taken by the hepatoportal circulatory system first to the liver (Figures c and d). There is no direct flow from the lymphatic system to other organs, so cancer cells within it – for example, melanoma cells – must enter the venous system to be transported to distant organs. Rarely, routes other than blood and lymphatic vessels are used in metastasis. Transcoelomic spread across the abdominal cavity occurs for gastric tumours that metastasize to the ovaries (known as Krukenberg tumours). Spread within the cerebrospinal fluid is thought to be responsible for the metastasis of medulloblastoma up and down the spinal column.

Lung metastases

Bone metastases

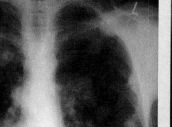

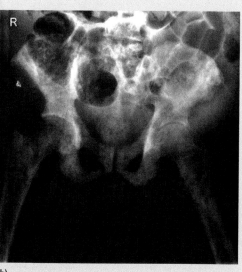

(a)

(b)

Liver metastases (ultrasound images)

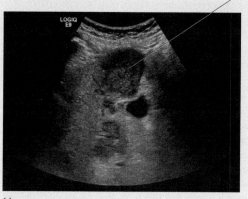

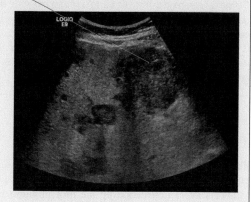

(c)

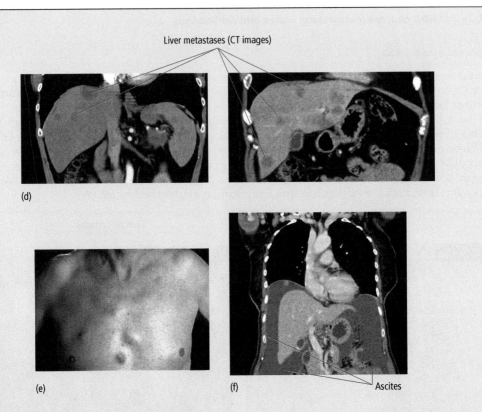

Liver metastases (CT images)

(d)

(e)   (f)   Ascites

Figure (a) Lung metastases. Plain chest radiograph showing multiple rounded metastases of varying sizes in a man with a metastatic testicular non-seminomatous germ cell tumour. Other tumours that commonly metastasize to the lungs include lung, breast, renal and thyroid cancers and sarcomas. (b) Bone metastases. Mixed sclerotic and lucent bone metastases of prostate cancer. (c) Ultrasound images of liver metastases. (d) CT images of liver metastases. (e) Patient with multiple cutaneous metastases from non-small cell lung cancer. (f) Sub-diaphragmatic peritoneal deposit and extensive ascites. The patient had advanced ovarian cancer and the peritoneal deposits have travelled from the primary site in the ascitic fluid. This is known as transcoelomic spread or spread across a body cavity (from "koilōma", the Greek word for a hollow or cavity).

Where cancers metastasize

Certain cancers tend to metastasize to particular organs and this cannot be accounted for by blood flow alone. The basis for this tissue tropism has been found to relate to chemokine and chemokine receptor expression. Breast cancer cells express high levels of the CXCR4 chemokine receptor. Lung tissue expresses high levels of a soluble ligand for the CXCR4 receptor. Therefore, breast cancer cells that are taken to the lung find a strong chemokine receptor "match", which may lead to chemokine-mediated signal activation. By contrast, in other organs where breast cancers less commonly metastasize, there are low levels of the ligand.

8. Inflammation promotes the growth of cancers

Although cancers generally have ways of avoiding destruction by the host immune system (see hallmark 9. Cancers avoid destruction by the host immune system), they still often induce a local inflammatory response. It was thought that this inflammatory response was part of the host's attempt to eradicate the cancer cells. Instead it appears that the inflammatory cytokines actually promote tumour growth, proliferation and angiogenesis. Rather like autoimmune disease it seems that this is another own goal of the immune system.

Additional capabilities of cancers (emerging hallmarks)

9. Cancers avoid destruction by the host immune system

Cancers employ a number of strategies to escape the host immune system so that they can survive and grow. They have acquired ways of avoiding both the innate and adoptive immune systems and this is why for most cancers, immunotherapy is ineffective.

10. Cancer cells deregulate cellular metabolism

Cancer cell proliferation is enabled by changes in energy metabolism to fuel growth. In many circumstances cancer cells switch from normal aerobic glycolysis to the much less efficient anaerobic metabolism. Although the rationale behind this metabolic switch in cancer cells is unclear, it may account for the resistance of some tumours to the effects of radiotherapy.

Genome instability

DNA damage or mutation will normally result in cell cycle arrest followed by DNA repair or apoptosis. Interference in this process may occur either by deficient DNA damage recognition and repair or abnormal gatekeeping of the cell cycle arrest/apoptosis response. This will result in the uncorrected accumulation of a large number of genetic abnormalities, which is referred to as "genomic instability". It is thought that this allows cells to acquire the six capabilities that characterize the cancer cell phenotype and physiology (Figures 2.8 and 2.9).

DNA repair

Environmental damage to DNA occurs commonly and eukaryotes have developed several techniques for repairing both double strand breakages and single strand errors in DNA.

1. Repair of double strand breaks in DNA:
   - homologous recombination using the sister chromatid as a template
   - non-homologous end joining (NHEJ)

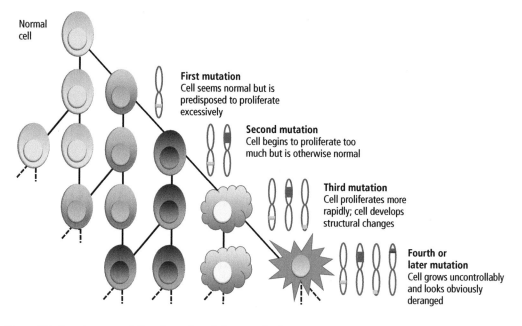

Normal cell

First mutation
Cell seems normal but is predisposed to proliferate excessively

Second mutation
Cell begins to proliferate too much but is otherwise normal

Third mutation
Cell proliferates more rapidly; cell develops structural changes

Fourth or later mutation
Cell grows uncontrollably and looks obviously deranged

Figure 2.8 Stepwise accumulation of genetic mutations contributing to oncogenic phenotype.

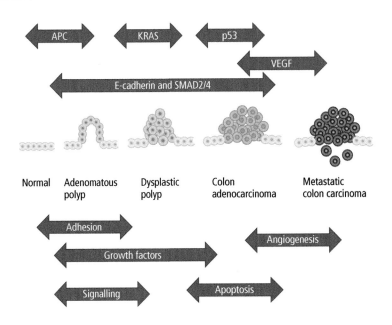

Normal   Adenomatous   Dysplastic   Colon   Metastatic
          polyp   polyp   adenocarcinoma   colon carcinoma

Figure 2.9 Colon cancer development from normal mucosa to metastatic carcinoma associated with stepwise acquisition of oncogenic mutations. APC, adenomatous polyposis coli gene; KRAS, Kirsten rat sarcoma viral oncogene homologue; p53, tumour protein 53 (TP53); SMAD, *Homo sapiens* homologue of *Drosophila* protein mothers against decapentaplegic (MAD); VEGF, vascular endothelial growth factor.

2. Repair of single strand mutations in DNA:
   - nucleotide excision repair (NER) for bulky adducts, pyrimidine dimmers and photoproducts
   - mismatch repair (MMR) for single mispaired bases and short deletions
   - base excision repair (BER) for alkylated bases or loss of a single base

Hereditary mutations of the enzymes involved in DNA repair will predispose to malignancy as they confer genome instability (Table 2.2).

DNA damage recognition

Another group of enzymes are required to recognize damaged DNA, leading to cell cycle arrest to allow DNA repair to be completed before the damage is replicated and passed on to the progeny cells. A number of cancer-predisposing syndromes are associated with inherited mutations of these enzymes. Examples include p53, whose inactivation is an early step in the development of many cancers. Patients with the Li–Fraumeni syndrome carry one mutant germline p53 allele and are at high risk for the development of

Table 2.2 Hereditary DNA repair syndromes

DNA damage	DNA repair mechanism	Examples of defect of DNA repair	Examples of cancers associated with defects
Double strand DNA breakage	Homologous (sister chromatid) repair	BRCA1 (hereditary breast and ovarian cancer)	Breast and ovarian cancers
	Non-homologous end joining (NHEJ)	XRCC4 (X-ray repair complementing defect gene) (lethal)	None (lethal defect)
Single strand DNA breakage	Nucleotide excision repair (NER)	XP (xeroderma pigmentosa)	Skin cancers, leukaemia and melanoma
	Mismatch repair (MMR)	MSH and MLH (hereditary non-polyposis colon cancer)	Colon, endometrium, ovarian, pancreatic and gastric cancers
	Base excision repair (BER)	MYH (hereditary non-polyposis colon cancer)	Colon cancers

sarcomas, leukaemia and cancers of the breast, brain and adrenal glands.

Epigenetic changes

Most of the discussion above about the molecular mechanisms of malignancy has described somatic and occasional germline mutations of DNA that lead to aberrant proteins that in turn contribute to onco-genesis. This argument follows the central dogma of molecular biology introduced by Francis Crick in the late 1950s, which stated that information flows in a unidirectional course from DNA sequence via RNA sequence to protein sequence. Although there are recognized exceptions to the central dogma, such as retroviruses and prions, it remains broadly true. How-ever, some inheritable changes in phenotype or gene expression arise by mechanisms other than changes in the sequence of DNA bases. These inheritable changes passed on from a cell to her daughters are called epigenetic changes and perhaps the most ob-vious of these is cell differentiation.

The term epigenetics was introduced by the British developmental biologist Conrad Hal Waddington in 1942 as a metaphor for cell differentiation and de-velopment from a progenitor stem cell. Waddington likened differentiation to a marble rolling down a landscape of hills and valleys to reach a final desti-nation. The destination (cell fate) was determined by the landscape (epigenetics) and the marble could not travel back to the top (terminal differentiation). To-day the term refers to modification of DNA and chro-matin that influences gene transcription, alteration of post-transcriptional RNA and finally to protein degradation.

DNA methylation

Perhaps the most recognized epigenetic modification of DNA is nucleotide base methylation, typically the addition of a methyl group to the cytosine pyrimi-dine ring. In vertebrates, DNA methylation usually oc-curs in a CpG dinucleotide. Unmethylated CpGs are grouped in clusters called "CpG islands" that occur in the 5′ regulatory regions of many genes. DNA methy-lation of CpG islands inhibits gene transcription by impeding the binding of transcriptional proteins and by binding methyl-CpG-binding domain (MBD) pro-teins. MBD proteins recruit additional proteins, such as histone deacetylases (HDACs), which modify hi-stones to form compact, inactive chromatin termed silent chromatin. Since epigenetic changes such as DNA methylation are inherited during cell replica-tion, maintenance of the pattern of DNA methyla-tion is required following each cycle of DNA replica-tion and this is achieved by DNA methyltransferases using the conserved DNA strand as the template (Fig-ure 2.10). DNA methylation of tumour suppressor genes has been found to be a common mechanism of epigenetic gene silencing in cancers.

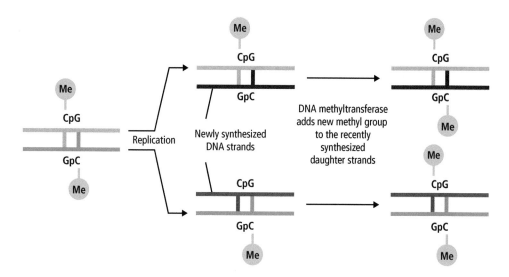

Figure 2.10 DNA methylation is passed on during cell replication to progeny cells by DNA methyltransferase enzymes that methylate CpG islands. CpG refers to the DNA dinucleotide sequence CG joined by the phosphate backbone of DNA.

Chromatin modification

Chromatin is composed of DNA and proteins, chiefly the histone proteins around which the DNA is wound. There are six classes of histones organized into core histones (H2A, H2B, H3 and H4) and linker histones (H1 and H5). The core histones, which are highly conserved through nature, share N-terminal amino acid sequences that are the sites for post-transcriptional modification, for example, acetylation and methylation. These histone modifications alter the binding of the DNA to the nucleosome and modify RNA polymerase activity and hence gene expression. In general, tightly bound DNA is less expressed. Numerous enzymes have been identified that are involved with the modification of histone protein leading to alterations of chromatin structure and regulation of gene expression. These include histone methyltransferase (HMT) and histone acetyltransferase (HAT); other enzymes catalyze the removal of these modifications including HDAC (Figure 2.11). Acetylation of histone tails reduces their binding affinity for DNA, allowing access for RNA polymerase and enhancing gene transcription. HDAC, therefore, by reversing histone tail residue acetylation suppresses gene expression, including tumour suppressor gene expression contributing to oncogenesis. A number of HDAC inhibitors have been studied including valproate and more recently vorinostat or suberoylanilide hydroxamic acid (SAHA), which is licensed for the management of cutaneous T-cell non-Hodgkin's lymphoma.

RNA interference

Post-translational interference of messenger RNA (mRNA) transcripts can also modify the expression of genes without altering the DNA sequence. Two types of small RNA molecules, microRNA (miRNA) and small interfering RNA (siRNA), can bind to specific complementary sequences of RNA or DNA and either increase or decrease their activity, for example by preventing an mRNA from producing a protein (Figure 2.12). RNA interference was originally identified in petunia plants. Botanists attempting to produce darker and darker petunia flowers inserted additional genes of an enzyme that catalyzes pigment synthesis. However, the transgenic plants produced white or variegated white flowers and this was subsequently found to be due to post-transcriptional inhibition of gene expression brought about by rapid mRNA degradation. The eventual explanation of this gene silencing phenomenon was identified in *Caenorhabditis elegans* by Craig Mello and Andrew Fire in 1998 who demonstrated that double-stranded RNA caused the gene silencing. They called this RNA interference (RNAi) and won the Nobel Prize in 2006 for this work. Both the role of RNAi in the epigenetic generation of cancers and the potential of RNAi as a therapeutic approach are the focus of fevered research.

Protein degradation

A further form of epigenetic modification that contributes to the cellular phenotype is the destruction of

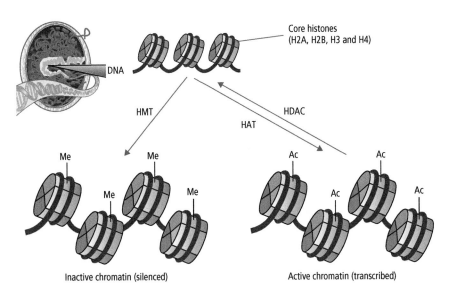

Figure 2.11 Mechanism of chromatin modification. Ac, acetyl; HAT, histone acetyltransferase; HDAC, histone deacetylase; HMT, histone methyltransferase; Me, methyl.

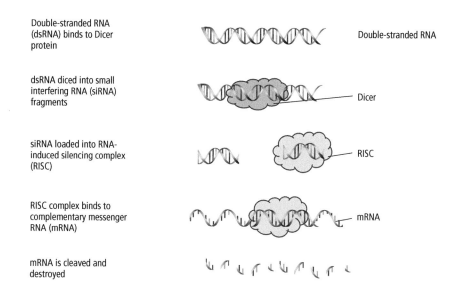

Double-stranded RNA (dsRNA) binds to Dicer protein

Double-stranded RNA

dsRNA diced into small interfering RNA (siRNA) fragments

Dicer

siRNA loaded into RNA-induced silencing complex (RISC)

RISC

RISC complex binds to complementary messenger RNA (mRNA)

mRNA

mRNA is cleaved and destroyed

Figure 2.12 Mechanism of RNA interference.

proteins chiefly by proteasomes. Proteins are tagged for degradation by a small protein called ubiquitin and this reaction is catalyzed by enzymes including the product of the gene disrupted in Von Hippel–Lindau syndrome and Fanconi's anaemia. At least four ubiquitin molecules attach to the condemned protein in a process called polyubiquitination and the protein then moves to a proteasome, where the proteolysis occurs (Figure 2.13). Epigenetic regulation of protein degradation could contribute to oncogenesis in a variety of ways. Gankyrin, a component of the proteasome, is overexpressed in hepatocellular cancers. Bortezomib, a new treatment for myeloma, acts by inhibiting proteasome function.

Genetic causes of cancer

Hereditary causes of cancer

The causes of cancer may be usefully divided into genetic and environmental factors. The genetic factors are either germline mutations that are present in every cell of the body or somatic alterations only found in the tumour cells. Germline mutations may be either inherited, in which case they follow a familial pattern or may be new sporadic mutations that neither parent has. Some of the germline mutations have been outlined as mutator phenotypes (DNA repair and damage recognition genes) above. Other germline cancer-predisposing mutations occur in tumour suppressor genes and oncogenes.

Oncogenes

The first clue to the identification of specific genes involved in the development of cancer came from the study of tumour viruses. Although cancer is generally not an infectious disease, some animal leukaemias, lymphomas and solid tumours, particularly sarcomas, can be caused by viruses. Oncogenes were identified following the discovery by Peyton Rous in 1911 that sarcomas could be induced in healthy chickens by injecting them with a cell-free extract of the tumour of a sick chicken. This was due to transmission of Rous sarcoma virus (RSV), an oncogenic retrovirus with just four genes:

- (*gag* group-specific antigen), which encodes the capsid protein
- (*pol* polymerase), which encodes the reverse transcriptase
- (*env* envelope), which encodes the envelope protein
- *src*, which encodes a tyrosine kinase

It is the *src* gene that is necessary for cell transformation and is therefore an oncogene – literally a gene capable of causing cancer. In the late 1970s Harold Varmus and Michael Bishop discovered that a homologous proto-oncogene (c-SRC) is present in the normal mammalian genome (the human *src* locus is on chromosome 20q12-q13) and has been hijacked by the retrovirus. The prefix v- denotes a viral sequence and the prefix c- a cellular sequence. In 1956, 55 years after his discovery of RSV and at the age of 87, Peyton Rous was (finally) awarded a Nobel

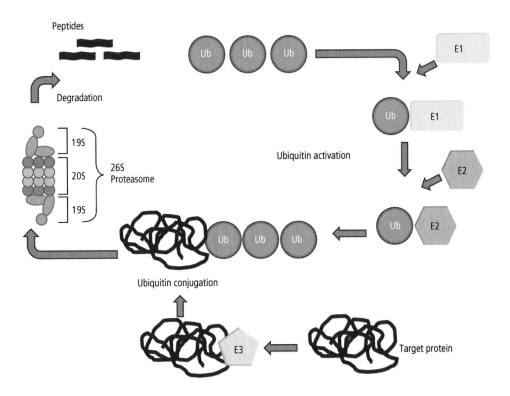

Figure 2.13 Proteasome pathway of protein ubiquitination and degradation. E, ubiquitination enzymes; Ub, ubiquitin.

Prize, whilst Bishop and Varmus only waited 10 years from their discovery to the award of their Nobel Prize in 1989. Around 50 oncogenes have been identified by their presence in transforming retroviruses (e.g. erbB, H-RAS, JUN) and further oncogenes have been discovered by positional cloning of chromosomal translocations (e.g. Bcl-2, BCR-ABL) and by transfection studies (e.g. N-RAS, RET). Most oncogenes contribute to cancer's autonomy in growth factors, either as plasma membrane receptors (e.g. RET, PTCH), signal transduction pathways (e.g. PTEN, NF1 and 2, VHL) or transcription factors (e.g. c-MYC, WT1) (Table 2.3).

Tumour suppressor genes

In contrast to oncogenes, tumour suppressor genes act as cell cycle brakes, slowing the proliferation of cells, and mutations in these genes also contribute to cancer. Germline mutations of tumour suppressor genes behave as autosomal-dominant familial cancer predispositions. Tumour suppressor genes require the loss of both functional alleles to support a cancer (unlike oncogenes where one mutant allele suffices).

In 1971 Alfred Knudson proposed the two hit model of tumour suppression to account for the differences between familial and sporadic retinoblastoma in children. In familial cases, tumours arose at a younger age and were more frequently bilateral. Knudson hypothesized that these children had inherited one defective retinoblastoma gene allele, followed by loss of the function of the second allele in the cancer cells through a somatic mutation (Figures 2.14 and 2.15). Tumour suppressor genes, like oncogenes, also involve a variety of functional categories, including cell cycle regulation (e.g. p53, Rb), DNA repair and maintenance (e.g. BRCA1 and 2, MLH1, MSH2), as well as signal transduction (e.g. NF1, PTEN) and cell adhesion (e.g. APC) (Table 2.2).

The Maths of Cancer or "How long have I had it?" (Figure 2.16)

20 doublings = 10^6 cells (million)

30 doublings = 10^9 cells (billion) weigh 1 g = earliest detectable

35 doublings = $10^{10.5}$ cells = usual number at diagnosis (3 cm diameter)

40 doublings = 10^{12} cells (trillion) weigh 1 kg = usual number at death

Table 2.3 Table of hereditary cancer predisposition syndromes

Syndrome	Malignancies	Inheritance	Gene	Function
Breast/ovarian	Breast, ovarian, colon, prostate	AD AD	BRCA1 BRCA2	Genome integrity
Cowden	Breast, thyroid, gastrointestinal, pancreas	AD	PTEN	Signal transduction (tyrosine phosphatase)
Li–Fraumeni	Sarcoma, breast, osteosarcoma, leukaemia, glioma, adrenocortical	AD	p53	Genome integrity
Familial polyposis coli	Colon, upper gastrointestinal	AD	APC	Cell adhesion
Hereditary non-polyposis colon cancer (Lynch type II)	Colon, endometrium, ovarian, pancreatic, gastric	AD AD AD AD	MSH2 MLH1 PMS1 PMS2	DNA mismatch repair
MEN 1 (multiple endocrine neoplasia 1)	Pancreatic islet cell, pituitary adenoma	AD	MEN1	Transcription repressor
MEN 2 (multiple endocrine neoplasia 2)	Medullary thyroid, phaeochromocytoma	AD	RET	Signal transduction (receptor tyrosine kinase)
Neurofibromatosis 1 (Figure 2.15)	Neurofibrosarcoma, phaeochromocytoma, optic glioma	AD	NF1	Signal transduction (regulates GTPases)
Neurofibromatosis 2	Vestibular schwannoma	AD	NF2	Cell adhesion
von Hippel–Lindau	Haemangioblastoma of retina and central nervous system, renal cell, phaeochromocytoma	AD	VHL	Ubiquination
Retinoblastoma	Retinoblastoma, osteosarcoma	AD	RB1	Cell cycle regulation
Xeroderma pigmentosa	Skin, leukaemia, melanoma	AR AR AR AR	XPA XPC XPD XPF	DNA nucleotide excision repair
Gorlin	Basal cell skin, brain	AD	PTCH	Signal transduction (repressor of hedgehog signalling)

AD, autosomal dominant; AR, autosomal recessive; GTPase, guanosine triphosphatase.

The cell cycle takes 16–24 hours to complete. For Burkitt's lymphoma the growth fraction is 0.29 (i.e. 29% of the cells are actively dividing at any one time) and hence the doubling time is about 2 days. In contrast, the growth fraction for non-small cell cancer of the lung is under 0.02 and the doubling time is around 130 days. To get to death (10^{12} cells) can take just 3 months for BL but for NSCLC to get to 10^9 (just detectable on CT) takes 10.5 years. In reality most lung cancers are found when they are 3 cm in diameter or $10^{10.5}$ cells, after 35 doublings (12.3 years).

Environmental causes of cancer

The multitude of environmental factors that are associated with the development of malignancy may be usefully divided into:

- Physical (radiation)
- Chemical (chemical carcinogens)
- Biological (infections)

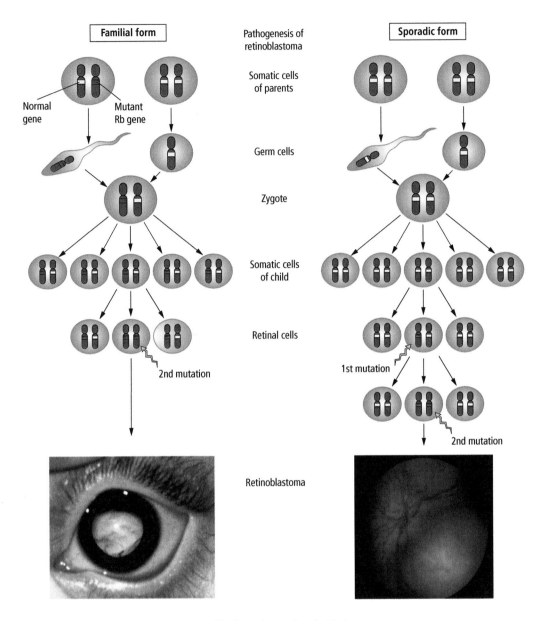

Figure 2.14 Knudson's two-hit hypotheses of familial and sporadic retinoblastoma.

Radiation

The major physical carcinogen is radiation. Radiation is ubiquitous and may either be ionizing (e.g. γ-rays from cosmic radiation and isotope decay, α-particles from radon, X-rays from medical imaging) or non-ionizing (e.g. ultraviolet (UV) light from the sun, microwave and radiofrequency radiation from mobile phones, electromagnetic fields from electricity generators and pylons, ultrasound radiation from imaging). Ionizing radiation ejects electrons from atoms yielding an ion pair and requires 10–15 eV (electronvolts). Ionizing radiation may be either electromagnetic (X-rays, γ-rays) or particulate (α-particles, neutrons). Non-ionizing radiation does not yield an ion pair but can still excite electrons resulting in chemical change.

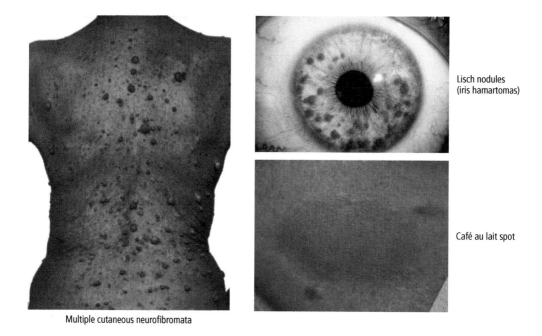

Lisch nodules
(iris hamartomas)

Café au lait spot

Multiple cutaneous neurofibromata

Figure 2.15 Multiple dermal neurofibromata typical of peripheral neurofibromatosis or type 1 NF, previously known eponymously as von Recklinghausen's disease. It is due to hereditary mutation of the NF1 neurofibromin gene on chromosome 2p22, which encodes a guanosine triphosphatase (GTPase) activating protein involved in the signal transduction cascade.

Ultraviolet radiation

UV radiation is electromagnetic radiation with a wavelength shorter than visible light (400–700 nm) but longer than X-rays (10–0.01 nm). It is subdivided into three wavelength bands:

- UVA (313–400 nm)
- UVB (290–315 nm)
- UVC (220–290 nm)

UVC has the most potent effects on DNA, which absorbs most strongly at 254 nm. However, UVC is

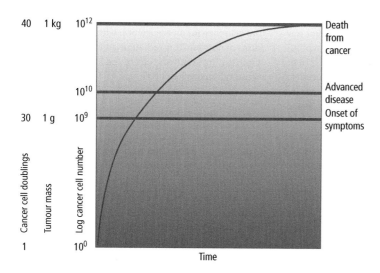

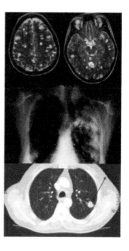

Figure 2.16 The maths of cancer.

Humans are exposed to broad range of electromagnetic frequencies

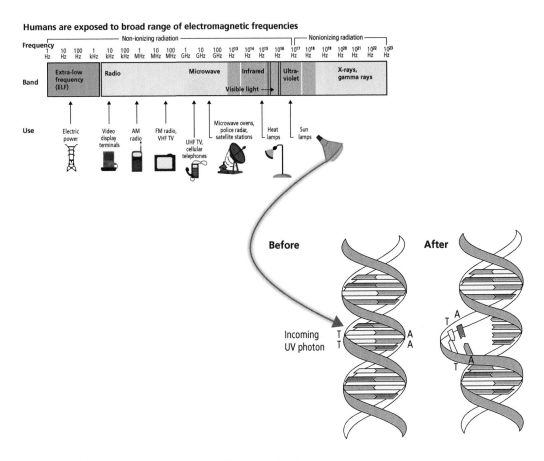

Figure 2.17 UV-light-induced thymidine dimers. T, Thymine; A, Adenine.

quickly absorbed by the atmosphere and hence UVB is considered to be the greater environmental hazard. Most UV radiation is absorbed by atmospheric ozone in the stratosphere and this ozone layer is being depleted in part due to chlorine in chlorofluorocarbons (CFCs), resulting in increasing UV exposure levels. Ultraviolet light is responsible for vitamin D activation and suntans. One of the major lesions induced in DNA by UV radiation is the thymidine dimer, a covalent bonding of adjacent thymidine residues on the same DNA strand (Figure 2.17). This causes local distortion of the double helix that is repaired by the NER pathway. The seven identified xeroderma pigmentosa genes encode essential components that undertake NER and hence xeroderma pigmentosa predisposes to UV-induced skin malignancies. Melanin pigment in the skin normally absorbs UV radiation, thus protecting the skin. Basal cell and squamous cell skin cancers increase with cumulative UV exposure, whilst

the relationship is less straightforward for melanoma. The evidence for an association with cancer for other forms of non-ionizing radiation (microwave, radiofrequency, ultrasound and electromagnetic radiation) is weak and inconsistent.

Ionizing radiation
Natural sources

Exposure to natural sources of ionizing radiation varies in different populations. Higher altitude and further latitude from the equator are both associated with higher cosmic radiation exposure composed of very high energy particles that are thought to originate outside our solar system including from supernovae. In addition, various regions have higher natural background levels from radon. Radon is a colourless, odourless gas formed from decay as part of the uranium-238 series. The radon-222 isotope, along

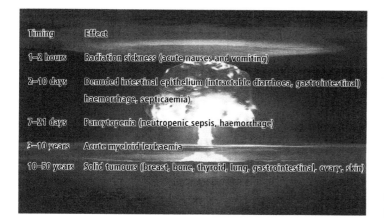

Timing	Effect
1–2 hours	Radiation sickness (acute nausea and vomiting)
2–10 days	Denuded intestinal epithelium (intractable diarrhoea, gastrointestinal) haemorrhage, septicaemia)
7–21 days	Pancytopenia (neutropenic sepsis, haemorrhage)
3–10 years	Acute myeloid leukaemia
10–50 years	Solid tumours (breast, bone, thyroid, lung, gastrointestinal, ovary, skin)

Figure 2.18 How atomic bombs kill.

with a number of its progeny, is an α-particle emitter. Radon gas levels are normally quoted in Bq/m^3 (1 becquerel (Bq) is one decay per second) and the average indoor levels in the United Kingdom are about 20 Bq/m^3. Local geology (igneous granite) with high levels of uranium produces high levels of radon in soil gas, but for it to escape to the surface the soil must be highly porous. In the United Kingdom, radon levels are particularly high in Devon and Cornwall, Derbyshire and Northamptonshire. From the results of eight case-control studies, it is believed that radon exposure accounts for a small fraction of lung cancers with a 14% increased risk for a person living for 30 years in a house with levels of 150 Bq/m^3.

Nuclear warfare

Most of the information on the induction of cancers by ionizing radiation comes from exposed populations, including Japanese people exposed to atomic bombs at Hiroshima ("Little Boy" was a uranium-235-enriched bomb dropped by Enola Gay) and Nagasaki

("Fat Man" was a plutonium-239 bomb dropped by Bockstar). The estimated populations of the two cities at the time of bombing was 560,000 and approximately 200,000 people died within the first few months of the acute effects of blast, burns and radiation exposure (Figure 2.18). The Radiation Effects Research Foundation has followed 86,000 survivors or hibakusha and, up to 1990, 7827 had died of cancer. The excess risk of leukaemia was seen especially in those exposed as children and was highest during the first 10 years after the bombing. However, the excess risk of solid tumours occurred later and still persists (Table 2.4).

Table 2.4 Cancer deaths in the hibakusha (survivors of Hiroshima and Nagasaki atomic bombs)

	Total number of deaths	Estimated number of deaths due to radiation	Percentage of deaths attributable to radiation
Leukaemia	176	89	51
Solid tumours	4687	339	7
Total	4863	428	9

Box 2.3 Chernobyl

On 26 April 1986, nuclear reactor number 4 at Chernobyl exploded in the world's worst nuclear accident. Over 10^{19} Bq of radioactive isotopes were released, including 5.2 × 10^{18} Bq of β-emitting isotopes of iodine that concentrate in the thyroid gland. An increase in thyroid cancer in children was first reported in 1990 but an excess of other tumours has not (yet?) been reported. Fallout from Chernobyl affected millions of people living within a few hundred kilometres from the reactor and caused a 30–100-fold increase in the incidence of thyroid cancer, especially in children. The younger the child at exposure, the greater the risk is. The increase so far is almost entirely papillary carcinoma of the thyroid and the dominant subtype has solid papillary morphology. At a molecular level, these tumours show rearrangement of the RET oncogene by inversion or translocation with partner genes to yield constitutively active c-RET tyrosine kinases.

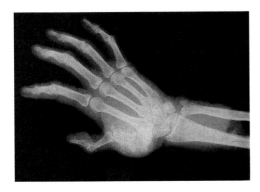

Figure 2.19 Osteosarcoma of the first metacarpal 15 years after radiotherapy for arthritis (no longer used). This radiograph shows cortical destruction, a soft tissue mass with internal calcification and periosteal reaction.

Table 2.5 Diagnostic imaging radiation doses

Imaging procedure	Radiation dose	Equivalent to natural background radiation for:
Chest X-ray	0.02 mSv	3 days
Chest CT scan	8 mSv	3.6 years or one transatlantic flight
Abdominal CT scan	10 mSv	4.5 years
Intravenous urogram	2.5 mSv	14 months
Brain CT scan	2.3 mSv	1 year
Mammogram	0.7 mSv	3 months

Medical radiation

The hazards of medical ionizing radiation may be difficult to determine as ionizing radiation-induced tumours are not identifiable by a particular signature DNA mutation (unlike the thymidine dimers induced by UV radiation). Some tissues, such as breast, thyroid and bone marrow, are more susceptible to the carcinogenic effects of ionizing radiation, although tumours have been described in every organ site following radiation exposure (Figure 2.19). Well-described examples of iatrogenic tumours include acute leukaemias induced by radiation treatment for ankylosing spondylitis prescribed in the late 1930s in the United Kingdom. Similarly, 20,000 Israelis received radiation for *Tinea capitis* (ringworm) in the 1950s and by the 1980s there was a significantly increased risk of meningioma. Similar increases in tumours have been observed in patients treated with radiotherapy, including men treated for prostate cancer, women treated for cervical cancers and Hodgkin's disease survivors. Diagnostic imaging radiation doses are shown in Table 2.5.

Occupational radiation

The first victims of occupational exposure to radiation included Marie Curie (the first woman to win a Nobel Prize and the only person to win two Nobel prizes in different scientific fields: physics 1903 and chemistry 1911) and her daughter Irène Joliot-Curie (also a Nobel laureate in chemistry 1935), who both died of leukaemia. In the 1920s, watch dials were hand painted with radium-based luminous paint. The female radium dial painters often licked their paint brushes to give them a sharp point and ingested the radium. Up to 3% of these women subsequently developed osteosarcomas after a latency of 5–10 years. These "radium girls" successfully sued their employer

Box 2.4 **Units of radiotherapy**

The simplest metaphor for radiation doses is rainfall.

- The amount of rain falling is the activity (Bq)
- The amount of rain hitting you is the absorbed dose (Gy)
- How wet you get is dose equivalent (Sv)

The becquerel (Bq) is the SI unit of radioactivity and 1 Bq is equivalent to one nuclear decay per second. It is named after Henri Becquerel who shared the Nobel Prize with Marie and Pierre Curie for the discovery of radioactivity. The Hiroshima bomb produced 8×10^{24} Bq.

The gray (Gy) is the SI unit of absorbed radiation dose for ionizing radiation. One gray is the absorption of 1 joule (J) of ionizing radiation by 1 kg of matter, usually human tissue. It is named after Hal Gray, a British pioneer of radiation biology and physics who also established the Gray Laboratories at Mount Vernon Hospital.

The sievert (Sv) is the SI unit of radioactive dose equivalence and reflects the biological effects in the tissue of radiation rather than its physical attributes. The equivalent dose will depend on the absorbed dose (measured in grays) as well as the type of radiation, as well as the time and volume and part of body irradiated. It is named after Rolf Sievert, a Swedish medical physicist. A dose of 3 Sv will lead to a lethal dose (LD) 50/30 or death in 50% of cases within 30 days and over 6 Sv survival is very unusual.

and this litigation resulted in the introduction of industrial safety standards and health and safety regulations at work. Similarly, pitchblende (uranium oxide) and uranium miners in Czechoslovakia, Sweden, Newfoundland and Colorado who have been exposed to radon are at increased risk of lung cancers.

Chemical carcinogenesis

Cancer is essentially a genetic disease arising from mutations of genes that affect the control of normal cell function (proto-oncogenes and tumour suppressor genes) or from polymorphic genes that govern enzyme systems that activate or detoxify environmental carcinogens (phase I and phase II enzyme reactions). Carcinogenic mutations can arise in several ways: genotoxic environmental factors (e.g. radiation and many chemical carcinogens), spontaneous DNA aberrations occurring during normal cell replication or hereditary germline mutations. Chemical carcinogenesis was shown to be a multistep process following studies in the 1940s using polycyclic aromatic hydrocarbons (PAHs) and a murine skin cancer model system. This identified three steps – initiation, promotion and progression – that involve separate biological processes. Chemical carcinogens may operate at any or all three stages. The minority of chemical carcinogens act directly on DNA (e.g. alkylating agents), whilst the majority are pro-carcinogens that require metabolic activation to the ultimate carcinogen forms. Many ultimate carcinogens are potent electrophiles, capable of accepting electrons (e.g. epoxides derived from polycyclic hydrocarbons, vinyl chloride and aflatoxins, the N-hydroxylated metabolites of azo dyes and the alkyldiazonium ions derived from nitrosamines).

Initiation

The key feature of initiation is the need for cell replication without repair of the chemically induced DNA damage. Initiation is irreversible, usually involves simple DNA mutations that are "fixed" by cell division and results in no morphological changes to the cells. Single exposure to a carcinogen may be sufficient for initiation. For example, aflatoxin B1 is one of a family of mycotoxin contaminants of food crops such as grain and groundnuts (peanuts). It is produced by *Aspergillus flavus*, which favours hot and humid conditions and is therefore most likely to contaminate food in Africa and Asia. Aflatoxin B1 is oxidized by hepatic P450 microsomal enzymes into aflatoxin B1 2,3-epoxide, which binds to DNA bases forming mutagenic adducts that preferentially induce GC to TA

transversions. These transversions have been identified frequently in codon 249 of the p53 gene in hepatocellular carcinomas in patients from southern Africa and China who are exposed to high levels of aflatoxin B1 and may also have hepatitis B virus (HBV) infection.

Promotion

Promotion is a reversible process requiring multiple exposures to the carcinogen, usually with a dose-response threshold. Promotion does not usually involve DNA mutations (non-genotoxic carcinogenesis) but provides a chemically mediated selective growth advantage. Thus, promotion results in the clonal expansion of cells. In the 1940s it was noted that 5% of mice treated with benzopyrene developed tumours but this figure rose to 80% when croton oil was added. Croton oil alone, however, produced no tumours. Subsequently, it was found that tetradecanoylphorbol acetate (TPA), a natural component of croton oil (from the seeds of *Croton tiglium*, a tree cultivated in India, which resemble castor seeds), interacts with the protein kinase c signal pathway, stimulating growth and thus acting as a promoter. TPA is the most widely used tumour promoter in cellular experimental models of oncogenesis. Similarly, oestrogens are believed to act as carcinogenic promoters. Indeed, transplacental diethylstilboestrol (DES) was shown to induce vaginal clear-cell adenocarcinomas in young women whose mothers had been treated with DES during pregnancy.

Progression

Progression is an irreversible step that results in morphologically identifiable cellular changes and frequently involves multiple complex DNA changes, such as chromosomal alterations. Progression and the accumulation of multiple genetic abnormalities that characterize cancer cells may occur spontaneously or may be driven by chemical carcinogens. Since individual cells may acquire these genetic changes, progression leads to heterogeneity of the cell population. Ultimately some cells will acquire a mutator phenotype and the six genetic attributes that characterize a cancer cell.

Diet and cancer

A role for dietary constituents has been described for a number of cancers and the evidence for some of these relationships is more robust than for others. Alcohol intake has been convincingly associated with

Box 2.5 A brief epidemiological history of smoking and cancer

Tobacco was one of the "gifts" from the New World to the Old along with syphilis and potatoes. Nicotine is named after Jean Nicot, a 15th century French ambassador to Lisbon, who was a great advocate of smoking and who in 1559 sent tobacco to Catherine de Medici, the then Queen of France. Tobacco was subsequently introduced to England by Sir Walter Raleigh in 1586. Smoking was actively encouraged amongst soldiers in the Thirty Years War, Napoleonic campaigns, Crimean War and, most notably, the First World War. Smoking reduces fear and anxiety and suppresses appetite and these were deemed beneficial to soldiers.

Early epidemiological links with non-lung cancers

In 1761, John Hill, a London doctor, wrote up several cases of nasal cancer amongst heavy tobacco snuff users and, in 1795, Thomas van Soemmering suggested a link between pipe smoking and lip cancer. The American Civil War Yankee general and later US President, Ulysses S. Grant, died in 1885 of throat cancer described with some pathos by Mark Twain in the first volume of his autobiography, and this Twain attributed to excessive smoking. In an early cohort study in the 1920s, Dr R. Abbe observed that, of 90 patients with oral cancer, 89 were smokers.

Epidemiological links with lung cancer

In 1939, Dr Franz Muller of the University of Cologne performed what is generally recognized as the earliest case-control study of smoking, which showed that a very high proportion of lung cancer patients were heavy smokers. However, the results were dismissed as unreliable because Hitler was a fanatical antismoker. Shortly after the Second World War, Austin Bradford Hill, Edward Kennaway, Percy Stock and Richard Doll set out to investigate links between smoking and lung cancer, at a time when 90% of adult males in the United Kingdom smoked, using a case-control dose–response strategy. Their case-control study was performed in 1948 in 20 London hospitals, interviewing two controls with gastric or colonic cancer as controls for each lung cancer patient. In all analyses, there was a dose–response relationship between the number of cigarettes smoked and the risk of lung cancer. This was published in 1950 in the *British Medical Journal*.

In 1951, Doll and Hill set up a prospective cohort study of 60,000 doctors on the medical register who were recruited via a letter in the *BMJ*; 40,000 replies were received and, in the following 2.5 years, there were 789 deaths, including 36 from lung cancer. There was a significant increase in the risk of lung cancer with increased tobacco consumption (see table below). However, they noted that the only two doctors who definitely died of smoking had died after setting fire to their beds whilst smoking in bed! This relationship was maintained in a 1993 update of the original cohort, which now includes 20,000 deaths (883 from lung cancer) and the relative risk for smoking >25 g tobacco a day was 20-fold.

	N	Tobacco 1 g/day	Tobacco 15 g/day	Tobacco >25 g/day
Lung cancer deaths	36	0.4/10,000	0.6/10,000	1.1/10,000
All deaths	789	13/10,000	13/10,000	16/10,000

Similar findings were reported in the early 1950s in the United States by Ernst Wynder, a medical student, and Evarts Graham, a thoracic surgeon, who, in 1950, published "Tobacco smoking as a possible etiologic factor in bronchiogenic carcinoma: a study of 684 proven cases" in the *Journal of the American Medical Association*. Evarts, a chain smoker, did not take enough heed of his own findings and also died of lung cancer.

an increased risk of oral, oesophageal and hepatic cancers. In contrast, dietary fat was believed to play an important role in breast cancer development based on animal studies, migrant studies and a few case-control trials. This led to great enthusiasm for reduced dietary fat intake to reduce the incidence of breast cancer. However, results from large prospective studies have failed to confirm a strong relationship between dietary fat intake and breast cancer. Two paths may contribute to dietary carcinogenesis. First, foodstuffs may include dietary genotoxins formed by contaminating moulds, products

Table 2.6 Cancers attributed to infection

Infection	Cancer	Number of cancer cases worldwide per year
RNA viruses		
Human T-cell leukaemia virus	Leukaemia	3000
Hepatitis C virus	Hepatocellular cancer	110,000
DNA viruses		
Human papillomavirus	Cervical cancer, anal cancer, oropharyngeal cancer	360,000
Hepatitis B virus	Hepatocellular cancer	230,000
Epstein–Barr virus	Burkitt's lymphoma, Hodgkin's disease, nasopharyngeal cancer	100,000
Human herpesvirus 8	Kaposi's sarcoma	45,000
Bacteria		
Helicobacter pylori	Gastric cancer, gastric lymphoma	350,000
Helminths		
Schistosoma haematobium	Bladder cancer	10,000
Liver flukes	Cholangiocarcinoma	1000

HIV, human immunodeficiency virus.

of storage or fermentation of food, products of cooking and food additives (e.g. aflatoxin contamination of food). Second, endogenous genotoxins, such as reactive oxygen species, may be formed and higher calorific intake may yield more genotoxins.

Carcinogenic infections

The association between infection and cancer is usually attributed to Peyton Rous, who described the acellular transmission of sarcoma between chickens in 1911. However, 6 years earlier, Goebel had reported a link between bladder tumours and bilharzia (schistosomiasis). It is estimated that 15% of cancers globally are attributable to infections (11% viruses, 4% bacteria and 0.1% helminths) (Table 2.6).

Oncogenic human DNA viruses
Human papillomavirus

The papillomaviruses are non-enveloped, icosahedral, double-stranded DNA viruses. Around 100 genotypes have been identified and >30 of these infect the female genital tract. Some genotypes are associated with benign lesions, such as warts (e.g. HPV-6 and -11), whilst others are known as high-risk genotypes and are associated with invasive cancer (e.g. HPV-16, -18, -31, -33, -45, -51, -52, -58 and -59) (Table 2.7). The prevalence of infection varies between populations but is 20–30% in women aged 20–25 years and

Table 2.7 Human papillomavirus (HPV) genotypes and associated conditions

Human disease	HPV genotype
Skin warts	HPV-1, -2, -3, -7 and -10
Epidermodysplasia verruciformis	HPV-5, -8, -17 and -20
Anogenital warts: exophytic condylomas	HPV-6 and -11
Anogenital warts: flat condylomas	HPV-16, -18, -31, -33, -42 and -43
Respiratory tract papillomas	HPV-6 and -11
Conjunctival papillomatosis	HPV-6 and -11
Focal epithelial hyperplasia	HPV-13 and -32

Table 2.8 Serological markers of hepatitis B virus infection

	HBsAg	HBeAg	Anti-HBe	Anti-HBs	Anti-HBc	Anti-HBc IgM
Acute infection	+	+/−	+/−	−	+	+++
Highly infectious carrier	+++	+	−	−	+	−
Low infectious carrier	+	−	+	−	+	−
Past infection	−	−	+	+	+	−
Past immunization	−	−	−	+	−	−

declines to 5–10% in women over 40 years old. HPV is sexually transmitted and the main determinant of infection is the number of sexual partners. Most infections are cleared spontaneously but a small proportion persist and are believed to be the origin of cervical dysplasia and invasive cancers. Latent infection is associated with cervical intraepithelial neoplasia (CIN), which is graded 1–3 according to the severity of cytological changes. The histological equivalents of these lesions are called squamous intraepithelial lesions, which may be low or high grade. Over 99% of invasive cervical cancers have detectable HPV DNA present and HPV can transform cells in culture. The molecular basis of papillomavirus-induced neoplasia is attributed to two viral oncogenes, E6 and E7. HPV E6 inactivates p53 and E7 degrades Rb protein. High-risk HPV genotypes have also been associated with anal, penile, vaginal and vulval cancers. In addition, HPV is thought to play a role in the development of a number of other malignancies, including head and neck cancers, conjunctival squamous cancers, oesophageal cancers and possibly cutaneous squamous cell cancers.

Studies have suggested that the detection of HPV in the cervix may be more sensitive for detecting CIN than conventional cytological screening. Prophylactic HPV vaccines that induce neutralizing antibodies may prevent infection and the associated malignancies. Most of the vaccines have used virus-like particles constructed of major capsid proteins without viral DNA or enzymes present. A nationwide HPV vaccination programme for teenage girls was started in the United Kingdom in 2008.

Hepatitis B virus

HBV is a double-stranded DNA virus that includes a single-stranded DNA region of variable length. The virus possesses a DNA-dependent DNA polymerase as well as a reverse transcriptase and replicates via an RNA intermediate. HBV has three main antigens: the "Australian antigen" is associated with the surface (HBsAg), the "core antigen" (HBcAg) is internal and the "e antigen" (HBeAg) is part of the same capsid polypeptide as HBcAg. All of these antigens elicit specific antibodies and are used diagnostically (Table 2.8).

Hepatitis B is one of the most common infections worldwide with 2 billion people having been infected and 300–350 million chronic carriers (Table 2.10). Hepatitis B is the ninth most common cause of death worldwide. Acute hepatitis B infection may be associated with extrahepatic immune-mediated manifestations and 1–4% of patients develop a fulminant form. Following acute infection, up to 10% will develop chronic hepatitis, either chronic persistent hepatitis, which is asymptomatic with modest elevation of transaminases and little fibrosis or chronic active hepatitis, which causes jaundice and cirrhosis and is associated with a 100× increased risk of hepatocellular cancer 15–60 years after infection. It is uncertain how hepatitis B leads to cancer, although the X protein of hepatitis B may interact with p53 causing disruption of the cell cycle control or the virus may act indirectly by causing increased hepatic cell turnover associated with cirrhosis.

Although treatment with α-interferon and antiviral agents (e.g. lamivudine, tenofovir, telbivudine, entecavir, adefovir) may lead to clearance of hepatitis B in chronic infection, recombinant subunit vaccines have been available since the early 1980s. The introduction of a mass immunization programme in Taiwan has been associated with a dramatic reduction in liver cancer in children.

Epstein–Barr virus

Epstein–Barr virus (EBV) (or human herpesvirus 4 (HHV-4)) is a ubiquitous double-stranded DNA gamma-herpesvirus. It was first identified by Epstein and his colleagues by electron microscopy of a cell line derived from a patient with Burkitt's lymphoma in 1964. Burkitt's lymphoma had been described only a few years earlier in 1956 by Dennis Burkitt, a surgeon working in Uganda. The subsequent finding that EBV was the cause of infectious

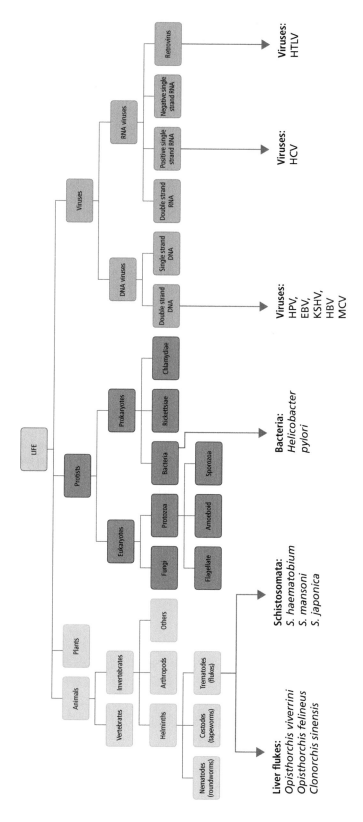

Figure 2.20 The onco tree of life. HPV, Human Papillomavirus; EBV, Epstein Barr virus; KSHV, Kaposi sarcoma herpesvirus; HBV, Hepatitis B virus; HCV, Hepatitis C virus; MCV, Merkel cell polyoma virus; HTLV, Human T cell leukemia virus.

Table 2.9 Diseases associated with Epstein–Barr virus infection

Non-malignant
Infectious mononucleosis
X-linked lymphoproliferative syndrome
(Duncan's syndrome)
Oral hairy leukoplakia
Malignant
Burkitt's lymphoma
Nasopharyngeal cancer
Post-transplant lymphoproliferative disorder
Hodgkin's disease
Primary cerebral lymphoma
Primary effusion lymphoma (with HHV8)
Leiomyosarcoma in children with HIV
Nasal T/NK non-Hodgkin's lymphoma

mononucleosis arose serendipitously when a laboratory technician in Philadelphia developed mononucleosis and was found to have acquired antibodies to EBV. EBV infects over 90% of the world's population and is transmitted orally. In normal adults, from 1 to 50 per million B lymphocytes are infected by latent EBV. A carcinogenic role for EBV has been confirmed for several types of lymphoma (Burkitt's lymphoma, Hodgkin's disease and immunosuppression-associated non-Hodgkin's lymphoma) and nasopharyngeal cancer (Table 2.9). EBV is estimated to be responsible for 100,000 cancers per year in the world.

Primary infection of epithelial cells by EBV is associated with the infection of some resting B lymphocytes. The majority of infected B cells have latent virus with a small percentage undergoing spontaneous activation to lytic infection. During lytic infection EBV replicates in the cell and when the progeny virions are released the host cell is destroyed. In contrast, during latent infection there is neither virus replication

nor host cell destruction. Most infected B lymphocytes have latent virus expressing at most ten of the >80 genes of EBV. The roles of these latent genes include maintenance of the episomal virus DNA, growth and transformation of B cells and evasion of the host immune system. A number of these latent genes are thought to contribute to the oncogenicity of EBV. For example, latent membrane protein 1 (LMP-1) mimics a constitutively activated receptor for TNF and BHRF1 and BALF1 are viral homologues of the anti-apoptotic protein bcl-2 that leads to evasion of programmed cell death. Thus, in contrast to retroviruses, which generally possess a single oncogene, EBV uses a number of genes that contribute to the steps towards cancer.

Human herpesvirus 8 (HHV-8/KSHV)

Kaposi's sarcoma (KS) was originally described over a century ago and four forms have subsequently been recognized. The first is classic KS and is usually found on the lower legs of elderly men of Mediterranean or Jewish descent without any immunosuppression. A second form, endemic or African KS, is found in all age groups in sub-Saharan Africa, where even before the HIV epidemic it was as common as colorectal cancer is in Europe. A third form associated with iatrogenic immunosuppression was recognized in patients who had received an allogeneic organ transplant. The fourth and most common form of the disease is associated with acquired immune deficiency syndrome (AIDS). All forms of KS are associated with HHV-8 (also known as Kaposi sarcoma herpesvirus (KSHV)), which that was identified in 1994. In addition, this virus is most prevalent in the populations at risk of KS. HHV-8 is also implicated in the pathogenesis of two rare lymphoproliferative diseases, primary effusion lymphoma and multicentric Castleman's disease (Figure 2.21). Like EBV, HHV-8

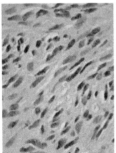

Kaposi's sarcoma

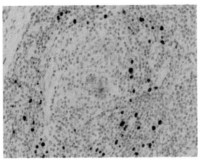

Multicentric Castleman's disease

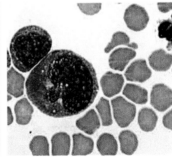

Primary effusion lymphoma

Figure 2.21 KSHV-related tumours. Immunohistochemistry staining for KSHV latent nuclear antigen (LANA) shows the presence of virus in spindle cells of Kaposi's sarcoma and the plasmablasts in multicentric Castleman's disease. KSHV, Kaposi's sarcoma herpesvirus (also known as Human herpesvirus (HHV8)).

Table 2.10 Comparison of HIV and hepatitis B and C viruses

	HCV	HBV	HIV
Global prevalence	3%	33%	0.5%
Global prevalence	170 million	2 billion	34 million
Chronic infection	150 million	350 million	34 million
Deaths per year	350,000	1 million	1.7 million
Annual death rate	0.40%	0.49%	5%

includes a number of cellular gene homologues that are thought to contribute to its oncogenic potential.

Oncogenic human RNA viruses
Hepatitis C virus

Hepatitis C virus was identified in 1989 as the cause of transfusion-acquired non-A, non-B hepatitis by Houghton, Choo and Kuo. HCV is a single-stranded RNA virus belonging to the flavivirus genus along with yellow fever and dengue. The prevalence of HCV varies geographically from 1–1.5% in Europe and the United States to 3.5% in Africa and transmission is chiefly parenteral, particularly by blood transfusion prior to the introduction of blood product screening. In contrast to HBV, 85% develop persistent HCV and 65% progress to chronic liver disease including hepatocellular cancer for which the relative risk is 20-fold (Table 2.10). The oncogenic mechanism for HCV remains unclear. Unlike retroviruses, there is no evidence of genome integration but cancer is preceded by cirrhosis and it is hypothesized that the virus induces a cycle of inflammation, repair and regeneration and thus indirectly contributes to the formation of cancer. There are at least six genotypes of HCV and the diagnosis is usually made by enzyme immunoassay for anti-HCV antibodies and confirmed by polymerase chain reaction (PCR) for HCV RNA. Treatment with pegylated interferon, ribavarin and bocepravir or telapravir leads to clearance of the virus in 50–80% depending in part upon the HCV genotype. Promising specific protease and polymerase inhibitors are now available for HCV but not really affordable.

Human T-cell leukaemia virus type 1

Human T-cell leukaemia virus type 1 (HTLV-1) is the main cause of adult T-cell leukaemia/lymphoma, a malignancy characterized by hypercalcaemia, lymphadenopathy, hepatosplenomegaly and myelosuppression. It is associated with a particularly poor prognosis and occurs almost exclusively in areas where HTLV-1 is endemic, such as the Caribbean, Japan and West Africa or in immigrants from these regions and their offspring. HTLV-1 is also associated with tropical spastic paraparesis and uveitis. HTLV-1 is an enveloped retrovirus that integrates into the host cellular genome. The virus is able to immortalize human T lymphocytes and this property is attributable to a specific viral oncogene, *tax*. Tax is a trans-activating transcription factor that can also lead to repression of transcription. Adult T-cell leukaemia/lymphoma develops in 2–5% of HTLV-1 infected people and is more common in those infected at a younger age.

Oncogenic bacteria
Helicobacter pylori

Helicobacter pylori is a spiral, flagellated, Gram-negative bacteria that colonizes the human gastrointestinal tract. It causes gastritis leading to peptic ulceration, although many infections are asymptomatic. The discovery of *H. pylori* and the recognition of its place in the pathogenesis of peptic ulcer disease are chiefly due to Barry Marshall, who, in order to prove his point, swallowed a solution of the organism and developed acute gastritis 1 week later. It is believed that half of the world population is chronically infected with *H. pylori*. Prospective sero-epidemiological data suggest that *H. pylori* infection is associated with a two fold to fourfold increase in the risk of gastric cancer as well as an increase in gastric low-grade mucosa-associated lymphoid tissue (MALT) lymphoma. As with the hepatitis viruses, the mechanism of oncogenesis is obscure but is believed to be an indirect result of chronic inflammation and consequential epithelial cell proliferation. The combination of two antibiotics with either a bismuth preparation or a proton pump inhibitor for 14 days eradicates *H. pylori* in 80% patients. However, re-infection is common. *H. pylori* is very prevalent and the time interval between *H. pylori* infection and gastric cancer is thought to be several decades. For these reasons, it may prove very difficult to assess the value of eradication interventions in reducing cancer risk.

Oncogenic helminths
Schistosomes

Schistosomes are parasitic blood flukes or flatworms (platyhelminths) belonging to the trematode class whose intermediate hosts are snails. Three species infect humans: *Schistosoma haematobium*, *Schistosoma mansoni* and *Schistosoma japonica*. Humans are infected by contact with fresh water where the parasite cercaria form penetrates the skin. It is estimated that 200 million people are infected with schistosomes

Table 2.11 Global distribution of schistosomiasis

Species	Geographical distribution	Number of humans infected
Schistosoma haematobium	North Africa, Middle East, sub-Saharan Africa	114 million
Schistosoma mansoni	Sub-Saharan Africa, Middle East, Brazil	83 million
Schistosoma japonica	China, the Philippines, Indonesia	1.5 million

(Table 2.11). Acute infection may produce swimmer's itch dermatitis and tropical pulmonary eosinophilia, although most people remain asymptomatic. The development of adult worms, days to weeks after infection, may cause Katayama fever, a systemic illness of fevers, rigors, myalgia, lymphadenopathy and hepatosplenomegaly. Chronic infection leads to granuloma formation at the sites of egg deposition, in the bladder for *S. haematobium* and in the bowel and liver for *S. mansoni* and *S. japonica*. The late sequelae include squamous cell carcinoma of the bladder in the case of *S. haematobium* and probably hepatocellular cancer with *S. japonica*. A single oral dose of praziquantel resolves the infection.

Liver flukes

Three species of food-borne liver flukes of the trematode class cause illness in humans. Infection is acquired by eating raw or undercooked freshwater fish and the flukes migrate to the biliary tree and mature in the intrahepatic bile ducts. There are two intermediate hosts in the life cycle – snails and fish. As many as 17 million people are estimated to be infected (Table 2.12). Cholangiocarcinoma has been recognized as a complication of chronic infection, and case-control studies have found a fivefold increased

Table 2.12 Global distribution of liver fluke infection

Species	Geographical distribution	Number of humans infected
Opisthorchis viverrini	Northern Thailand, Laos	9 million
Opisthorchis felineus	Kazakhstan, Ukraine	1.5 million
Clonorchis sinensis	China, Korea, Taiwan, Vietnam	7 million

risk with liver fluke infection. The oncogenic mechanism is again unclear although chronic inflammation is believed to play a role. The antihelminth drug praziquantel is the treatment of choice.

Worldwide contributions to cancer

The current world population is six billion and the global burden of cancer is estimated to be 10 million new cases and 6 million deaths annually. Projections for 2020, when the global population is estimated to have risen to 8 billion are 20 million new cases and 12 million deaths annually. Tobacco contributes to 3 million cases of cancer (chiefly lung, head and neck, bladder), diet to an estimated 3 million cases (upper gastrointestinal, colorectal) and infection to a further 1.5 million cases (cervical, stomach, liver, bladder and lymphomas) globally. Prevention by tobacco control, dietary advice and affordable food and infection control and immunization could have a major impact in reducing the global burden of cancer. The differences in outcome for tumours between the developed and the developing worlds are most marked for the rare but curable cancers where access to therapy dramatically improves survival (e.g. acute leukaemias, Hodgkin's disease and testicular cancers). Small differences are recorded where screening programmes aimed at early detection are effective (e.g. cervical and breast cancers), whilst there are little differences in outcome in the common tumours where prevention has a major role (e.g. lung, stomach and liver cancers). These observations have led to a World Health Organization (WHO) list of priorities to reduce global cancer that starts not with scientific research or expensive chemotherapy, but with tobacco and infection control (Table 2.13). In an optimistic scenario the implementation of these priorities could reduce the estimated cancer incidence of 20 million in 2020 to 15 million and could reduce the expected mortality of 12 million to 6 million.

Table 2.13 WHO cancer priority ladder

1. Tobacco control
2. Infection control
3. Curable cancer programme
4. Early detection programme
5. Effective pain control
6. Sample cancer registry
7. Healthy eating programme
8. Referral guidelines
9. Clinical care guidelines
10. Nurse education
11. National cancer network
12. Clinical evaluation unit
13. Platform technology focus for region
14. Clinical research programme
15. Basic research programme
16. International aid programme

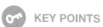 KEY POINTS

- The molecular changes of cancer are classified into six hallmarks, two enabling and two emerging characteristics
- Genetic and epigenetic modifications account for the molecular biology of cancer
- The causes of cancers can be classified into hereditary germline mutations and environmental factors including radiation, chemical and infectious agents
- Many of the causes of cancers are modifiable by lifestyle interventions
- The routes of cancer spread and the final destination of metastases varies according to the primary tumour site

3

The principles of cancer treatment

Learning objectives

✓ Distinguish different treatment strategies for cancer including palliative care with examples

✓ Compare surgery, radiotherapy, chemotherapy, endocrine, immunological and targeted treatments and their toxicities

✓ Explain the mechanisms of action of anti-cancer therapies

Appropriate care

The care of people with cancer requires careful deliberation and consultation with the patient. The appropriate care will depend upon the prognosis, the effectiveness and toxicity of any therapy and finally, most importantly, on the patient's wishes. To empower patients to participate in this decision-making process requires them to be fully informed and the clear delivery of this information is essential. A number of resources are available to supplement the information divulged by clinicians to their patients. These include many web-based resources as well as patient information leaflets published by charities including Macmillan and Cancer Research UK (CRUK) as well as individual tumour-type patient groups such as Breast Cancer Breakthrough and Prostate Cancer UK. It is increasingly appreciated that the management of patients with cancer requires a multidisciplinary approach involving a team of professionals including surgeons, clinical and medical oncologists, palliative care physicians, radiologists, histopathologists, specialist oncology and palliative care nurses, clinical psychologists, counsellors, dieticians, occupational therapists, physiotherapists, social workers and clinical geneticists.

The aims of therapy should be clearly identified before embarking on a course of treatment. Treatment may either be curative, aiming to prolong the quantity of life or palliative, aiming to improve the quality of life. When considering the management of individual tumour types, the maxim that prevention is better than cure should be recalled. Cancer prevention and screening are essential if the global burden of malignancy is to be minimized.

During the last quarter of the 20th century, the role of chemotherapy, radiotherapy and endocrine therapy after primary surgery for localized breast cancer was recognized. These additional treatments are defined as adjuvant therapies. Thus, adjuvant therapy is treatment after the primary tumour has been removed surgically and in the absence of detectable residual disease. Whilst large clinical trials demonstrated the advantages of adjuvant therapy to a population of women with breast cancer, the benefits for each individual cannot be specified; the statistics relate to the group as a whole. Oncologists observing the success of adjuvant treatments have progressed to the investigation of the role of primary or neoadjuvant treatments. Neoadjuvant therapy, usually chemotherapy

Oncology: Lecture Notes, Third Edition. Mark Bower and Jonathan Waxman.
© 2015 by John Wiley & Sons, Ltd. Published 2015 by John Wiley & Sons, Ltd.
Companion Website: www.lecturenoteseries.com/oncology

or endocrine therapy, is delivered prior to surgery or radiotherapy to downsize the tumour, thus demonstrating the sensitivity of the tumour and potentially reducing the extent of the surgical resection or radiation field.

Cancer staging

In order to work out what treatments are feasible for a person with cancer, the extent of spread of the cancer needs to be established as this is one of the most important influences on survival.

How to stage a tumour

In addition to the histological grade of a tumour, an important criterion in treatment decisions and the major determinant of outcome is the extent of spread or stage of a cancer (Figure 3.1). Staging a tumour is essentially an anatomical exercise that uses a combination of clinical examination and radiology. A uniform staging system is employed for most tumour sites that is based upon the size of the primary Tumour, the presence of regional lymph Nodes and of distant Metastases. The details of this **TNM** classification vary between different tumour sites. As always, there are exceptions, including the staging system for lymphomas that was originally set out following a conference at the University of Michigan in Ann Arbour. It

is known as the Ann Arbour Staging System, and most radiologists assume that it is named after a person rather than a town, so this is a chance to score points at X-ray meetings.

Radiology techniques

Staging depends to a large extent upon radiology, and this is the most commonly used tool to evaluate the response of cancers to therapies. Anatomical imaging by plain films, computed tomography (CT), ultrasound and magnetic resonance imaging (MRI) are the standard methods. Using the correct terms impresses other clinicians and may make a trip to the radiology department less daunting for junior doctors requesting an investigation. X-rays measure radiodensity (radiolucency and radio-opacity) and ultrasound measures echogenicity and echoreflectivity, whilst CT scans report attenuation values measured in Hounsfield units and MRI reports signal intensity.

Computed tomography

CT scanning is the production of three-dimensional images using X-rays that have been directed through tissues and the images produced depend on the density of the tissues. CT was developed in the 1970s by Sir Godfrey Hounsfield and Allan McLeod Cormack who shared the Nobel Prize in 1979. The first CT scanner built at EMI Central Research Laboratories is said to have been funded by the success of the

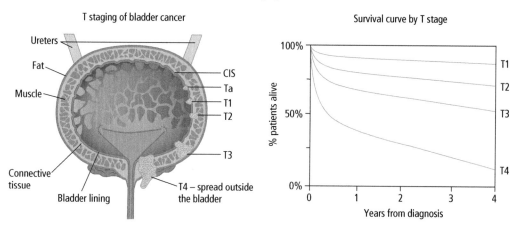

Figure 3.1 T-stage classification for bladder cancer and influence on survival. CIS, carcinoma *in situ*; Ta, non-invasive papillary tumour; T1, tumour invades subepithelial connective tissue; T2, tumour invades superficial muscle; T3, tumour invades deep muscle or perivesical fat; T4, tumour invades prostate, uterus, vagina, pelvic wall or abdominal wall.

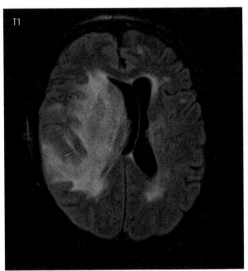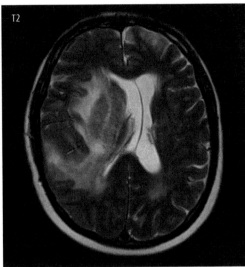

Figure 3.2 T1 (left) and T2 (right) MRI scans demonstrating a large right basal ganglia glioma with midline shift, compression of the right lateral ventricle and peritumoural oedema.

Beatles who were signed to the EMI label. CT measures the attenuation of different tissues to ionizing radiation and calculates a mean value for a volume of tissue known as a voxel. This is displayed on a two-dimensional image as a single pixel. The attenuation is calculated relative to water, which has a Hounsfield unit (HU) value of 0, so high attenuation tissues have a positive HU value (e.g. bone +400 HU) and low attenuation tissues a negative HU value (e.g. fat −120 HU). Different window settings are used to look at different ranges of the Hounsfield greyscale. For example, in the bone windows setting, the lungs will look uniformly black, whilst in the lung windows, the bones look uniformly white. Intravenous iodinated contrast agents improve the sensitivity and specificity of CT but are contraindicated in patients with asthma, allergies to contrast or poor renal function.

Magnetic resonance imaging

Unlike CT, MRI does not use ionizing radiation but instead a powerful magnetic field aligns the spin of protons, especially hydrogen atom protons, in water and fat. A radiofrequency pulse then energizes the protons, and the gradual release of this energy from the protons as they relax back to their original magnetic alignment may be detected as radiofrequency signals. The signal intensity relates to the concentration of mobile hydrogen nuclei in tissues. T1

(longitudinal relaxation or spin–lattice) and T2 (transverse relaxation or spin–spin) relaxation time constants depend on the physical properties of the tissues. If you want to impress the neuroradiologists (not always a useful ploy in the authors' experience), water such as cerebrospinal fluid is black (low signal intensity) on T1 images and white (high signal intensity) on T2 images (Figure 3.2). Whilst CT is a good tool to examine tissues composed of high atomic weight elements such as bone, MRI is better suited to non-calcified tissues. For similar reasons, CT contrast agents usually are composed of high atomic number atoms such as iodine or barium, whilst MRI contrast agents such as gadolinium are paramagnets that have magnetic properties only in the presence of an externally applied magnetic field. MRI is generally superior for imaging the brain, whilst CT is better for solid tumours of the chest and abdomen, as it is faster and generates fewer motion artefacts. MRI is also better suited to patients who may require many examinations because it does not carry the risks of ionizing radiation. MRI is, however, contraindicated in patients with metallic objects such as pacemakers *in situ* and it is also quite claustrophobic and noisy in the scanner.

Positron emission tomography

Positron emission tomography (PET) is a functional imaging modality that detects γ-rays emitted by

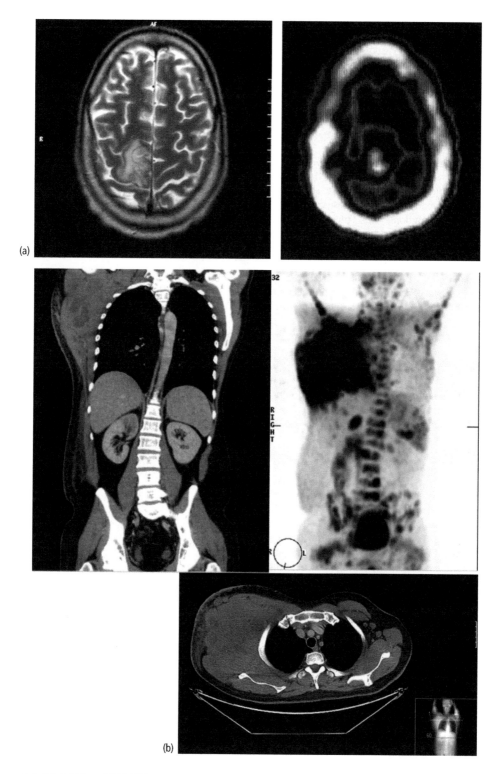

Figure 3.3 (a) T2-MRI and FDG-PET scan showing an FDG avid parietal primary cerebral lymphoma. (b) CT and FDG-PET scans demonstrating a huge right axillary and anterior chest wall mass due to Burkitt lymphoma. The FDG-PET also demonstrates extensive involvement of other nodal groups, bones and the right kidney upper pole (stage 4B). FDG, Fluorodeoxyglucose; PET, positron emission tomography.

Table 3.1 Commonly used isotopes in nuclear imaging in oncology

Isotope	Half-life	Tracer	Oncological use
^{99}Tc (technetium)	6 hours	Methylene diphosphonate (MDP)	Bone scan
^{111}In (indium)	67 hours	Octreotide	Neuroendocrine tumours
^{131}I (iodine)	8 days	Sodium iodide	Thyroid cancer
^{131}I (iodine)	8 days	Meta-iodobenzylguanidine (MIBG)	Phaeochromocytoma & neuroblastoma
^{67}Ga (gallium)	68 hours	Gallium citrate	Lymphoma

positrons (positively charged electrons) emitting radionuclide tracers. Positrons have a short half-life and are generated by cyclotrons. Common positron-labelled radionuclides include fluorine (^{18}F), carbon (^{11}C), oxygen (^{15}O) and nitrogen (^{13}N). In oncology, the most frequently used tracer is ^{18}F-fluorodeoxyglucose (FDG), a short half-life glucose analogue that is taken up into actively metabolizing cells including cancer cells and following intracellular phosphorylation is trapped in these cells. Hence, the distribution in the body of FDG reflects glucose uptake within the body. This means that PET scanning may differentiate between residual masses and active disease in lymphoma. As a consequence, FDG-PET scanning is used in both staging and monitoring cancer treatment (Figure 3.3). PET scanning techniques continue to progress through the use of novel tracers, such as choline in prostate cancer, which has greater specificity for the cancer than FDG.

Radio-isotope scanning

In addition to PET scanning, other functional images may be used in the diagnosis and staging of specific cancers, using isotope-labelled radionuclide tracer elements (Table 3.1 and Figure 3.4). The isotope-labelled tracers that are used diagnostically may also be used therapeutically. Bone scintigraphy uses bis-phosphonates labelled with ^{99}Tc and is more sensitive than X-rays for detecting metastases, though surprisingly the tracer reflects blood flow at the site of the supposed metastases and so there is a differential diagnosis for tracer uptake, which may include Paget's disease and osteoarthritis.

Performance status

In addition to the histological grade and the stage of a cancer, the general health of patients will determine how long they survive and may influence treatment decisions. Scales that measure the performance status or functional capacity of patients include: the Eastern

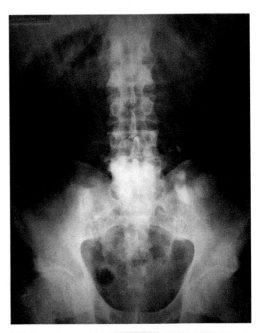

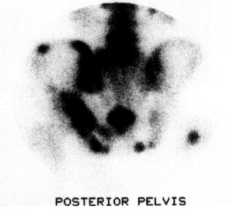

POSTERIOR PELVIS

Figure 3.4 Plain pelvic radiograph (above) and corresponding area of technetium pyrophosphate bone scan (below) of a patient with sclerotic bone metastases from prostate cancer.

Table 3.2 Functional capacity grading (ECOG) and Karnofsky performance scales

ECOG functional capacity grading

0	Asymptomatic
1	Symptomatic but fully ambulant
2	Symptomatic; ambulant >50% waking hours
3	Symptomatic; confined to bed >50% waking hours
4	Symptomatic; bed bound

Karnofsky performance status score (%)

100	Normal; no complaints; no evidence of disease
90	Able to carry on normal activity; minor signs or symptoms
80	Normal activity with effort; some signs or symptoms
70	Care for self; unable to carry on normal activity or do active work
60	Requires occasional assistance, but able to care for most of needs
50	Requires considerable assistance and frequent medical care
40	Disabled; requires special care and assistance
30	Severely disabled; hospitalization indicated but death not imminent
20	Very sick; hospitalization necessary; active supportive treatment necessary
10	Moribund; fatal processes progressing rapidly

Co-operative Oncology Group (ECOG) grading system, which is also known as the WHO or Zubrod score and the Karnofsky scale (Table 3.2). The performance status, however estimated, is an important prognostic indicator for almost all tumour types.

Table 3.3 Survival rates for various diseases

	Stroke	Heart failure	Prostate cancer	Breast cancer
5-year survival rate	50%	62%	50–99%	73–89%

Prognosis: it is not cancer, is it doc?

Although a very significant stigma is attached to the diagnosis of cancer, for most of the general population the fear outweighs the reality and comparison with other more palatable illnesses yield results that are not always expected (Table 3.3).

Surgical oncology

Surgery has six major roles in the management of people with cancer:

1. Cancer prevention
2. Cancer diagnosis and staging
3. Treating cancer
4. Management of oncological emergencies
5. Palliation of cancer symptoms
6. Surgical reconstruction following cancer therapy

Surgical oncology is the oldest discipline for the management of cancer and originates with attempts at curative resections. Surgical oncology enjoyed a golden era at the end of the 19th century and early 20th century prior to the World War I (Table 3.4).

Table 3.4 Landmarks in radical surgical oncology

Year	Surgeon	Operation
1881	Albert Billroth	Subtotal gastrectomy
1890	William Halsted	Radical mastectomy
1897	Carl Schlatter	Total gastrectomy
1898	Johann von Mikulicz	Oesophagogastrectomy
1900	Ernest Wertheim	Radical hysterectomy
1906	W. Ernest Miles	Abdominoperineal excision of rectum
1913	Franz Torek	Oesophagectomy
1913	Wilfred Trotter	Partial pharyngectomy
1933	Evarts Graham	Pneumonectomy
1935	A. O. Whipple	Pancreaticoduodenectomy

Box 3.1 Cancer staging, see also Table 8.2, p. 129.

Cancer staging

T(umour) staging of breast cancer

T1

Tumour ≤2 cm

Diagram showing stage
T1 breast cancer
Copyright © CancerHelp UK

T2

Tumour 2–5 cm across

Diagram showing a stage
T2 breast cancer
Copyright © CancerHelp UK

T3

Tumour >5 cm across

Diagram showing a stage
T3 breast cancer
Copyright © CancerHelp UK

1 cm

2 cm

4 cm

6 cm

T4

T4 is divided into four groups:
T4a – The tumour has spread into the chest wall
T4b – The tumour has spread into the skin and the breast may be swollen
T4c – The tumour has spread to both the skin and the chest wall
T4d – Inflammatory carcinoma – this is a cancer in which the overlying skin is red, swollen and painful to the touch (see below).

Lymphoma staging

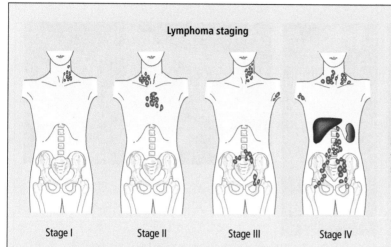

Stage I   Stage II   Stage III   Stage IV

A = without symptoms
B = with symptoms including unexplained weight loss (≥10% in 6 months prior to diagnosis), unexplained fever, and drenching night sweats.

Stage I	one lymph node area
Stage II	two or more lymph node areas but confined to one side of the diaphragm
Stage III	lymph nodes above and below the diaphragm – spleen involvement is included
Stage IV	outside the lymph node areas, e.g. bone marrow, liver and other extranodal sites

Two worked examples of lymphoma staging

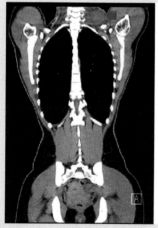 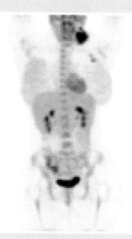 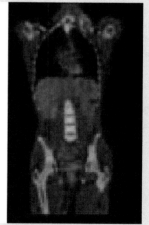

CT scan   FDG-PET   Fused CT/PET

FDG-PET and CT images of patient with left supra-clavicular lymph node mass of Hodgkin's lymphoma (◀). She was asymptomatic and this was the only site of disease (Stage IA)

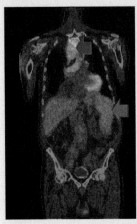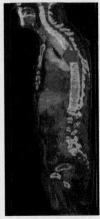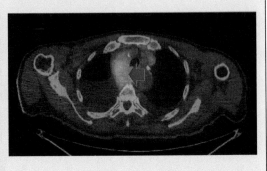

FDG-PET images of patient with mediastinal lymph nodes (◀) and splenic involvement by Hodgkin's lymphoma (◀). He had significant weight loss and night sweats (Stage IIIB).

Subsequent advances in surgical oncology included the development of endocrine surgery for metastatic disease. Surgical hormone ablation for the management of breast cancer was pioneered over 100 years ago by George Beatson, a Glaswegian surgeon who gave his name to Scotland's largest cancer centre (Table 3.5).

Surgical cancer prophylaxis

The prevention of cancer by surgery has expanded greatly in recent years with the identification of individuals at high risk of developing malignancies because they have inherited germline genetic mutations associated with cancer predisposition. However, perhaps the most widespread example of surgical cancer prevention is the role of orchiopexy in the management of undescended testes. Undescended testes are the most common birth defect of the male genitalia, affecting up to 3% of live births. Although in many cases the testes will descend to the scrotum during the first year of life, undescended testes are associated with a 4–40-fold increased risk of malignancy, especially testicular seminoma. Orchiopexy, surgery to move the undescended testis into the scrotum, has been shown to reduce infertility, although it remains controversial whether it also reduces the risk of malignancy. Nevertheless, it certainly makes the detection of testicular tumours easier to recognize and diagnose at an earlier stage.

Familial adenomatous polyposis (FAP) is an autosomal dominant disorder characterized by the development of multiple polyps in the colon, which may undergo transformation to malignant tumours. Most patients with FAP will develop a colonic cancer by the age of 40 years, so prophylactic colectomy is generally recommended before the age of 25 years. Similarly, risk-reducing prophylactic mastectomy may be advocated for women with inherited mutations of BRCA genes (Table 3.6).

Surgical diagnosis and staging of cancer

Oncological diagnosis hinges on histopathology and surgeons play a major role along with interventional radiologists in obtaining tissue specimens. Whilst aspiration cytology and fine-needle biopsies can be undertaken radiologically or endoscopically, more extensive incision or excision biopsies require surgical

Table 3.5 Landmarks in endocrine surgery for advanced cancer

Year	Surgeon	Operation
1896	George Beatson	Oophrectomy for breast cancer
1941	Charles Huggins and Clarence Hodges	Orchidectomy for prostate cancer
1951	Rolf Luft and Herbert Olivecrona	Hypophysectomy for breast cancer
1952	Charles Huggins and D. M. Bergenstal	Adrenalectomy for breast cancer

Table 3.6 Prophylactic surgery

Indication	Prophylactic operation
Cryptorchidism	Orchiopexy
Polyposis coli/chronic ulcerative colitis	Colectomy
Familial medullary thyroid cancer (MEN 2 and 3)	Thyroidectomy
Familial breast cancer (BRCA 1 and 2)	Mastectomy
Familial ovarian cancer (BRCA 1 and 2)	Oophrectomy

BRCA, breast cancer; MEN, multiple endocrine neoplasia.

involvement. Careful specimen orientation and inking prior to histological sectioning may be required to assess the status of tumour margins. The optimal surgical approach and biopsy technique for tumour sampling must take into account concerns about contaminating new tissue planes with cancer cells that could jeopardize subsequent therapy. For example, thoracoscopic pleural biopsy of mesothelioma may result in needle-track metastases along the path of surgical instrumentation. The risk of this surgical spread of the cancer is reduced in mesothelioma by postoperative radiotherapy to the biopsy track. Surgery had a major role in the staging of tumours prior to the development of improved radiological techniques and a staging laparotomy was routine care in the management of Hodgkin's disease until the late 1980s. Surgical staging retains a role in the management of ovarian epithelial cancer and the surgical placement of radio-opaque titanium clips (that are non-ferrous and thus safe in the MRI scanner) may guide postoperative radiotherapy in some tumours.

Surgical treatment of cancer

The surgical treatment of cancer includes definitive curative surgery (with or without adjuvant treatments), debulking operations, metastasectomy and endocrine ablation surgery for advanced diseases, although the latter is largely historical as pharmacological hormone manipulations have taken over most of this role. It is really important to avoid unnecessary surgery in patients with extensive unresectable cancer whilst ensuring that patients with potentially curative tumours are not denied surgery. The treatment of cancer by multidisciplinary teams including radiologists,

pathologists, physicians and surgeons is designed to ensure the right patients have the right operations at the right time. For example, this approach aims to guarantee that patients who are candidates for neoadjuvant down-staging therapy prior to surgery are not wheeled straight into the operating theatre.

Most early curative surgery aimed to remove tumours *en bloc*, that is, with the draining lymph nodes. In recent times, surgeons have developed the use of more conservative function-preserving operations. Examples of the latter include wide local excision rather than mastectomy and partial nephron-sparing nephrectomy rather than radical nephrectomy for small renal tumours. A further development in surgery for skin tumours was introduced by Dr Frederic Mohs in the 1930s when he was still a medical student at the University of Wisconsin-Madison. Mohs' surgery for skin tumours involves sectioning the tumour and mapping its surgical margins during the operation to ensure completeness of tumour resection. Instead of using a breadknife and the pathologist looking at each slice, the Mohs' technique is more like a vegetable peeler with the pathologist examining each peeling for residual cancer involvement during the surgery. Whilst this is a more laborious technique, it is especially valuable for tumours at specific anatomical sites such as the eyelids and in recurrent disease (see Fig. 32.6, p. 262).

Debulking operations that do not result in complete surgical removal of the tumour are not always futile. They can provide important clinical benefits in selected tumour types, including ovarian cancer and primary brain tumours, and are usually followed by either chemotherapy or radiotherapy. Debulking surgery forms part of the treatment algorithm in several uncommon tumours such as thymomas and pseudomyxoma peritonei. Mucin secretion into the abdominal cavity by mucinous adenocarcinomas most commonly arising in the appendix is the usual cause of pseudomyxoma peritonei. The term "myxoma" is derived from the Greek for mucin, but the etymology of the medical terms myxoma and pseudomyxoma seem to have got mixed up. Myxomas are benign pedunculated connective tissue tumours usually arising in the atria of the heart and are not mucinous, whilst pseudomyxoma peritonei fills the abdominal cavity with true jelly-like mucin.

The surgical resection of secondary deposits may seem perverse since the presence of metastases implies systemic dissemination of the cancer. Nevertheless, surgical oncologists have embraced this approach enthusiastically, mainly on the basis of relatively weak evidence from uncontrolled retrospective series that have been interpreted as demonstrating a survival benefit. The resection of lung, liver and brain metastases has become a part of the routine treatment strategy for a number of types of cancer. The most common indication for surgical metastasectomy is for hepatic secondaries from colorectal cancer. The rationale for this approach is based upon reported 5-year survivals of around 30% in patients undergoing surgery compared to around 10% in those who received chemotherapy. However, there are no randomized controlled studies that support hepatic metastasectomy and the case series are inevitably confounded by selection and reporting bias. Similarly, pulmonary metastasectomy has been widely adopted for osteogenic sarcomas, soft tissue sarcomas, renal cell tumours and melanomas, and cerebral metastasectomy has also been advocated in a similar spectrum of malignancies. In contrast to metastasectomy, the surgical resection of residual masses following the completion of chemotherapy forms part of the multidisciplinary treatment of advanced non-seminomatous germ cell tumours to remove residual differentiated teratoma that could relapse at a later date. Finally, surgical endocrine ablation is nowadays rarely indicated for metastatic cancer although surgical castration is occasionally performed for advanced prostate cancer.

Surgery for oncological emergencies

Surgery has an important role in the optimal management of oncological emergencies, in particular, metastatic spinal cord compression where rapid surgical decompression reduces neurological disability (see Cord compression in Chapter 46). Surgical decompression and spinal column stabilization should be offered to patients with a good prognosis and needs to be undertaken as swiftly as possible, preferably before patients lose the ability to walk. The optimal neurosurgical approach will depend upon the anatomical site of compression and the stability of the spine. If spinal metastases involve the vertebral body or threaten spinal stability, posterior decompression should always be accompanied by internal fixation with or without bone grafting.

Surgical palliation of cancer

The palliation of tumour-associated obstruction, fluid accumulation and bleeding may require surgical intervention, although the placement of shunts and stents is now more frequently undertaken by endoscopists and interventional radiologists. Plastic or metal stents are used to relieve obstruction of

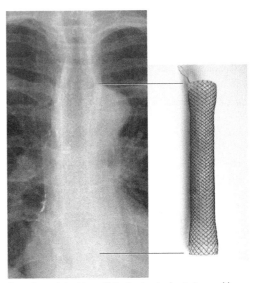

Oesophageal stent to palliate dysphagia due to inoperable oesophageal cancer

Figure 3.5 Oesophageal stent to palliate dysphagia.

the bowel, oesophagus, bronchial tree, biliary ducts and ureters and even patients with advanced malignancy benefit (Figure 3.5). Diathermy or laser coagulation of tumour-related haemorrhage similarly is a valuable palliative intervention that can often be undertaken endoscopically. Surgical relief of bowel obstruction may be indicated when stenting is not feasible but usually requires either colostomy or ileostomy depending upon the level of the obstruction. Fistulae are abnormal passageways connecting two epithelial-lined organs not normally connected and include rectovaginal, enterovaginal, colovesical and vesicovaginal or combinations of these. Fistulae may be either related to locally advanced disease or may be a consequence of radiotherapy. Fistula surgery is complex and demanding, requiring surgical expertise and often prolonged recovery, so it is usually reserved for cancer patients in remission. The surgical placement of shunts to prevent the reaccumulation of ascites (usually peritoneal–venous shunts, e.g. LeVeen shunt) and pleural effusions (usually pleuroperitoneal shunts, e.g. Denver shunt) may be indicated for symptom palliation. Surgical oncologists may also be called upon to perform surgery for ulcerating and necrotic locally advanced cancers such as toilet mastectomy for fungating breast tumours. Orthopaedic surgeons frequently operate on pathological bone metastases either as a form of secondary prevention or following pathological fractures (Figure 3.6).

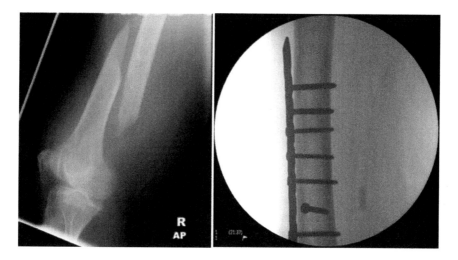

Figure 3.6 Pathological spiral fracture through right femoral shaft metastasis from prostate cancer repaired with a distal femoral plate.

Internal fixation of bones with lytic metastases are especially important in weight-bearing bones with large deposits occupying more than half the bone cortex that are at a high risk of fracturing. Surgeons thus have an important role in the palliation of symptoms in advanced malignancy, and their input into the multidisciplinary team should not be seen as just to establish the diagnosis and surgically resect curable cancers.

Surgical reconstruction following cancer therapy

The aggressive treatment of bulky tumours often leaves major residual defects and in combination with plastic surgeons, the discipline of surgical oncology has developed reconstructive surgery to reduce some of the effects of tumour resections. Plastic surgeons have developed a reconstructive ladder of increasingly complex wound management to deal with some of these residual deficits (Table 3.7). Reconstructive surgery is not, however, the exclusive responsibility of plastic surgeons. For example, orthopaedic surgeons have developed sophisticated procedures for limb reconstruction following sarcoma surgery using bone grafts and prostheses. Maxillofacial surgeons reconstruct mandibles with free-flap fibula transplants following surgery for oral cavity cancers. ENT surgeons medialize vocal cords with silicon injection to overcome the hoarse voice associated with recurrent laryngeal nerve palsy caused by mediastinal tumours. Breast reconstruction following mastectomy often

Table 3.7 Reconstructive ladder of increasingly complex wound management coined by plastic surgeons

1. Healing by secondary intent
2. Primary closure
3. Delayed primary closure
4. Split-thickness graft
5. Full-thickness skin graft
6. Tissue expansion
7. Random pattern graft
8. Pedicled flap
9. Free flap with vascular microsurgery

involves the insertion of a tissue expander that is progressively injected with saline over the ensuing weeks until a suitable size and shape has been achieved, when it may be replaced by a more permanent implant. The second most common breast reconstruction procedure involves flaps of tissues from other parts of the body such as the back, abdomen, buttocks or thigh. These flaps may be pedicled, leaving the original blood supply or may be free flaps with vascular microsurgery to connect to a new blood supply. A latissimus dorsi muscle flap can be performed without significant loss of function and retaining its original blood supply. Abdominal flaps usually take tissue from the lower abdomen, for example, the transverse rectus abdominis myocutaneous (TRAM) flap that leaves the abdominal wall weakened. More recent abdominal flaps attempt to retain abdominal wall strength by using a muscle-sparing deep inferior epigastric perforator (DIEP) flap or superficial inferior epigastric artery (SIEA) flap. These require greater microsurgical skill. Other autologous tissue donor sites for breast reconstruction include superior gluteal artery perforator (SGAP) and inferior gluteal artery perforator (IGAP) flaps from the buttocks.

Radiotherapy

Radiotherapy involves the use of high-energy ionizing radiation to cause DNA damage and ultimately cell death. The damage induced by ionizing radiation may be lethal or sub-lethal to the tumour cells. In sub-lethal cell injury, damage to cellular proteins and organelles causes microscopic changes in the cell characterized down the microscope by swelling of mitochondria and endoplasmic reticulum and cloudiness of the cytoplasm known as hydropic degeneration. Cells may repair sub-lethal damage by removing damaged proteins and organelles by a cell stress response and autophagy and replace them with newly synthesized components. In contrast, lethal damage results in either cell necrosis or apoptosis.

Ionizing radiation acts by ejecting an electron from an atom to yield an ion pair. This may lead to direct damage to DNA via molecular excitation or indirectly via the hydrolysis of water into free radicals with an open electron shell configuration characterized by the presence of an unpaired electron (Figure 3.7). These free radicals are highly reactive, usually short-lived chemicals such as the neutrally charged hydroxyl radical (OH·) derived from water, which has an *in vivo* half-life of about 10^{-9} seconds. The other common free radical formed from water is superoxide (O_2^-) with one unpaired electron, which is responsible for the

"oxidative burst" or oxygen-dependent intracellular killing of ingested bacteria by phagocytes and is detoxified by the enzyme superoxide dismutase.

The measurement of radiation

Radiation is like rain:

- The amount of rain falling is the activity (measured in Becquerel – Beq)
- The amount of rain hitting you is absorbed dose (measured in Gray - Gy)
- How wet you get is dose equivalent (measured in Sievert – Sv)

The dose of radiotherapy is defined as the amount of energy deposited in tissues and is measured in Grays (Gy) after Hal Gray, a British pioneer of radiation biology and physics who also established the Gray Laboratories at Mount Vernon Hospital. One Gray is the dose absorbed when 1 J (joule) is deposited in 1 kg of tissue. Each Gray per cell causes approximately 10,000 damaged DNA bases, 1000 damaged deoxyribose sugars, 1000 single strand breaks, 40 double strand breaks, 150 DNA–protein cross-links and 30 DNA–DNA cross-links. Radiation can have an effect at any point in the cell cycle, although it is only at the time of mitosis that cell death occurs. Therefore, there can be a time lag of days, weeks or even months between the radiotherapy and the full effects of the treatment becoming manifest. Typical radiotherapy doses for solid epithelial tumours are 60–80 Gy. This is delivered as multiple fractions over time for several reasons. Dose fractionation allows normal cells to recover from sub-lethal damage between fractions, whilst tumour cells are less efficient at repairing damage. Dose fractionation also ensures that tumour cells in different phases of the cell cycle are exposed to radiation since it causes greatest damage in the G2 and M phases. The exact scheduling and fractionation of radiotherapy varies but in general doses of around 2 Gy are delivered on a daily basis 5 days a week. In some circumstances, more frequent dosing has been shown to be more efficacious but is of course more demanding on resources. For example, continuous hyperfractionated accelerated radiotherapy (CHART) involves radiotherapy delivered three times a day, every day of the week, usually for a fortnight.

Radiotherapy utilizes X-rays, electron beams and β- or γ-radiation produced by radioactive isotopes. X-rays are produced when a high-energy electron beam that is produced by heating an electrode in a vacuum, strikes matter. The energy of X-rays can be changed by altering the voltage input to the cathode of the X-ray tube that accelerates the electrons.

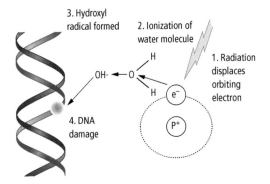

Figure 3.7 How radiation damages DNA.

Box 3.2 A brief lesson in fundamental particles

According to the standard model of quantum theory, the universe is made up of fermions (quarks and leptons) and bosons (force carriers). There are three sets of quark pairs and three sets of lepton pairs and for every particle there is a corresponding antiparticle, denoted by a bar over the symbol. Quarks are named after a quote in James Joyce's Finnegan's Wake "Three quarks for Muster Mark!", and they carry three types of colour charge (which have nothing to do with visible colours). Quarks do not exist in isolation but are confined in colour charge neutral hadrons. Two types of hadrons exist, mesons that are formed from a combination of a quark and an antiquark and baryons that are formed of three quarks. Protons are baryons formed of three quarks (uud) that carry a net +1 electrical charge, whilst neutrons are baryons with no net electrical charge (udd) and pi-mesons are formed by a quark (u) and an antiquark ($\bar{d}$) and carry a +1 electrical charge.

Four forces or interactions are known: strong force, weak force, electromagnetic force and gravitational force. The force carriers or bosons for all but gravity have been identified. The strong nuclear force (also known as the colour charge) that holds protons and neutrons together in atomic nuclei is mediated by gluons exchanging colour charges with quarks. The weak nuclear force is responsible for lepton decay and β-radiation and is mediated by W^+, W^- and Z bosons. The electromagnetic force is, of course, mediated by photons whilst the force carrier particle for gravity has not been observed but nevertheless has been named graviton. The Higgs boson particle theorized in 1964 and finally realized in 2012 was the final missing piece to complete the standard model and accounts for the masses of elementary particles (except photons and gluons).

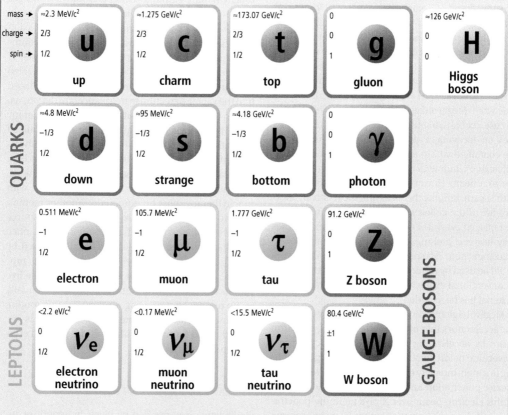

Figure 3.8 A brief lesson in particle physics.

Diagnostic radiology uses low-voltage equipment (e.g. 50 kV), producing X-rays of longer wavelength that are less penetrating. Therapeutic X-rays are produced by higher-voltage machines (30–50 MeV) producing shorter wavelength, more penetrating X-rays.

Radiotherapy is delivered in three ways: external beam radiotherapy, brachytherapy and radioisotope therapy. External beam radiotherapy involves the use of isotope sources or linear accelerators to deliver radiation from a distance. In the case of brachytherapy, the radioactive source is a solid radioactive nuclide emitting γ-rays, which is placed within the tumour or closely applied to the tumour. Finally, radioactive isotopes that are preferentially taken up in the target organ may be administered orally or intravenously; for example, oral iodine-131 is given for the treatment of thyroid tumours and intravenous strontium-89 in palliative treatment of bone metastasis.

External beam radiotherapy

Superficial voltage machines operate at 50–150 kV, and their energy does not penetrate more than 1 cm below the surface of the skin. They are used chiefly to treat superficial skin cancers. Orthovoltage machines that yield X-rays of 200–300 kV of energy penetrate to a depth of 3 cm. Metastases in bones close to the skin surface (ribs, sacrum) are frequently treated on these machines. Megavoltage radiotherapy machines usually use a cobalt-60 source that produces X-rays of 1.25 MeV on decaying to nickel-60. The cobalt-60 sources are contained within a protective lead shield and an adjustable window in this shield allows regulation of the γ-ray beam. However, there is considerable scatter of the beam, limiting the focus and the relatively short half-life of the cobalt source means that it needs to be replaced every 3–4 years and that treatment times may become prolonged as the cobalt nears the replacement date. It is speculated that cobalt-60 sources could be used by terrorists to produce a "dirty" bomb, a conventional explosive device to which radioactive material has been added.

Megavoltage machines have been replaced by linear accelerators that produce a high-energy electron beam by accelerating electrons down a cylindrical waveguide before they bombard a fixed target, resulting in a high-intensity electron beam (4–20 MeV) with greater penetration and less scatter. The advantages of this electron beam over X-rays lie in the penetration and decay characteristics that allow an electron beam to deliver its high energy to deep-seated tumours whilst sparing normal tissues in its pathway (Figure 3.9).

The accurate shaping of the radiation field to encompass the cancer but minimize damage to normal tissues really began with the introduction of the multileaf collimator composed of over 100 metal leaves, 5 mm thick and each aligned parallel to the radiation field. As each leaf may be moved independently to block part of the field, the resulting radiation field may be shaped and sculpted to suit the target. A further refinement of this process, known as intensity-modulated radiotherapy (IMRT), involves moving the multileaf collimator during the dose so that another level of fine tuning of the field can be achieved (Figure 3.10). One more recent development is image-guided radiation therapy (IGRT) that links the carefully shaped field with a continuous image of the patient. This process can overcome, for example, movement artefacts generated by the patient (hopefully still) breathing.

Brachytherapy

Brachytherapy employs sealed radionuclide sources that are implanted directly into a tumour or body cavity to deliver localized radiotherapy (Table 3.8). Examples of brachytherapy include radioactive iridium-192 needles or wires implanted into tumours of the breast, tongue and floor of the mouth. Sealed caesium-137 radioactive sources may also be placed into the vagina or rectum to treat cancers of the vagina, cervix, lower uterus, rectum or anus. Brachytherapy seeds are increasingly being used to treat localized prostate cancer (Figure 3.11). The major disadvantage of brachytherapy is the risk to staff handling the radioactive sources and caring for the patients. The radioactivity exposure of all staff involved with brachytherapy must be monitored. Another method used to reduce exposure is to place inactive source holders while the patient is anaesthetized and once they have been correctly located (as determined by X-ray), the patient is allowed to recover from the procedure. With the patient in a shielded room, the live radioactive source is then introduced, either manually or by remote control using a selectron. This routine is termed manual or remote after-loading and is frequently used for tumours of the upper vagina, cervix and endometrium.

Radioisotope therapy

Radioactive isotopes can be given by mouth or injection and are taken up by a particular tissue where they remain. Radioisotope therapy can only be used where a tumour is in a tissue that will preferentially

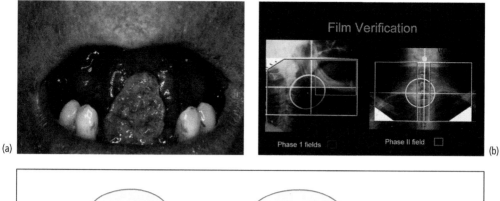

(a)

Film Verification

Phase 1 fields ☐   Phase II field ☐

(b)

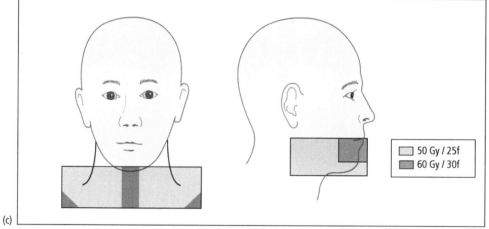

☐ 50 Gy / 25f
☐ 60 Gy / 30f

(c)

Figure 3.9 (a) Squamous cell cancer of the oral cavity. (b) Radiological verification of the radiotherapy fields. (c) The planned radiotherapy fields.

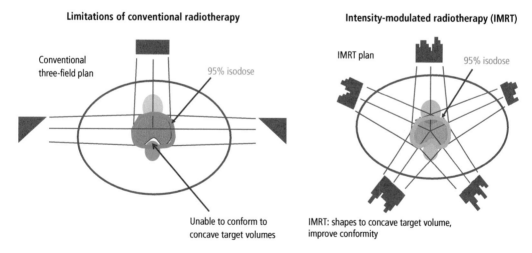

Limitations of conventional radiotherapy

Conventional three-field plan

95% isodose

Unable to conform to concave target volumes

Intensity-modulated radiotherapy (IMRT)

IMRT plan

95% isodose

IMRT: shapes to concave target volume, improve conformity

Figure 3.10 Comparison of conventional and intensity-modulated radiotherapy planning.

Table 3.8 Radionuclides used for brachytherapy

Source	Half-life	Mean X-ray energy	Form
Cobalt-60	5.3 years	1.25 MeV	Pellets (beads, tubes, needles)
Caesium-137	30 years	0.66 MeV	Tubes, needles
Iridium-92	74 days	0.37 MeV	Wires, hairpins, cylinders
Iodine-125	60 days	0.03 MeV	Grains, seeds

Prostate cancer brachytherapy
(radioactive seed implantation)

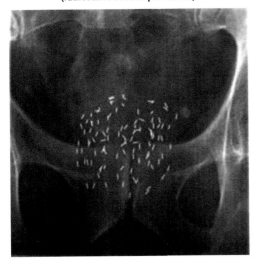

Figure 3.11 Prostate brachytherapy seeds *in situ* seen on pelvic X-ray.

accumulate a specific isotope, leaving other tissues unaffected (Figure 3.12). Examples are the thyroid, which will take up radioactive iodine and bone that naturally accumulates phosphorus or will take up bone-seeking radiochemicals such as rhenium-186 hydroxyethylidene diphosphate (^{186}Re-HEDP) (Table 3.9). A disadvantage with this approach is that the

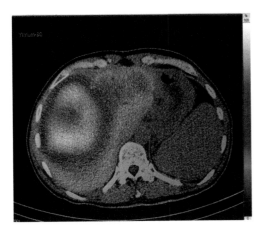

Figure 3.12 Selective internal radiation therapy (SIRT) using microspheres loaded with radioisotopes (in this case Yttrium-90) injected into the hepatic arteries to treat inoperable liver cancer. The microspheres are about one-third the size of a human hair width.

Table 3.9 Table of systemically administered radionuclides used in oncology

Radioisotope	Decay	Uses in oncology
Iodine-131	Beta: 192 keV Gamma: 364 keV Half-life: 8 days β- and γ-emitter	Used in treating thyroid cancer and in imaging the thyroid gland
Phosphorus-32	1.71 MeV Half-life: 14 days β-emitter	Used in the treatment of polycythemia vera
Rhenium-188	2.12 MeV Half-life: 17 hours β-emitter	Used to irradiate coronary arteries via an angioplasty balloon and in relieving the pain of bone metastases
Samarium-153	Beta: 825 keV Gamma: 103 keV Half-life: 47 hours β- and γ-emitter	Used in relieving the pain of bone metastases
Strontium-89	1.481 MeV Half-life: 50 days β-emitter	Used in relieving the pain of bone metastases

source cannot be recovered, limiting the degree of control over the total exposure to radiation.

Toxicity of radiotherapy

External beam radiotherapy is usually given as repeated daily dose fractions rather than as a single large dose of radiotherapy, which would lead to severe damage to the normal tissues. Even with fractionation, normal tissues have a maximum tolerated dose as indicated in Table 3.10. The area to be irradiated is referred to as the radiation field. This is marked out on the skin before treatment, and such markings often persist after treatment as tattooed dots. These radiotherapy tattoos are assiduously sought by clinical medical exam candidates, but in real life, most patients will tell you that they have had radiotherapy if you ask them nicely. In general, radiation-related side effects occur within the field of treatment although a few systemic manifestations such as fatigue and nausea may occur. The toxicity of radiotherapy increases with both the volume of tissue irradiated and the dose given. The transient side effects that develop during

Table 3.10 Table of normal tissue tolerance of radiotherapy

Tissue	Radiation effect	Dosage (Gy)
Testis	Sterility	0.2
Eye	Cataract	10
Lung	Pneumonitis	20
Kidney	Nephritis	25
Liver	Hepatitis	30
Central nervous system	Necrosis	50
Gastrointestinal tract	Ulceration, haemorrhage	60

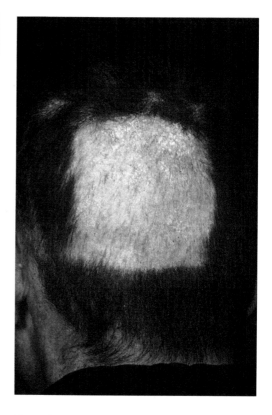

Figure 3.13 Clearly demarcated scalp alopecia due to radiotherapy.

treatment tend to reflect the acute damage to normal healthy tissue. Careful planning of the beam size and shielding of surrounding tissue, ensuring that radiation fields give effective tumour eradication with an acceptable level of toxicity, is, therefore, a prerequisite of successful therapy.

Radiotherapy-related side effects can be usefully divided into early and late toxicities (Table 3.11). Early toxicity occurs in hours to weeks and includes both systemic effects such as nausea, lethargy and myelosuppression (when a large volume of bone marrow is within the treated area; e.g. whole femur or pelvis radiation). Localized skin toxicity is a common early side effect that may be local erythema

Table 3.11 Table of adverse early and late reactions to radiotherapy

Timing	Tissue	Reaction
Early reactions	Skin	Dermatitis
	Oral mucosa	Stomatitis
	Bladder	Cystitis
	Oesophagus	Oesophagitis
	Bowel	Diarrhoea, ulceration
	Bone marrow	Myelosuppression
Late reactions	Central nervous system	Necrosis
	Kidney	Nephritis
	Liver	Hepatitis
	Lung	Pneumonitis and fibrosis
	Vascular endothelium	Fibrosis

progressing to ulceration and desquamation in the more severe cases. Other early side effects depend on the anatomy of the radiotherapy field, for example, alopecia with cranial irradiation (Figure 3.13), oropharyngeal mucositis with head and neck radiotherapy and diarrhoea, proctitis and cystitis with pelvic fields. These early reactions occur in tissues that are rapidly dividing and are usually present during or shortly after the course of radiotherapy and in most cases are reversible. Late side effects may take months or years to manifest themselves and once again depend upon the site being irradiated. These late tissue reactions occur when slowly dividing cells attempt division and are less frequently reversible. In some cases, the effects are believed to be mediated by fibrosis of the vascular endothelium. Examples of late reactions include necrosis in the central nervous system leading to transverse myelitis and paralysis with spinal cord radiation fields, radiation-induced pneumonitis (Figure 3.14), nephritis and osteomyelitis. Finally, radiotherapy is carcinogenic and may induce secondary tumours.

Radiation pneumonitis

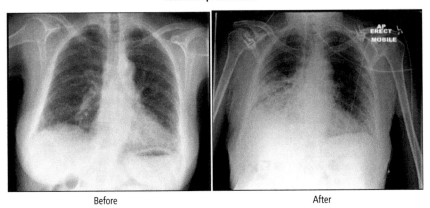

Before   After

Figure 3.14 Radiation pneumonitis with alveolar infiltrates and basal consolidation following irradiation of right breast cancer.

Radiosensitivity and radioresistance

Tumour resistance to radiotherapy appears to be an intrinsic property of that cancer, rather than an acquired attribute selected for by treatment, as in the case of chemotherapy. Indeed, the radiation sensitivities of many types of tumours are relatively predictable. The response of tissues both malignant and normal to fractionated radiation depends upon the "5 Rs":

- Repair
- Reassortment
- Repopulation
- Reoxygenation
- Radiosensitivity

In this context, repair is recovery from sub-lethal damage and is dependent on DNA repair mechanisms. Reassortment refers to the cell cycle phase of the tumour cells. Cells in G2 and M phases are most susceptible to radiotherapy, so after a first dose, cells in G1 and S will make up a greater proportion of the live tumour cells. Depending on the timing of the subsequent fraction of radiotherapy, these cells may have progressed or "reassorted" to G2 and M phases with increased sensitivity. Repopulation is the ability of tumour cells to grow and divide between doses of radiotherapy; this is a particular problem with prolonged fractionation and delayed fractions. Hypoxic cells are relatively radioresistant, and after the first fractions of radiotherapy, the death of sensitive cells reduces the competition for oxygen in the tumour, and cells that were hypoxic previously become reoxygenated and hence more susceptible to radiation. Different cell lineages are more or less radiosensitive, and these differences are in part intrinsic and independent of environmental factors. Amongst the factors that influence the radiosensitivity of tumours are the DNA repair genes, the production of free radical scavenging molecules (e.g. glutathione-S-transferases, superoxide dismutases, glutathione peroxidase), genes controlling apoptosis and cell cycle regulatory genes.

Chemotherapy

Drug discovery

The origins of chemotherapy for cancer lie in the use of biological warfare during the First World War, most hauntingly described in Wilfred Owen's poem "Dulce et decorum est". Following the extensive use of chlorine gas in trench warfare, the German Army first released mustard gas at Ypres on the night of 12–13 July 1917. Mustard gas had been synthesized in 1854 by Victor Meyer and was noted to be a vesicant in 1887. As a weapon of mass destruction, mustard gas, or Yperite as it was then known, had the advantages over chlorine of requiring smaller doses, being almost odourless and remaining active in the soil for weeks. The British gas casualties from 1914–1918 reveal the greater fatalities with mustard gas. Mustard gas exposure causes a severe blistering rash and conjunctivitis followed by myelosuppression after around 4 days. During the Second World War, the only use of mustard gas resulted in an own goal when the Luftwaffe sunk the USS *John Harvey* off Bari harbour in southern Italy in 1943. The ship was carrying 2000 M47A1 bombs containing a total of 100 tonnes of mustard gas, and the American sailors who survived developed conjunctivitis and skin blistering followed by a steep fall in their white cell counts, as documented by the naval surgeon Colonel Stewart Alexander. Meanwhile at Yale University, Alfred Gilman and Louis Goodman were using the closely related nitrogen mustard (mechlorethamine) initially in murine lymphoma models. In 1944, the first patient with lymphosarcoma (high-grade non-Hodgkin's lymphoma) was treated, and although Mr J. D., a 48-year-old silversmith, achieved a temporary remission of his tumour, he later died of bone marrow failure.

The subsequent development of chemotherapy following this fortuitous finding as a by-product of biological warfare, owes much to luck and trial and error rather than design. One serendipitous discovery was made by Barnett Rosenberg, a physicist at Michigan State University in 1965. He studied the effects of electric currents on *Escherichia coli* by using platinum electrodes in a water bath and found that they stopped dividing but not growing, leading to bacteria up to 300 times longer than normal. This was found to be due to cisplatin, a product from the platinum electrodes, which was interfering with DNA replication. By the end of the 1960s, a number of cytotoxic drugs from natural sources had been identified. In 1971, President Nixon, losing the war in Vietnam, declared war on cancer, signing the Cancer Act and establishing a drug discovery programme at the National Cancer Institute (NCI). This project trawled though thousands of natural chemicals in search of potential cytotoxic agents. It was not until the 1990s that rational drug design targeting known tumour-related features emerged. Examples of this include trastuzumab, a monoclonal antibody raised against erbB2/neu/Her-2 in breast cancer and imatinib, which inhibits the adenosine triphosphate (ATP) binding site of brc-abl fusion protein kinase in chronic myeloid leukaemia. In 2013, over 125,000 cancer patients in England were treated with systemic anticancer therapy receiving over 538,000 cycles of treatment.

Mechanisms of cytotoxic drugs

Amongst the many classifications of cytotoxic agents is a functional classification of cytotoxics (Table 3.12).

Alkylating agents

Alkylating agents transfer an alkyl group to purine (adenine and guanine) bases of DNA. Bifunctional alkylating agents form covalent bonds between two different bases, resulting in interstand or intrastrand cross-links, whilst monofunctional alkylating agents cannot form cross-links but cause adducts. Both forms of DNA alteration inhibit DNA synthesis, so alkylating agents act chiefly during the S phase of the cell cycle. Bifunctional agents can act on more than one base and are more cytotoxic, whilst monofunctional agents are more mutagenic and carcinogenic. One of the mechanisms of tumour resistance to alkylating agents is enzymatic removal of alkyl groups from purine bases and enhanced repair of cross-links.

Antimetabolites

Antimetabolites are structurally similar to natural compounds and in general interfere with cellular enzymes. These agents inhibit the metabolism (usually synthesis) of compounds necessary for DNA, RNA or protein synthesis. They include (1) purine analogues, (2) pyrimidine analogues, (3) folic acid analogues and (4) others, for example, hydroxyurea. Most antimetabolites have their greatest activity during the S phase.

Intercalating agents

Intercalating agents disrupt the steric integrity of the DNA double helix. The exact mechanisms of this action remain uncertain, although anthracycline antibiotics intercalate into the DNA major groove between base pairs of the DNA double helix and this action is non-covalent with no base sequence specificity. Platinum agents also intercalate and form intrastrand links similar to those formed by alkylating agents.

Spindle poisons

Antimicrotubule drugs can be divided into two groups, those that stabilize microtubules by inhibiting depolymerization (e.g. taxanes) and those that are depolymerizing agents that inhibit polymerization of tubulin (e.g. vinca alkaloids). Spindle poisons inhibit the mitotic spindle function and therefore act in the M phase of the cell cycle. Tubulin exists as α-tubulin and β-tubulin monomers in dynamic equilibrium with tubulin polymers or microtubules. Resistance to spindle poisons may occur by mutations of β-tubulin, and these point mutations do not confer cross-resistance between taxanes and vincas. An early spindle cell poison included colchicine used for acute gout, familial Mediterranean fever and rarely psoriasis. Although colchicine, like vincas causes depolymerization, it binds to a distinct site and is not used as a cytotoxic.

Table 3.12 A functional classification of cytotoxics

Functional group	Chemical group	Examples
Alkylating agents	Nitrogen mustards	Chlorambucil
		Cyclophosphamide
		Melphalan
	Nitrosoureas	BCNU (carmustine)
		CCNU (lomustine)
		Streptozotocin
	Tetrazine compounds	Dacarbazine
		Temozolomide
	Aziridines	Mitomycin C
		Thiotepa
	Methane sulphonic esters	Busulphan
Antimetabolites	Purine analogues	6-Mercaptopurine
		6-Thioguanine
	Pyrimidine analogues	Cytarabine
		Gemcitabine
	Dihydrofolate reductase inhibitors	Methotrexate
		Ralitexed
	Thymidylate synthetase inhibitors	5-Fluorouracil
	Ribonucleotide reductase inhibitors	Hydroxyurea
Intercalating agents	Platins	Cisplatin
		Carboplatin
		Oxaliplatin
	Antibiotics	Doxorubicin
	Anthracyclins	Daunorubicin
	Anthraquinones	Mitoxantrone
	Others	Bleomycin
		Mitomycin C
		Actinomycin D
Spindle cell poisons	Vinca alkaloids	Vincristine
		Vinblastine
		Vinorelbine
	Taxanes	Paclitaxel
		Docetaxel
Topoisomerase inhibitors	Topoisomerase I inhibitors: camptothecins	Topotecan
		Irinotecan
	Topoisomerase II inhibitors: epipodophyllotoxins	Etoposide
		Teniposide

Topoisomerase inhibitors

Topoisomerases prevent DNA strands from becoming tangled by cutting DNA and allowing it to wind or unwind. There are two mammalian classes of topoisomerases: topoisomerase I breaks single strands of DNA, whilst topoisomerase II breaks both strands of DNA. Topoisomerase I inhibitors act by inhibiting the religation step of the nicking–closing reaction, trapping topoisomerase I in a covalent complex with DNA. Topoisomerase I inhibitors act in the S phase and belong to the camptothecin group. Camptothecin was discovered by the NCI screening of plant-derived compounds and was isolated from a Chinese small tree *Camptotheca acuminata*. Topoisomerase II is inhibited both by DNA intercalators (e.g. anthracyclines) and by non-intercalators (e.g. epipodophyllotoxins).

Chemotherapy resistance

The major obstacle to successful cures with chemotherapy is the development of drug resistance by tumours. Indeed, the intrinsic resistance of some tumour cell types accounts, in part, for the variable sensitivity of different cancers to chemotherapy (Table 3.13). In some circumstances drug resistance is to a single drug only, whilst in other cases there is

Table 3.13 Sensitivity and curability of selected cancers treated with chemotherapy

Chemosensitivity	Tumour
Sensitive and curable	Leukaemias Lymphomas Germ cell tumours Childhood tumours
Sensitive and normally incurable (radical palliation)	Small cell lung cancer Myeloma
Moderately sensitive (palliation or adjuvant treatments)	Breast cancer Colorectal cancer Ovarian cancer Bladder cancer
Low sensitivity (chemotherapy of limited use)	Kidney cancer Melanoma Adult brain tumours Prostate cancer

cross-resistance between different drugs. The latter mechanism is due to the expression of molecular efflux pumps in tumour cell membranes. The most commonly found pump in multiresistant tumour cells is P-glycoprotein (Pgp) or the multidrug resistance protein (MDR). This transmembrane protein pumps natural toxins out of cells (including most chemotherapy agents) and is normally present in selected cells of the body such as renal proximal tubule cells, the apical mucosal cells of the colon and the canilicular surface of hepatocytes. Overexpression of Pgp/MDR by cancer cells confers a survival advantage in the presence of chemotherapy by inducing tumour resistance.

Cytotoxic-specific drug resistance can be achieved by a number of mechanisms, including efficient repair of DNA, reduced drug uptake, increased drug efflux, decreased intracellular activation of the drug, increased intracellular inactivation of the drug, activation of biochemical pathways that bypass the pathway being blocked by the cytotoxic drug and finally compensation for blocked enzyme pathways by increased enzyme production. An example of the last form of drug-specific resistance occurs with methotrexate, an antifolate antimetabolite that inhibits dihydrofolate reductase (DHFR). The first ever cancer cures with chemotherapy alone were reported with methotrexate for choriocarcinoma in 1963. In resistant tumour cells, there is amplification of the DHFR gene, with many thousands of copies of the gene leading to higher levels of DHFR to overcome the inhibitory actions of methotrexate.

How chemotherapy is used

Cytotoxic drugs are rarely used as single agents but are usually administered in combinations in an attempt to improve treatment efficacy by reducing the development of drug resistance, based on similar principles in the management of infectious diseases such as tuberculosis. A number of considerations are applied to the design of chemotherapy combinations. Only drugs that have proven activity as single agents should be included and preference should be given to drugs with non-overlapping toxicities and different modes of action. Cycles or pulses of chemotherapy given intermittently are designed to allow for recovery of normal tissues between doses without enabling the tumour cells to repopulate. Although this goal is frequently desirable, in recent years a number of continuous infusion chemotherapy regimens have been developed. The importance of a good acronym for a chemotherapy regimen should not be underestimated. No single regimen has remained the gold standard of care for as long as the CHOP regimen for non-Hodgkin's lymphoma, easily seeing off competition from the likes of ProMACE-CytaBOM. With greater experience of the benefits and disadvantages of chemotherapy, its safety has improved and the indications for its use have expanded. As with radiotherapy and endocrine treatments, chemotherapy is increasingly used in an adjuvant context (Table 3.14).

In some circumstances chemotherapy, resistance may be overcome by escalating the dose of cytotoxic drugs. In many circumstances, the dose-limiting toxicity (DLT) of chemotherapy is myelosuppression, and if this can be avoided, doses may be doubled or more before reaching the next DLT, which is often mucosal damage. Autologous (from the patient him/herself) and allogeneic (from a donor) bone marrow transplantation (BMT) was developed to this end. Prior to

Table 3.14 Cancers effectively treated by neoadjuvant and adjuvant chemotherapy

Therapy	Tumour
Cancers effectively treated by neoadjuvant chemotherapy	Soft tissue sarcoma Osteosarcoma Locally advanced breast cancer
Cancers effectively treated by adjuvant chemotherapy	Wilms' tumour Osteosarcoma Breast cancer Colorectal cancer

Table 3.15 Cancers effectively treated by high-dose chemotherapy and stem cell transplantation

Disease	Stage	Transplant	Approx. 5-year disease-free survival
CML	Stable phase	Allogeneic	30%
ALL	Second remission	Allogeneic/autologous	40%
AML	First remission	Allogeneic/autologous	50%
High-grade non-Hodgkin's lymphoma	Responsive relapse	Autologous	45%
Hodgkin's disease	Responsive relapse	Autologous	45%
Neuroblastoma	High-risk first line	Allogeneic/autologous	50%
Neuroblastoma	Relapsed	Allogeneic/autologous	25%
Non-seminomatous germ cell tumour	Responsive relapse	Autologous	50%
Myeloma	First line	Allogeneic/autologous	30%

ALL, acute lymphoblastic leukaemia; AML, acute myeloid leukaemia; CML, chronic myeloid leukaemia.

high-dose chemotherapy, progenitor stem cells are harvested either from multiple bone marrow aspirations (BMT) or now more often from peripheral blood following growth factor stimulation (peripheral blood stem cell transplant (PBSCT)). These stem cells are immature haematopoietic cells capable of repopulating the bone marrow. The patient then receives the conditioning high-dose chemotherapy and/or radiotherapy, and subsequently the stem cells are reinfused as a transfusion. This approach has an appreciable mortality of 20–50% in the case of allogeneic BMT and of 5% with autologous PBSCT. However, stem cell transplantation has a defined role in the management of a number of malignancies (Table 3.15).

Side effects of chemotherapy

The main actions of chemotherapy are focused on killing rapidly dividing cancer cells and hence many of their toxicities arise because of the effects on normal cells with high rates of turnover. Indeed, the side effects of chemotherapy may be divided into the predictable toxicities that are common, often dose related and usually related to the mechanism of action of the drug. In contrast, idiosyncratic side effects are usually rarer, unrelated to dose or mechanism of action but tend to be drug specific. The predictable effects of chemotherapy on fast dividing normal cells (bone marrow, gastrointestinal tract epithelium, hair follicles, spermatogonia) will be a consequence of inhibition of cell division and are especially found with cell cycle phase-specific cytotoxics. In contrast, the side effects on slow-growing cell types will occur most frequently with drugs that are not cell cycle specific, such as the alkylating agents that introduce DNA mutations

into these cells, resulting in secondary leukaemias and other tumours.

The side effects of chemotherapy may be divided into three time groups: (1) immediate effects that occur within hours, (2) delayed effects that occur within days, weeks or months but are generally manifested whilst the full course of chemotherapy treatment is ongoing and (3) late effects that occur months, years or decades after the chemotherapy has ceased. The top five side effects ranked by patients according to severity are nausea, fatigue, hair loss, concern about the effects on friends and family and finally vomiting. The immediate toxicities include nausea and vomiting, anaphylaxis, extravasation and tumour lysis. The delayed side effects are the most abundant and include alopecia, myelosuppression, stomatitis and the majority of the unpredictable toxicities. The late effects of chemotherapy include infertility and secondary malignancies.

Early side effects

Nausea and vomiting

Vomiting is a central reflex initiated in the vomiting centre of the medulla that coordinates the contraction of the diaphragm and abdominal muscles with relaxation of the cardiac sphincter and the muscles of the throat. There are four inputs into the vomiting centre: the labyrinths (e.g. motion sickness), the higher cortical centres (e.g. fear, anticipation), the vagus nerve sensory input from the gastrointestinal tract, particularly the small bowel, and finally the chemoreceptor trigger zone (CTZ). The CTZ is located in the area postrema adjacent to the fourth ventricle where the

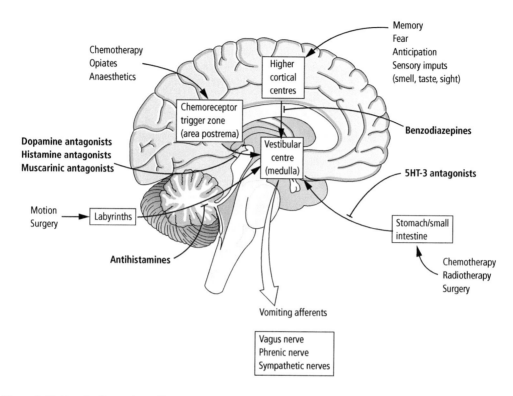

Figure 3.15 Neural pathways in vomiting.

blood–brain barrier is relatively deficient and chemicals in the blood and cerebrospinal fluid are sensed, stimulating the vomiting centre. The different inputs to the vomiting centre rely on different neurotransmitters, and this can be exploited pharmacologically in the control of symptoms (Figure 3.15). Chemotherapy chiefly acts on the gastrointestinal tract, causing serotonin (5-hydroxytryptamine (5HT)) release and acting via the afferent vagus nerve. It also stimulates the CTZ, which employs dopaminergic and muscarinic pathways. Occasionally, anticipatory vomiting is problematic, and this acts through the higher cortical centres using γ-aminobutyric acid (GABA) neurotransmission. In contrast, the labyrinthine pathways utilize histamine-1 receptors, and motion sickness is often successfully controlled with antihistamines.

The likelihood of being sick with chemotherapy depends upon the emetogenicity of the cytotoxics used as well as host-related factors. Cisplatin and mustine are amongst the most emetogenic, whilst vinca alkaloids rarely cause nausea. Younger age, women, patients who have been sick previously with chemotherapy and patients with a low alcohol intake are all more likely to suffer with chemotherapy-induced vomiting.

Acute vomiting within 6 hours of chemotherapy is best controlled by a combination of steroids and 5HT-3 receptor antagonists. Delayed vomiting occurring up to 5 days after the chemotherapy is best treated with steroids and dopamine antagonists. Anticipatory vomiting that occurs prior to receiving chemotherapy is treated with benzodiazepines.

Anaphylaxis

As with all medicines, anaphylaxis may occur with chemotherapy and the most common culprits are taxanes and asparaginase. The incidence of hypersensitivity with paclitaxel is so high that routine prophylaxis with steroids and antihistamines (H1 and H2) is administered to all patients receiving paclitaxel.

Extravasation

Extravasation is the inadvertent administration of chemotherapy into the subcutaneous tissue. This leads to pain, erythema, inflammation and discomfort, which if unrecognized and untreated can lead to tissue necrosis with the possibility of serious

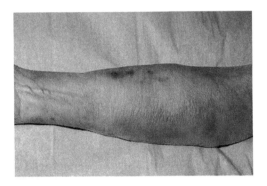

Figure 3.16 Extravasation of carboplatin chemotherapy showing swollen and red skin which was cold.

sequelae. The position, size and age of the cannulation site are the factors that have the greatest bearing on the likelihood of problems occurring (Figures 3.16, 3.17, 3.18 and 3.19) and the experience of the specialist administering the chemotherapy is crucial in this aspect. The likelihood of damage occurring is determined by the cytotoxic drug, with anthracyclines being especially likely to cause severe injury.

Tumour lysis

The rapid cytolysis of a large volume of cancer cells at the start of chemotherapy occasionally results in the tumour lysis syndrome or metabolic chaos. The destruction of tumour DNA leads to hyperuricaemia from the breakdown of nucleotide bases. The cytolysis causes hyperkalaemia by releasing intracellular potassium, and the breakdown of proteins and DNA causes hyperphosphataemia and secondary hypocalcaemia. Acute renal failure may be a consequence of the high levels of urate and phosphate, whilst the high levels of potassium may lead to cardiac arrhythmias. Tumour lysis only really occurs to a significant extent with acute leukaemias and high-grade lymphomas including Burkitt's lymphoma. Bulky tumours, poor renal function and high levels of urate before chemotherapy increase the risk of tumour lysis.

Uric acid is soluble at physiological pH but precipitates in the acidic environment of the renal tubules, leading to crystallization in the collecting ducts and ureters, leading to obstructive uropathy. Similarly, calcium phosphate is precipitated in the renal tubules and microvasculature producing nephrocalcinosis. The most important issue in the management of tumour lysis is its prevention by a combination of hyperhydration, allopurinol and urinary alkalinization to pH >7 with sodium bicarbonate to reduce urate precipitation in the renal tubules. Allopurinol is an inhibitor of xanthine oxidase, the enzyme that catalyzes the conversion of soluble xanthine (a product of purine catabolism) to uric acid. The treatment of established tumour lysis is an oncological

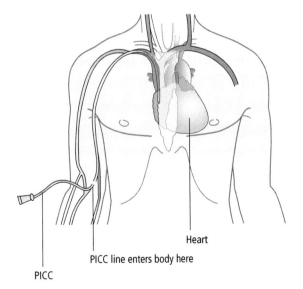

Heart

PICC line enters body here

PICC

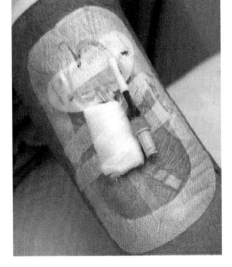

Figure 3.17 Peripherally inserted central catheter (PICC).

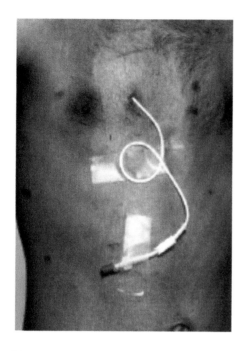
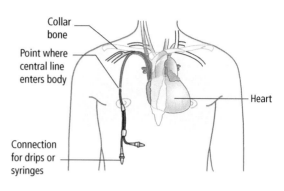

Collar bone

Point where central line enters body

Heart

Connection for drips or syringes

Figure 3.18 A patient with a Hickman line, a skin-tunnelled, long-term silicon catheter with a Dacron cuff about 2 cm above the exit site that acts as a barrier to micro-organisms and prevents catheter dislodgment. Hickman lines are used for continuous infusional chemotherapy or for patients with poor venous access. Hickman lines are placed in the radiology department using ultrasound guidance or in theatres under general anaesthetic.

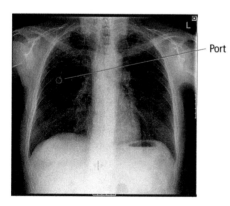

Port

Figure 3.19 Portacath for the delivery of chemotherapy.

emergency. The majority of patients who develop tumour lysis have chemosensitive tumours and are receiving a potentially curative treatment. These patients should be considered candidates for urgent haemodialysis. A relatively new addition to the treatment is recombinant urate oxidase (rasburicase), which converts insoluble urate to soluble allantoin (see Chapter 40).

Delayed side effects (predictable)

The main predictable delayed side effects of chemotherapy are alopecia, bone marrow suppression and gastrointestinal mucositis.

Alopecia and onychodystrophy

Hair loss with chemotherapy is both drug and dose dependent and is related to the frequency of cycle repetition. Long-term therapy may result in the loss of pubic, axillary and facial hair in addition to scalp hair. The loss of scalp hair often occurs in an acute episode while washing, usually 2–6 weeks after starting chemotherapy. It should be emphasized to patients that alopecia from chemotherapy is reversible, with hair regrowth beginning 1–2 months after completing chemotherapy. The hair may regrow a lighter

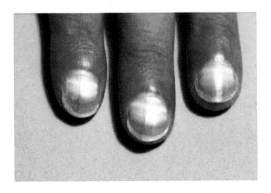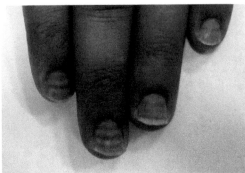

Figure 3.20 Beau lines. Horizontal lines in nails represent arrest of nail growth due to cycles of chemotherapy.

or darker colour and is often curlier initially. Doxorubicin and cyclophosphamide are the commonest culprits. Patients should be offered wigs, which are available from the National Health Service (NHS). Scalp cooling (below 22°C) may reduce alopecia by causing vasoconstriction and reducing circulation to hair follicles. The pharmacokinetic profiles of cytotoxics dictate that scalp cooling is only effective for anthracyclines. Concerns have been raised over the potential risk of developing scalp and cerebral metastases due to reduced drug circulation to these sites with scalp cooling. Along with alopecia, a frequent complication of chemotherapy is onychodystrophy or nail changes other than colour changes that usually make the nails brittle and prone to shedding (onycholysis) as well as fungal infection (onychomycosis). A common physical sign in patients who have received cyclical chemotherapy are Beau's lines, horizontal grooves or lines on the nail plate that indicate cycles of arrested nail growth with chemotherapy cycles (Figure 3.20).

Myelotoxicity of chemotherapy

The myelosuppressive effects of chemotherapy may affect the circulating red cells, white cells and platelets, and the manifestations in these three series are in part related to their circulatory lifespans. In circulation, the half-life of an erythrocyte is 120 days, of a leucocyte is 6–8 hours and of a platelet is 7 days.

There is a significant risk of severe myelosuppression if chemotherapy is initiated when the total white cell count is <3.0 × 10^9/L (or the neutrophil count is <1.5 × 10^9/L) and/or the platelet count is <150 × 10^9/L. These values are the usual cut-offs for administering a cycle of chemotherapy; however, it may be given at lower values in patients with haematological malignancies or if supportive therapy is anticipated and when non-myelosuppressive regimens are employed. Myelosuppression is the DLT for many cytotoxic agents; the main exceptions are vincristine, bleomycin, streptozotocin and asparaginase, which do not cause myelosuppression.

Thus, anaemia is rarely a DLT but is generally cumulative over successive cycles of chemotherapy. Anaemia is most troublesome with cisplatin because the nephrotoxicity of this agent may decrease erythropoietin production from the kidneys in response to anaemia. The symptoms of anaemia include fatigue, lethargy and exertional dyspnoea with haemoglobin levels in the range 80–100 g/L. Reduced exercise capacity progresses to dyspnoea and tachycardia at rest and complications including cerebrovascular (e.g. transient ischaemic attacks) and cardiovascular (e.g. angina) ischaemia as the haemoglobin falls below 80 g/L. The management of chemotherapy-induced anaemia is with transfusion, and in the case of cisplatin-induced anaemia, at least, erythropoietin may be beneficial (Box 3.3).

Box 3.3 Haematopoietic growth factors

The proliferation and maturation of blood cell lineages is determined by haemopoietic growth factors or colony-stimulating factors (CSFs). Bone marrow stromal cells produce many of these growth factors. Recombinant haemopoietic growth factors are administered to ameliorate chemotherapy-induced cytopenias. They are given parenterally to avoid proteolytic degradation in the gastrointestinal tract.

Erythropoietin

This growth factor is naturally produced by the kidney in response to hypoxia and stimulates red cell proliferation. It may be overproduced in renal cell carcinoma leading to paraneoplastic polycythemia. As well as its role in the treatment of anaemia of chronic renal failure, erythropoietin may be used to treat cytotoxic-induced anaemia, particularly where cisplatin is implicated.

Granulocyte colony-stimulating factor

Granulocyte colony-stimulating factor (G-CSF) is a lineage-restricted growth factor promoting granulocyte differentiation, whilst granulocyte–macrophage CSF (GM-CSF) is multifunctional, affecting granulocytes, monocytes, megakaryocytes and erythroid precursors but not basophils. Both CSFs are used in the treatment of chemotherapy- and radiotherapy-related neutropenia. Evidence-based guidelines are available that describe the rational use of G-CSF in four circumstances:

1 Primary prophylaxis (i.e. with the first cycle of chemotherapy): not routinely used, occasionally used for pre-existing neutropenia, for example, due to marrow infiltration.

2 Secondary prophylaxis: only for curable tumours with proven importance of maintaining dose intensity (germ cell tumours, choriocarcinoma, lymphoma).

3 Febrile neutropenia: data do not support routine G-CSF usage but indicate use in the presence of pneumonia, hypotension, multiorgan failure and fungal infection.

4 Peripheral blood stem cell mobilization prior to harvesting for high-dose therapy and stem cell rescue.

Thrombopoietin

Thrombopoietin (TPO) is constitutively produced by the liver and kidneys and acts on many stages of megakaryocyte growth and differentiation. Romiplostim, a fusion protein analogue of TPO and eltrombopag, a small molecule agonist of the TPO receptor have been licensed for use in idiopathic thrombocytopenic purpura (ITP), but their action may be too slow to reverse chemotherapy-induced thrombocytopenia.

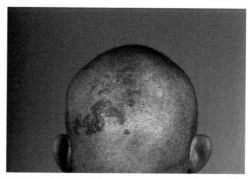

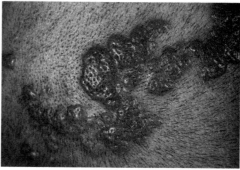

Figure 3.21 Herpes zoster scalp (with closeup below). Herpes zoster of left C2 distribution erupting as an opportunistic infection during a course of chemotherapy for Hodgkin's disease.

Neutropenia (neutrophil count $<1.0 \times 10^9$/L) is the commonest DLT of chemotherapy and is a frequent cause of treatment delays and dose reductions. Neutropenia is most often manifest as infection (Figure 3.21) and neutropenic sepsis is a medical emergency, which if left untreated is potentially fatal. It is frequently overlooked by untrained medical staff and delays in starting intravenous antibiotics can be fatal. Neutropenic sepsis is defined as a fever of 38.0°C or higher for at least 2 hours when the neutrophil count is below 1.0×10^9/L.

The treatment of neutropenic sepsis includes a thorough clinical history and physical examination to identify possible sources of infection. Initial management must include resuscitation measures for shock if present. An infection screen should be performed, including blood cultures from peripheral veins as well as from any central access catheters, a urine sample for microscopy and culture, a chest X-ray and a throat swab for culture. Treatment should not be delayed awaiting the results of cultures. The most common organisms associated with neutropenic sepsis are common bacterial pathogens. Empirical antibiotic treatment should be instituted with broad-spectrum bactericidal antibiotics and policies will be dictated by local antibiotic resistance patterns. The most common initial treatment regimens are a parenteral combination of an aminoglycoside with either a cephalosporin or a broad-spectrum penicillin.

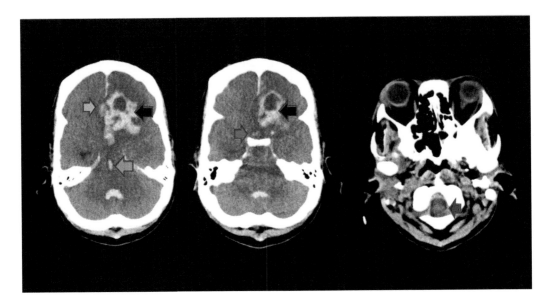

Figure 3.22 Fatal intraparenchymal **left frontal haemorrhage** with bleeding into the fourth ventricle (orange) and subarachnoid spaces. There is associated subfalcine (green), uncal (blue) and tonsillar (red) herniation. The patient had severe thrombocytopenia following induction chemotherapy for acute leukaemia.

Alternatively, monotherapy with a cephalosporin may be used. If there is no response within 36–48 hours, the antibiotic regimen should be reviewed in the light of culture results and consideration given to adding antifungal cover (e.g. amphotericin B). For patients with severe neutropenic sepsis as defined by hypotension, pneumonia or multiorgan failure, G-CSF should be administered. Following an episode of neutropenic sepsis, consideration should be given to reducing the chemotherapy dosage in subsequent cycles or if dose intensity has been shown to influence the outcome (e.g. germ cell tumours, Hodgkin's disease) secondary prophylaxis with G-CSF to reduce the duration of neutropenia should be considered (Box 3.3).

Thrombocytopenia is a common side effect of chemotherapy, particularly with carboplatin, that rarely causes clinical manifestations unless it is severe. Although petechiae and bruising may occur, major haemorrhage is very rare unless the platelet count falls below 20×10^9/L. At platelet counts below 10×10^9/L, there is an appreciable risk of gastrointestinal or cerebral haemorrhage, and prophylactic administration of pooled platelets is warranted (Figure 3.22). Growth factor support for thrombocytopenia is currently investigational only (Box 3.3), and chemotherapy dose delays and reductions may be necessary following low platelet nadir counts.

Gastrointestinal tract mucositis

Mucositis is a frequent delayed side effect of chemotherapy occurring in 40–50% of patients and is even more common in patients receiving chemo-radiotherapy or radiotherapy alone for head and neck cancers. It is thought that chemotherapy and radiotherapy damage basal epithelial cells in the intestinal mucosa leading to apoptosis, atrophy and ulceration. Once ulceration occurs, bacterial and fungal infection and activation of macrophages leads to further inflammation (Figure 3.23).

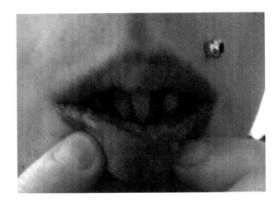

Figure 3.23 Mucositis.

Mucositis is associated with significant morbidity and mortality risk and chemotherapy dose reductions and delays. Sucking ice lollies during chemotherapy may reduce the incidence of mucositis with some cytotoxics by a mechanism analogous to the cold cap treatment for the prevention of alopecia. Various "magic mouthwashes" (usually a mild local anaesthetic and antiseptic combination) may provide symptomatic relief from mucositis. The time course of mucositis closely resembles that of neutropenia, typically occurring 7–14 days after the administration of chemotherapy. Recent developments in the management of mucositis also hint at comparisons with the investigational study of keratinocyte growth factors as treatment for mucositis. In a few cases, specific antidotes reduce the incidence of mucositis, such as folinic acid rescue after methotrexate.

Delayed side effects (idiosyncratic)

Many delayed side effects of chemotherapy are drug specific and are not immediately predictable from their mechanisms of action. The organs most frequently affected include the skin, nerves, heart, lungs and blood vessels.

Dermatological side effects

Dermatological complications include the already mentioned acute complications of extravasation and anaphylaxis as well as idiosyncratic delayed toxicities. These include hyperpigmentation, which occurs commonly with 5-fluorouracil and bleomycin and may follow the lines of the veins into which the chemotherapy has been administered. A hand and foot syndrome of painful redness, scaling or shedding of the skin of the palms and soles may occur with continuous infusions of 5-fluorouracil chemotherapy and also with liposomal anthracycline chemotherapy. In the latter case, the cytotoxics are delivered in a liposome to dramatically prolong their half-life, mimicking the pharmacokinetics of a continuous infusion regimen. A third unusual dermatological side effect of chemotherapy is radiation recall, an erythematous reaction of skin in the area of a previous radiation field. Indeed, this may occur even when the radiation treatment was decades earlier and is most commonly seen with gemcitabine chemotherapy.

Cardiological side effects

Acute arrhythmias can occur during chemotherapy infusions or shortly thereafter, and this rare occurrence happens most frequently with taxanes. Similarly, 5-fluorouracil rarely precipitates chest pain and acute myocardial infarction, pericarditis and cardiac shock. However, the most common cardiotoxicity of chemotherapy is a dose-related dilated cardiomyopathy seen with anthracyclines. This usually presents with heart failure within 8 months of the last anthracycline dose. Diuretics improve symptoms and the early use of an angiotensin-converting enzyme inhibitor can increase the left ventricular ejection fraction, improving prognosis, which, however, remains poor. This side effect limits the total cumulative dosage of anthracyclines that can be administered. The maximum cumulative lifetime doses of the anthracyclines have been established although cardiomyopathy may be seen at lower total doses and is likely to be due to an idiosyncratic reaction rather than a dosage-related side effect. There are different sensitivities to anthracyclines in children as compared with adults.

Neurological side effects

Although only a few cytotoxics penetrate the cerebrospinal fluid, many cytotoxics cause neurotoxicity. Peripheral neuropathy, the most frequent neurotoxicity of chemotherapy, is commonly seen with vinca alkaloids, taxanes and platinum derivatives. The longest nerves are most affected, so it presents as a symmetrical sensory loss over the feet and hands. This may progress to worsening paraesthesia, loss of tendon reflexes and eventually motor loss. Features usually slowly improve over several months following cessation of chemotherapy, although residual deficits may persist indefinitely. The same cytotoxics may be responsible for an autonomic neuropathy leading to abdominal pain, constipation, paralytic ileus, urinary retention, bradycardia and postural hypotension. Acute encephalopathy most commonly is associated with ifosfamide and symptoms include confusion, agitation, seizures, somnolence and coma. Cerebellar toxicity may follow cytarabine therapy and 5-fluorouracil. Cisplatin-induced ototoxicity is characterized by the progressive loss of high-tone hearing and tinnitus.

The inadvertent intrathecal administration of vinca alkaloids is fatal, and this catastrophic clinical error has arisen because of confusion of the drug with a cytotoxic agent intended to be given intrathecally (usually methotrexate). Several such incidents have occurred in NHS hospitals in the 1990s, representing an estimated rate of about three per 100,000 intrathecal chemotherapy treatments and resulting in the jailing of a junior doctor in 2001. Strict guidelines surrounding the administration of intrathecal chemotherapy are now in place to prevent this occurrence.

Pulmonary side effects

Chronic pulmonary toxicity and fibrosis occurs with a number of cytotoxics and the outcome is generally poor. Bleomycin is the most common culprit, and the risk increases with dose. Pulmonary fibrosis is much more common in patients who have received bolus dosages of bleomycin, which should be avoided; bleomycin should be given by slow intravenous infusion over hours. The most terrible toxicity that oncologists observe is that of a young man successfully treated for testicular cancer who becomes breathless and then dies from pulmonary fibrosis secondary to bleomycin treatment. The cardinal symptom of drug-induced pulmonary toxicity is dyspnoea associated with non-productive cough, fatigue, fever and malaise. Symptoms usually develop over several weeks to months. The chest X-ray classically shows reticulonodular infiltration at the bases and occasionally pleural effusions (Figure 3.24a). Lung function tests demonstrate a reduced diffusing capacity for carbon monoxide and restrictive ventilatory defects (Figure 3.24b). The usual treatment is with corticosteroids, although there is no evidence to support a benefit and the mortality is high. Patients are treated with oxygen and this makes the fibrosis worse.

Hepatic side effects

Many cytotoxic agents cause elevated serum transaminases and bilirubin, and fatty infiltration and cholestasis may occur as the toxic effect progresses. Hepatic veno-occlusive disease (VOD) results from the blockage of venous outflow in the small centrilobular hepatic vessels following damage to cells in the area of the liver surrounding the central vein. This rare side effect occurs with high-dose chemotherapy, often as part of stem cell transplantation. The clinical features are painful hepatomegaly, ascites, peripheral oedema, marked elevations in serum enzymes and bilirubin and hepatic encephalopathy. The onset is often abrupt, occurring during the first post-transplant week, and the clinical course is fatal in up to 50%.

Late side effects

Gonadal side effects

Chemotherapy causes a variety of toxic effects on male and female gonads leading to infertility. Most cytotoxic drugs given in late during pregnancy are

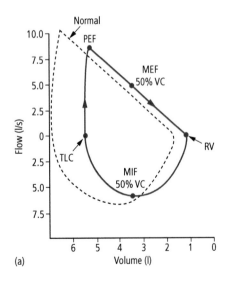

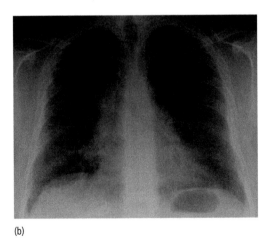

(a)   (b)

Figure 3.24 (a) Lung flow loop and (b) chest radiograph of a 35-year-old man treated with combination chemotherapy including bleomycin for advanced germ cell tumour of the testis. The chest radiograph demonstrates diffuse interstitial shadowing most prominent in the lower zones. The lung flow loop shows a restrictive deficit typical of bleomycin fibrosis. MEF, mid-expiratory flow; MIF, mid inspiratory flow; PEF, peak expiratory flow; RV, residual volume; TLC, total lung capacity; VC, vital capacity.

not teratogenic, but many will have teratogenic effects on the foetus if given in early pregnancy. If fertility is maintained or restored, there are concerns about the heritability of the cancer and at least a theoretical risk of mutagenic alterations to germ cells; however, large studies of the children of cancer patients have shown no increased risk. Efforts have been made to conserve fertility using luteinizing hormone-releasing hormone (LHRH) agonists, but these have failed.

Adult male gonadal toxicity

Male germ cells lie within the seminiferous epithelium and include stem spermatogonia, differentiating spermatogonia, spermatocytes, spermatids and sperm. The differentiating spermatogonia actively proliferate and are therefore highly susceptible to cytotoxic agents. In contrast, the Leydig cells, which are in the interstitium and produce androgens, and the Sertoli cells, which provide support and regulatory factors to the germ cells, do not proliferate in adults and so survive most cytotoxic therapies. Because later-stage germ cells (spermatocytes onwards) do not proliferate, they are not susceptible to chemotherapy – sperm counts do not fall immediately on starting chemotherapy but may take 2–3 months to decline; although minor falls in testosterone production may occur, only testicular radiation will produce significant testosterone deficiency. Men due to start chemotherapy should be offered sperm storage in order to enable them to father children in the future. Modern developments in *in vitro* fertilization are particularly relevant to the cancer patient. For those patients who were considered to be unsuitable for semen storage and remain azoospermic post treatment, the technique of intracytoplasmic sperm injection (ICSI) may be appropriate. Just remember, only one sperm is required to fertilize one ovum.

Adult female gonadal toxicity

In women, unlike men, the germ cells do not proliferate whereas the somatic cells do and this accounts for the different gonadal toxicity of chemotherapy in women and men. Female germ cells proliferate before birth as oogonia that arrest at the oocyte stage. At birth, a woman has 1 million oocytes, which are reduced to 300,000 at puberty. Oocytes are progressively lost by atresia, development and ovulation, until almost all are lost and menopause is reached. The interval from recruitment of primordial follicles to ovulation is 82 days, and when cytotoxics destroy maturing follicles, temporary amenorrhea results. However, if the number of remaining primordial follicles falls below the minimum number necessary for

menstrual cyclicity, irreversible ovarian failure occurs with permanent amenorrhea. This accounts for the increased risk of chemotherapy-induced menopause in older patients. Permanent ovarian failure is often accompanied by vasomotor symptoms, whilst temporary amenorrhoea, which may last up to 5 years after chemotherapy, is usually asymptomatic. As in men, alkylating agents are the major culprits causing permanent gonadal failure in women. At present, ovum storage remains an unreliable method for routine usage and requires ovarian stimulation prior to egg harvesting, which introduces a delay prior to starting chemotherapy and is relatively contraindicated in breast cancer. The storage of fertilized eggs (embryos) is more successful. The Roman Catholic Church still opposes all forms of *in vitro* fertilization and, under the papacy of Benedict XVI, condemned the practice in the 2008 magisterial instruction *Dignitas Personae*, further evidence of the deficiencies of the penultimate pope.

Teratogenicity of chemotherapy

Many cytotoxics are teratogenic in murine models, although data in humans are thankfully limited. All alkylating agents are teratogenic, with limited information suggesting a significant risk of malformed infants if exposed in the first trimester but no increased risk during the second and third trimesters. Methotrexate is, of course, a potent abortifactant during early pregnancy. No clear evidence is available to support the timing of pregnancy following chemotherapy although most clinicians advise a 2–5 year gap before pregnancy.

Carcinogenicity of chemotherapy

Many cytotoxic agents are genotoxic, and this not only accounts for their antitumour activity but also carries the risk of inducing cancers; alkylating agents are the most potent carcinogens in this group (Table 3.16). The risk of induced malignancies depends not only on the cytotoxics administered but also on the initial cancer diagnosis, with greatest risks in patients with Hodgkin's disease, where the second malignancy rate is 10–15% after 15 years. Two forms of secondary acute leukaemia following chemotherapy are widely recognized. Alkylating agents are carcinogenic with acute leukaemias occurring in up to 5% 3–5 years after exposure and associated with chromosome 5q or 7 deletions (Figure 3.25a). Survival after secondary acute myeloid leukaemia (AML) is poor, usually only a few months. There is also an increased incidence of solid tumours after alkylating

Table 3.16 Table of carcinogenic medicines

Carcinogenic drug	Associated tumour
Cytotoxics (especially alkylating agents and topoisomerase II inhibitors)	Acute myeloid leukaemia
Cyclophosphamide	Bladder cancer
Immunosuppression	Kaposi's sarcoma, post-transplantation lymphoproliferation
Oestrogens (unopposed)	Endometrial cancer
Oestrogens (transplacental)	Vaginal adenocarcinoma
Oral contraceptive pill	Hepatic adenoma
Androgenic anabolic steroids	Hepatocellular carcinoma
Phenacetin	Renal pelvis transitional cell cancer
Chloramphenicol	Acute leukaemia
Phenytoin	Lymphoma, neuroblastoma

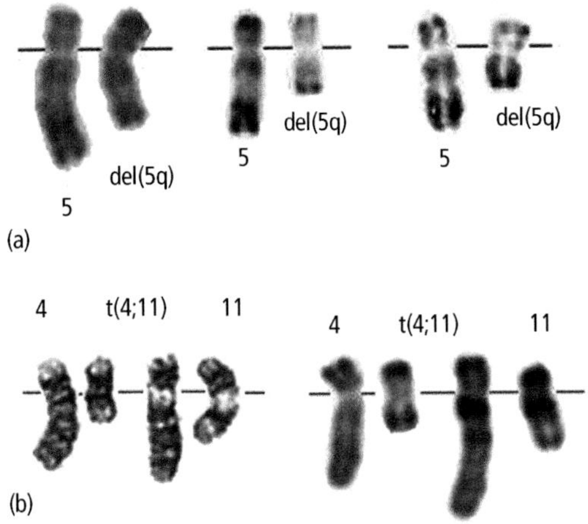

Figure 3.25 Chromosome translocation in secondary leukaemia. Partial karyotypes from patients with secondary acute leukaemia follow chemotherapy. (a) Deletions on the long arm of chromosome 5 are characteristic of alkylating-agent-related secondary acute myeloid leukaemias that typically arise 3–5 years after chemotherapy and may be preceded by myelodysplasia. (b) The t(4:11) reciprocal chromosomal translocation commonly found in acute leukaemias that occur 2–3 years after chemotherapy with topoisomerase II inhibitors.

agents. Secondary acute leukaemia also occurs in patients treated with topoisomerase II inhibitors (Figure 3.25b). These leukaemias occur early, 2–3 years after therapy, and are associated with translocations of 11q23 (MLL gene) or 21q22 (AML1 gene). Data on the development of secondary solid tumours are less clear, although cyclophosphamide is linked to a fourfold relative risk of bladder cancer and appears to be related to cumulative dose. Antimetabolites are generally not thought to be carcinogenic.

There is something quite horrible about the development of second cancers after curative treatment of a first cancer, and for this reason, effort has been expended in developing alternative treatment programmes that are not associated with increased cancer risk. The development of second cancers used to be a problem of particular poignancy in patients with Hodgkin's disease. This tumour commonly occurs in younger people who are returned to a normal life expectancy until the unpleasantness of their presentation with a second cancer. The alternative programme, which is in current use for the treatment of Hodgkin's disease, is called ABVD. This was originally introduced by a group of Italians, whose pronouncements about the effectiveness of ABVD chemotherapy were regarded with some scepticism by the medical community. However, a randomized trial organized in North America showed that the Italians were right, which surprised even the Italians.

Psychiatric dysfunction

It is generally thought that patients who have cancer would tend to be more depressed than the population without malignancy. However, this is far from the truth. So far from the truth that it is a completely incorrect view. There is no difference in the incidence of mental illness in people affected with cancer than in a normal population. There is controversy around the association between pre-morbid psychiatric conditions and the development of cancer. The only malignancy in which there has been shown to be an association is breast cancer, where early work described a link between pre-morbid depression and breast cancer. The link is slight. Patients with cancer go through a series of mental changes around the time of their diagnosis. Each of these stages may be protracted, even to the extent that the patient remains unable to grow beyond that particular phase. These symptoms are symptoms of a grief response, as seen in many other situations. Initially, patients deal with malignancy by denial. They next move to a grief response, progressing from there to acceptance of their own situations.

Delayed side effects in children

Growth disorders in children

Both growth disorders and mental changes are problems that come chiefly as a result of the use of radiotherapy in childhood. Irradiation of the chest in the treatment of Hodgkin's disease is associated with destruction of the growing plates of the vertebrae and ribs and dysmorphic appearance in later life. For this reason, treatment with spinal radiotherapy is generally avoided in leukaemia and lymphoma occurring in childhood, with chemotherapy being the preferred option.

Mental change in children

Cerebral radiotherapy given as part of prophylaxis for central nervous system recurrence of leukaemia may also cause significant problems. These problems are not generally of growth or of hormonal function, as the pituitary is relatively resistant to radiation. However, personality defects are described with increased incidence, as are global loss of cerebral function manifesting as a less than expected IQ, personality change and occasionally fits. Although relatively resistant to radiation therapy, pituitary function can be damaged with loss of the gonadotrophs leading to failure to achieve puberty. Loss of thyroid-stimulating hormone (TSH) production occurs with high-dosage radiotherapy and loss of posterior pituitary function with even higher dosages of radiation therapy.

Gonadal toxicity in children

The germinal epithelium in the prepubertal testis does not appear to be any more resistant to cytotoxic therapy than in the adult, and the sterilizing effects of chemotherapy on prepubertal boys may be predicted from data in adults. In contrast prepubertal girls are less susceptible to ovarian failure than adult women. Most chemotherapy regimens do not cause failure of pubertal development and menarche.

Endocrine therapy

Endocrine therapy (or hormonal manipulation) is an important part of managing cancers whose growth is dependent on hormones, namely breast and prostate cancers. The aims of endocrine therapy for cancer are to reduce the circulating levels of hormones or block their actions on the cancers. The origins of endocrine therapy for breast and prostate cancer come from surgical oophrectomy and orchidectomy.

Breast cancer

In order to grow, many breast cancers that produce oestrogen receptors rely on supplies of oestrogen (Figure 3.26). LHRH agonists such as goserelin cause downregulation of pituitary LHRH receptors and, via a decrease in luteinizing hormone/follicle-stimulating hormone (LH/FSH), lead to a reduced plasma oestradiol. This is used in the neoadjuvant, adjuvant and palliative setting in premenopausal women. Tamoxifen binds to oestrogen receptors and prevents oestradiol binding. It is used in the neoadjuvant, adjuvant and palliative setting in postmenopausal women. Aromatase inhibitors, such as anastrozole, bind and inhibit aromatase enzyme in peripheral tissues including adipose tissue, which converts androstenedione and testosterone and other androgens into oestradiol and oestrone. This is the major source of oestradiol synthesis in postmenopausal women. They are used in the palliative setting for women whose disease progresses on tamoxifen. All the above drugs can cause menopausal symptoms, namely hot flushes, sweats and vaginal dryness. Specific and important adverse effects of tamoxifen are thromboembolic disease and uterine carcinoma.

Prostate cancer

The growth of prostatic carcinoma is under the control of androgens, hence the aim of hormonal therapy is to reduce testosterone levels or prevent androgen binding to the androgen receptor. LHRH agonists cause downregulation of pituitary LHRH receptors and via a decrease in LH lead to a reduced serum testosterone and tissue dehydrotestosterone (Figure 3.26). There is also a direct effect at the level of the tumour cell. The adverse effects are impotence, loss of libido, gynaecomastia and hot flushes. Tumour flare, an increase in tumour size, which can cause symptoms such as increase in bone pain and spinal cord compression, can occur with the initial use of these drugs owing to the an initial increase in testosterone. Therefore, an anti-androgen such as bicalutamide, cyproterone acetate or flutamide should be prescribed for at least 2 weeks before LHRH agonists to prevent this happening. Anti-androgens act by blocking and preventing testosterone from attaching to the androgen receptor in prostate cancer cells (Figure 3.27). The adverse effects of anti-androgens are hepatotoxicity, gynaecomastia, diarrhoea and abdominal pain. Combined androgen blockade (or maximal androgen blockade) is a term used to describe the use of an LHRH agonist and androgen receptor antagonist together. These agents are used alone or in

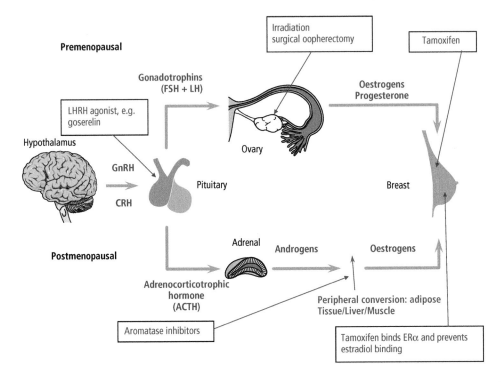

Figure 3.26 Endocrine therapy of breast cancer: Hypothalamic–pituitary–gonadal axis in women and potential therapeutic interventions. CRH, corticotrophin-releasing hormone; ERα, oestrogen receptor α; FSH, follicle-stimulating hormone; LH, luteinizing hormone; LHRH, luteinizing hormone-releasing hormone; GnRH, gonadotrophin-releasing hormone.

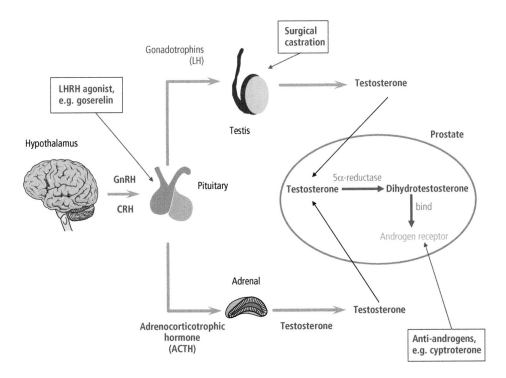

Figure 3.27 Endocrine therapy of prostate cancer: Site of actions of luteinizing hormone-releasing hormone agonists and anti-androgens on the hypothalamic–pituitary–testis axis. CRH, corticotrophin-releasing hormone; LH, luteinizing hormone; LHRH, luteinizing hormone-releasing hormone; GnRH, gonadotrophin-releasing hormone.

combination for either locally advanced or metastatic prostate cancer and provide a survival benefit as compared with monotherapy.

Immunological therapy

In as early as the 1700s, it was recorded that certain infectious diseases could exert a beneficial therapeutic effect upon malignancy. Most prominent among the clinicians aiming to take advantage of these observations was a New York surgeon, William B. Coley. He used a bacterial vaccine, the eponymous Coley's toxin, to treat inoperable cancers and in 1893 reported high cure rates. Although a central role for the immune system in the surveillance and eradication of tumours has been postulated since then, immunotherapy has only a minor place in the treatment of cancers. Support for any role of immunity in the control of cancer comes from a number of observations. For some malignancies, a dense infiltration of lymphocytes in the tumour imparts a better prognosis. Cultivating and re-infusing these tumour-infiltrating lymphocytes occasionally results in some regression of the tumour. Conversely, people with immunodeficiencies have higher rates of cancers; however, in general, these tumours are less common cancers that are caused by oncogenic viruses. Both passive and active specific immunotherapy and non-specific immunotherapy have a limited role in the management of cancer.

Passive specific immunotherapy

Passive immunotherapy with monoclonal antibodies is an established treatment for breast cancer and non-Hodgkin's lymphoma. Monoclonal antibodies are produced by a single clone of B-cells and may be humanized to reduce their immunogenicity. In 1975, Georges Kohler and Cesar Milstein developed a procedure to fuse myeloma cells with B-lymphocyte cells from the spleen of immunized mice. These fused hybridoma cell clones retained the ever-living characteristics of myeloma cells and the ability to secrete monoclonal antibodies against the antigen that the mouse was immunized with. Milstein and Kohler shared the 1984 Nobel Prize with Niels Jerne for this work. Cesar Milstein had left his native Argentina for Cambridge in 1963 following the military coup that deposed the moderate President Frondizi. He joins a long list of distinguished British Nobel laureates in physiology and medicine who arrived in Britain

as political asylum seekers, described in "Hitler's Gift" a great book by Jean Medawar and David Pyke, including Max Perutz (discoverer of the structure of haemoglobin), Hans Krebs (who described the citric acid cycle) and Ernst Chain (who, with Florey, developed the clinical application of Fleming's discovery of penicillin).

Several monoclonal antibodies are currently widely used in oncology and have been genetically modified to reduce the murine origins to prevent the development of host antibodies against the mouse sequences of the antibodies (Figure 3.28), for example, rituximab and trastuzumab (Box 3.4). Rituximab is a chimeric monoclonal antibody directed against CD20, a protein expressed on pre-B and mature B-cells. This is non-specific, as it will ablate both normal and malignant B-cells. However, the normal cells

---

Box 3.4 Name that antibody

Common suffix for all monoclonal antibodies:
– mab

Suffix sub-stem denotes the origin of the antibody:

-o-	mouse	ibritumomab, sulesomab
-xi-	chimeric	cetuximab, infliximab
-zu-	humanized	bevacizumab, trastuzumab
-u-	human	adalimumab

Suffix sub-sub-stem denotes disease or therapeutic area:

-anib-	angiogenesis inhibitor	ranibizumab
-ci-	cardiovascular	abciximab, bevacizumab
-le(s)-	inflammatory lesions	sulesomab
-li-	immunomodulator	infliximab, omalizumab
-tu-	tumour	cetuximab, trastuzumab
-vi-	viral	palivizumab

However, there are inconsistencies. For example, bevacizumab, which according to the sub-stem -ci- was perhaps originally expected to be used in cardiovascular disease, is used to treat patients with colorectal cancer and macular degeneration; bevacizumab, cetuximab and ranibizumab all inhibit angiogenesis but have different sub-stems.

Monoclonal Antibodies

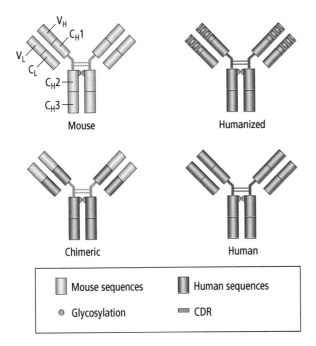

Mouse

Humanized

Chimeric

Human

Nomenclature:

| Mouse sequences | Human sequences |
| Glycosylation | CDR |

-mab = monoclonal antibody (mAb)

-ximab = chimeric mAb

-zumab = humanised mAb

Figure 3.28 Nomenclature and structure of chimeric and humanized monoclonal antibodies. CDR, complementarity determining regions; C, constant region; V, variable region; H, heavy chain; L, light chain.

are subsequently regenerated by the bone marrow from normal stem cells. It is effective in low-grade and follicular non-Hodgkin's lymphoma. Trastuzumab is a humanized monoclonal antibody directed against human epidermal growth factor receptor 2 (HER2), which is overexpressed in 30% of breast cancers and is associated with a poorer prognosis. It is used in metastatic breast cancer that is HER2 positive. Both these drugs can cause flu-like symptoms on infusion, such as chills and pyrexia. In addition, trastuzumab has been noted to be cardiotoxic, especially when given with anthracyclines.

Active specific immunotherapy

Active cellular immunotherapy involves the harvesting and *ex vivo* activation (in the test tube) of lymphokine-activated killer (LAK) cells (cytokine-primed immune cells) and is an experimental treatment for renal cancers and melanoma. Other trial active immunotherapies include tumour vaccines, and this technology is most often studied in the tumour types where occasional spontaneous regressions have been documented.

Non-specific immunotherapy

Global stimulation of the host cellular immune system in order to promote tumour rejection was probably the basis of Coley's adjuvant therapy. This has been replaced with the use of bacillus Calmette-Guerin (BCG), which is administered intravesically (via a catheter into the bladder) to prevent recurrence of superficial bladder cancers and interferons and interleukins.

Interferon

There are three human interferons:

- Interferon alpha (IFN-α) produced by leukocytes
- Interferon beta (IFN-β) produced by fibroblasts
- Interferon gamma (IFN-γ) produced by T lymphocytes

IFN-α is licensed for use currently and may act by enhancing the expression of human leucocyte antigen (HLA) antigens by tumour cells leading to increased recognition and lysis by cytotoxic T-cells and natural killer cells. Only IFN-α is used in the treatment of cancers, including hairy cell leukaemia, chronic myeloid leukaemia, melanoma, renal cell cancer and Kaposi's sarcoma. The adverse effects of IFN-α are flu-like symptoms, fatigue and myelosuppression.

Interleukin-2

Interleukin-2 (IL-2) is a cytokine produced predominantly by activated CD4+ helper T lymphocytes that have been stimulated by antigen. It acts via a cell surface receptor expressed also on activated T-cells, thus behaving as an autocrine growth factor. In response to IL-2, CD4+ helper T-cells are capable of differentiating from an initial common state (T_H0) into one of two apparently distinct types called T_H1 and T_H2. The T_H1 pathway is essentially cell-mediated immunity, with the activation of macrophages, natural killer cells, cytotoxic T-cells and a prolonged inflammatory response. The T_H2 pathway is essentially a humoral pathway, with the production of cytokines, which promote B-cell growth, and the production of antibodies. IL-2 causes the growth and proliferation of activated T-cells, thus expanding tumouricidal LAK cells, and may be used to treat melanoma and renal cell cancers. The adverse effects of IL-2 are fluid retention, multiorgan dysfunction and bone marrow and hepatic toxicity.

CTLA-4 and PD1 targeting

Cytotoxic T lymphocytes have an important role in destroying some tumours and a new protein receptor on their surface, called cytotoxic T-lymphocyte antigen 4 (CTLA-4) turns off this action. Targeting CTLA-4 with the monoclonal antibody ipilimumab prolongs life expectancy in advanced melanoma. Another molecule on cytotoxic T-cells, programmed death 1 (PD-1) characterizes dying off T-cells and monoclonal antibodies that target PD-1 have been shown to be effective in a number of cancers that are relatively resistant to cytotoxic chemotherapy.

Targeted therapies

Protein kinase inhibitor therapy

Protein kinase enzymes phosphorylate the amino acid residues of their substrates, usually tyrosine, serine or threonine. The human genome includes about 500 protein kinases and perhaps 30% of all human proteins may be modified by phosphorylation, which may result in functional changes. Phosphorylation of substrate proteins may alter their enzyme activity, cellular location or association with other proteins and this is especially important in cellular pathways such as signal transduction that are dysregulated in cancer cells. Protein kinase inhibitors are a relatively new and rapidly expanding class of drugs used in cancer treatment and include both monoclonal antibodies (-mabs) and small molecules (-nibs) (Table 3.17). In general, nibs target tyrosine kinase domains, whilst mabs target the ligand-binding domains of receptors. Many of these novel agents have been developed using knowledge of the biology of tumours to target-specific pathways in cancer cells. It was anticipated that this would have the added benefit of minimizing toxicity, although some unexpected side effects have emerged, such as the cardiotoxicity of trastuzumab.

Targeted therapies include an expanding and miscellaneous collection of other agents, including the

Table 3.17 Table showing the common protein kinase inhibitors used in oncology

Name	Target	Class	Clinical uses
Bevacizumab	VEGF	Monoclonal antibody	Colon cancer and NSCLC
Cetuximab	EGFR	Monoclonal antibody	Colon cancer and head and neck cancer
Dasatinib	BCR/ABL	Small molecule	CML
Erlotinib	EGFR	Small molecule	NSCLC
Gefitinib	EGFR	Small molecule	NSCLC
Imatinib	BCR/ABL	Small molecule	CML and GIST
Lapatinib	EGFR and Her2	Small molecule	Breast cancer
Sorafenib	Multiple target kinases	Small molecule	Kidney cancer and liver cancer
Sunitinib	Multiple target kinases	Small molecule	Kidney cancer and GIST
Trastuzumab	Her2	Monoclonal antibody	Breast cancer

BCR/ABL, breakpoint cluster region/Abelson murine leukaemia viral oncogene homologue; CML, chronic myeloid leukaemia; EGFR, epidermal growth factor receptor; GIST, gastrointestinal stromal tumour; NSCLC, non-small cell lung cancer; VEGF, vascular endothelial growth factor.

proteosome-targeting agent bortezomib, differentiating agents such as all-trans retinoic acid and arsenic trioxide and inhibitors of poly(ADP-ribose) polymerase (PARP) a DNA repair enzyme in breast cancer treatment.

Clinical trials

As new cytotoxic drugs are developed and other novel agents are found, it is essential to evaluate their potential in a structured fashion in clinical trials. A stepwise progression has been introduced that includes three phases of clinical trials:

- Phase I trials determine the toxicity, including the dose-limiting toxicities and the dose scheduling of a new agent. They enrol a small number of patients with resistant tumours.
- Phase II studies are designed to identify promising tumour types, using the dosing regimens established from the phase I trials.
- Phase III trials are larger randomized comparisons that allocate patients either to the new treatment or the established standard therapy.

In all phases of clinical trials, evaluations of response and toxicity are according to well-established standards. The side effects are measured using the Common Toxicity Criteria scale that rates the severity of side effects on a 4-point scale. The response to treatment is assessed using the Response Evaluation Criteria in Solid Tumours (RECIST) criteria, which are largely radiological and clinical measurements of the tumour size before and after treatment. A complete response is defined as the complete disappearance of all known disease, whilst a partial response roughly equates to a greater than 50% reduction in the size of measurable lesions with no new ones appearing. Although there is considerable debate as to whether these response criteria are appropriate for some of the novel therapies such as anti-angiogenic treatments, they are currently necessary for licensing approval of cancer drugs. The aims of clinical trials of a new agent include proving that it works, obtaining a license from the US Food and Drug Administration (FDA) and the European Medicines Evaluation Agency (EMEA) as well as making money. In most cases, all the goals are complementary; however, there are examples from the biotechnology boom of the 1990s where making money appeared to be the sole objective and venture capitalists made fortunes without a drug ever achieving clinical use or benefiting any patients.

Randomized clinical trials are needed to establish evidence-based treatment protocols as well as determining the value of new agents. Large clinical trials are a major focus of clinical activity in oncology and patients are actively encouraged to participate in studies. The principles that underlie clinical trial management are outlined in Box 3.5.

Palliative care

Although it is widely held that palliative care is only offered when there is no chance of cure, this attitude risks denying patients adequate analgesia and supportive care irrespective of their prognosis. The concept that palliative care to provide optimal symptom control and enhanced quality of life should only be available to those patients with advanced disease is ridiculous. The integration of palliative care into the early management of patients with cancer is recognized as benefiting patients and encouraging a more holistic attitude to their care. The discipline of palliative care throughout the globe owes much to the pioneering work of Dame Cecily Saunders. She started life as a nurse during the Second World War and subsequently worked as a social worker before training in medicine, which she viewed then as the only route to change the care of the dying. She advocated above all else that listening to patients as the best way to care for them. In 1967, she established the first hospice in the world, St Christopher's Hospice in London, in order to meet the needs of the dying patient, which are so often left unmet in a hospital. The hospice movement developed a comprehensive approach to dealing with the variety of symptoms experienced by patients with progressive debilitating illness, including promoting the safe use of opiate analgesia. This attitude has been developed to deliver whole-person care and to view the patient not in isolation but as part of a social unit that also includes family and friends.

Pain is the most feared and most common symptom of advanced malignancy, and emotional, spiritual and psychological components may intensify physical pain. In Mother Teresa's Home for the Dying, the homeless of Kolkata (formerly Calcutta) were denied any analgesia other than aspirin and often suffered unnecessarily with great pain in the pursuit of austere religion. The relief of pain should therefore be viewed as part of a comprehensive pattern of care encompassing all aspects of suffering. The physical component of pain cannot be treated in isolation, nor can a patient's anxieties be effectively addressed whilst they are suffering physically. It is obvious

Box 3.5 **Cancer trials**

Cancer screening

The value of a diagnostic test in clinical medicine depends upon whether the result means what you think it does and nowhere is this more relevant than in cancer screening. The usefulness depends upon three factors: the sensitivity of the test, the specificity of the test and the population prevalence of the cancer.

Sensitivity

The sensitivity of a test is the ability of a test to pick up a condition (the cancer):
- Sensitivity = number of true cases detected/all true cases.
  A test that is 95% sensitive will detect 95% of all cases (or, put another way, will miss 5% of cases).

Specificity

The specificity of a test is the probability that a negative test is a true negative (the person does not have the cancer):
- Specificity = number of true negatives detected/all true negatives.
  A 75% specificity means that the test will identify 75% people correctly as not having cancer, but 25% people without cancer will have a positive test result (false positive).

Usefulness

The practical usefulness of a test in a given population can be summarized using:
- Positive predictive value (the chance that a positive will be a true positive in that population) = true cases detected/all positive test results (true positives and false positives)
- Negative predictive value (the chance that a negative will be a true negative in that population) = true negative results/all negative test results (true negatives and false negatives)

Prevalence and incidence

- Prevalence = frequency of a condition in the community at a given point in time (e.g. the prevalence of cancer in children in the United States is one in 330 children <19 years)
- Incidence = frequency of a disease occurring over a period in time (e.g. in 2010, there were 49,564 new cases of breast cancer in women in the United Kingdom, giving a crude incidence of 157 new breast cancer cases per 100,000 females. The European age-standardized rate is lower at 125.9 per 100,000 females because the age of the women in the United Kingdom is older than the standardized European population and breast cancer rates are higher in older women)

Cancer treatments

Running a clinical treatment trial

Ethics
The Declaration of Helsinki outlines an international basis of ethical clinical research. The first version (1964) arose from the Nuremberg Code, which was established after the trial of the Nazi doctors who participated in human "experiments" during the Holocaust. It describes the rights of patients in clinical trials, including the right to abstain from a study, the access to adequate information about both potential benefits and hazards of involvement, the right to withdraw from the trial at any time and finally the desirability of giving written informed consent prior to enrolment. In the United Kingdom, research trials must be submitted to research ethics committees for review, and clinicians participating in clinical trials must be trained and accredited in Good Clinical Practice (GCP).

Trial design

After a new potential treatment has been discovered and tested in animals, it enters a stepwise series of clinical trials that enrol progressively more patients. For new cancer treatments, there are three classical phases of studies:

- Phase I trials determine the relationship between toxicity and dose schedules of treatment and usually enrol a small number of patients with advanced cancer with no alternative treatment options available.
- Phase II trials identify tumour types for which the treatment appears promising and generally recruit larger numbers of patients with a single tumour type who have undergone all established lines of treatment.
- Phase III trials assess the efficacy of treatment compared to standard treatment including toxicity. These larger usually randomized trials include a large number of patients who are randomized to the best current established "gold standard" therapy versus the new experimental treatment.

Randomization

Proper randomization should ensure unbiased comparisons by allocating patients to one arm of a study without allowing the patient or the doctor to choose. Hence, randomization controls for both known and unknown confounding factors. The first randomized controlled trial (RCT) was performed by the Medical Research Council in 1948 on the use of (single agent) streptomycin in tuberculosis, and Sir Austin Bradford Hill is credited with introducing this methodology (see also his role with Sir Richard Doll in establishing the role of smoking in lung cancer in Box 2.5).

Control

Controlled trials compare a "new" experimental therapy with an existing treatment – either active or placebo.

Blinding

In double-blinded trials, neither the patient nor the doctor knows which treatment is being administered.

Sample size

The number of patients (sample size) required in a trial will depend on the number of events (deaths or relapses) predicted in each arm and the difference that you wish to be able to demonstrate between the two arms of the trial. If you wish to detect a small difference between the two groups, more patients are needed.

Analysis

In an RCT, first patients are screened for eligibility (enrolled), then they are randomized to a treatment arm (allocation), then they receive the treatment and finally they are followed up. At each stage, some patients may drop out of the study for a variety of reasons. "Intention-to-treat" analysis compares outcomes between all patients originally allocated one treatment with all patients allocated to the other treatment, whilst "on-treatment" analysis only compared patients who actually received one treatment with those who actually received the other treatment.

Endpoints

Clinical trial endpoints in cancer trials include overall survival duration, disease-free survival, time to disease progression, response rate, quality-of-life measures, adverse effects and treatment toxicity. However, some patients receive subsequent lines of treatment at relapse and survival for some cancers in prolonged, so some trials use different end points. In addition to timed endpoints, many trials in solid cancers use measures of the size of the cancer or metastases as an endpoint where cancer shrinkage has been shown to correlate with survival. A standardized system for evaluating changes in the size of cancers has been established: the Response Evaluation Criteria In Solid Tumours (RECIST) criteria, which measure response in terms of radiological and clinical tumour shrinkage. The definitions broadly are:

- Complete response (CR): disappearance of all known cancer
- Partial response (PR): >50% reduction in measurable lesions and no new lesions
- Stable disease (SD): lesions unchanged (<50% smaller or <25% larger)
- Progressive disease (PD): new lesions or measurable lesions >25% larger

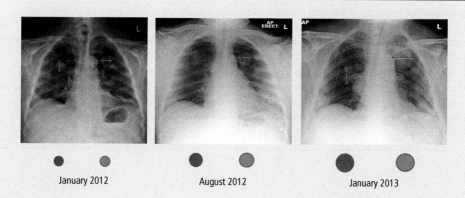

January 2012   August 2012   January 2013

Figure 3.29 Growing pulmonary metastases from colorectal cancer primary. Between January 2012 and August 2012, the lung metastases increased <25% (stable disease), but between January 2012 and January 2013, they had growth >25% (progressive disease).

Side effects

Similarly, a standardized system has been developed to describe and quantify the side effects of treatment in cancer clinical trials. The most widely used grading scale is the Common Terminology Criteria for Adverse Events (CTCAE), which grades side effects by severity on a 0–5 scale.

Interpreting the results

Evidence-based medicine

Over the last 2 decades, there have been numerous advances in evidence processing, including the production of streamlined guides to aid critical appraisal of the literature, evidence-based abstraction services, online and other forms of electronic literature searching, growing numbers of high-quality systematic reviews and frequently updated textbooks in paper and electronic formats. All these initiatives have contributed to the emergence of evidence-based medicine as the optimal framework for clinical management.

Meta-analysis

Combining published data into a meta-analysis to provide an evidence base for clinical management is widely advocated. A meta-analysis may provide a more precise, less biased and more complete assessment of the available information than individual studies. However, the preferential publication of striking results in small studies and non-publication of larger negative studies (publication bias) may skew meta-analyses. Thus, the reliability of a meta-analysis depends on the quality and quantity of the data that go into it. The Grading of Recommendations, Assessment, Development and Evaluation (GRADE) system requires systematic review of the literature and assessment of both the quality of the evidence and the strength of the recommendation.

Bias

Bias in a study is a design flaw that results in an inevitable likelihood that the wrong result may be obtained. Bias cannot be controlled for at the analysis stage.

Potential biases in screening for cancer

Screening should reduce mortality, but the following three biases which all make screening look better than it is should be considered:
- *Lead time bias*: the diagnosis of disease is made earlier in the screened group, resulting in an apparent increase in survival time, although the time of death is the same in both groups.

- *Lag time bias*: the probability of detecting disease is related to the growth rate of the tumour. Aggressive, rapidly growing tumours have a short potential screening period. More slowly growing tumours have a longer potential screening period and are more likely to be detected when they are asymptomatic, causing an apparent improvement in survival in the screened group.
- *Overdiagnosis bias*: The detection of very slow-growing tumours in the screened group produces an apparent increase in the number of cases of cancer. These slow-growing cancers may not reduce the lifespan in the screened population. In contrast, these indolent tumours may remain silent in the control population, as they may never cause symptoms. Thus, overdiagnosis bias increases apparent survival and reduces disease-related mortality in the screened group.

Daily care plan review

COMMUNICATE with patient/family to clarify aims of care and update family on a regular basis and following any change in management. In particular, consider and explain resuscitation, hydration, sedation and use of medications
DOCUMENT significant conversations in the notes and ensure contact numbers for key family members
- This may include preferences around place of care, support needs and specific issues such as tissue donation

REVIEW INTERVENTIONS AND MEDICATIONS – focus on comfort and dignity
- Consider and explain interventions based on a balance of benefits and burdens, including prescription of fluids (IV or s/c), decreasing frequency/stopping of observations
- Communicate decisions with patient (where possible) and family
- If the patient has an ICD, contact cardiac physiologist for advice

MAINTAIN EXCELLENT BASIC CARE – frequent assessment, action and review
- Regular mouth and eye care (remove contact lenses if necessary). Turning for comfort as appropriate
- Encourage and support oral food / hydration as patient is able
- Check bladder and bowel function
- Ensure dignity and compassion in all care

ASSESS SYMPTOMS REGULARLY – frequent assessment, action and review
- Prescribe medications as required for anticipated symptoms, e.g. pain, nausea, agitation, respiratory secretions (advice can be found on intranet – 'Symptom management guidelines for dying patients')
- Medications may be required via subcutaneous syringe pump if symptomatic/no longer tolerating oral meds
- Advice available from the palliative care team

IDENTIFY SUPPORT NEEDS OF FAMILY
- Ensure contact numbers and contact preferences updated for key family members
- Explain facilities available, e.g. accommodation, parking permits, folding beds if available
- Consider single room for patient if available

IDENTIFY SPIRITUAL NEEDS – for both patient and family
- Document specific actions required
- Refer to chaplaincy as appropriate

CARE AFTER DEATH
- Timely certification of death (often important for bereaved families)
- Family bereavement booklet
- Inform GP and other involved clinicians

Figure 3.30 Example of a daily care plan.

under these circumstances that a multidisciplinary approach is required. In addition to pain relief, expertise in the management of other common symptoms is essential, including constipation, diarrhoea, nausea, vomiting, dyspnoea and fatigue. In some circumstances, surgery or radiotherapy may provide valuable symptomatic palliation, for example, for the relief of spinal cord compression. Moreover, in selected circumstances, palliative chemotherapy is indicated even if the term seems to be a clinical oxymoron.

Until recently, the delivery of palliative care has been hospice based. However, the hospice concept has now extended to both the acute hospital and community settings, where specialist teams work in partnership with primary care teams in the delivery of palliative care. Community-based palliative care may enable patients to die at home or at least remain at home for as long as possible, which has long been known to be the favoured option of most patients.

Care at the end of life has been the focus of a great effort in recent years to improve the final days and hours of a person's life. In the late 1990s, in order to address the unmet needs of the (predictably) dying cancer patient, the Royal Liverpool University Hospital and Liverpool's Marie Curie Hospice developed the Liverpool Care Pathway (LCP). The LCP was an aid for the multi-disciplinary team to ensure that unpleasant medical interventions are discontinued, comfort measures introduced and appropriate continuing medicines are provided to ensure relief of symptoms. However, in 2012, the media (inevitably led by the Daily Mail) heavily attacked the LCP, claiming that it was used for euthanasia of the elderly and criticized the financial incentives paid to NHS hospital trusts for hitting targets associated with using the LCP. These financial rewards have been removed, and most NHS hospitals have replaced the LCA with a less prescriptive and more individualized approach to end-of-life care. Nevertheless, the principles for caring for dying patients still starts with the recognition that a patient's condition is deteriorating and the exclusion of reversible causes such as opiate toxicity, infection and hypercalcaemia. Once it has been identified that a patient is actively dying, a holistic assessment of the needs of both the patients and the carers should be initiated. This should include a clear discussion with the patient and their family, explaining that death is potentially imminent and the concerns of the patient and family should be carefully addressed. Documentation of the agreed individualized care plan and conversations should be completed, and the care plans should be regularly reviewed at least daily and care plans re-evaluated.

An example of the daily care plan review is shown in Figure 3.30.

 KEY POINTS

- Cancer treatment depends upon the prognosis, efficacy and toxicity of the therapy
- Prognosis is determined in general by tumour stage, grade and the performance status of the patient
- Surgery has a role in cancer prophylaxis, diagnosis, primary treatment, oncological emergencies, symptom palliation and reconstruction
- Radiotherapy may be delivered as external beam, brachytherapy or isotope therapy in either a curative or palliative context
- Cytotoxic chemotherapy works by targeting DNA, its bases and tubulin and may be classified into alkylating agents, antimetabolites, intercalating agents, spindle poisons and topoisomerase inhibitors
- The toxicities of chemotherapy are divided into early delayed and late effects that generally can be predicted from their mechanisms of action
- Endocrine treatments are useful in hormone sensitive tumours such as breast, prostate and thyroid cancer
- Targeted treatments with monoclonal antibodies (-mabs) and protein kinase inhibitors (-nibs) are increasingly being prescribed for the management of diverse cancers

4

Cancer and people

Learning objectives

✓ Recognize psychological distress and psychosocial problems that affect cancer patients

✓ Apply techniques for breaking bad news

✓ Describe burnout and coping strategies used by clinicians caring for cancer patients

✓ Evaluate complementary and alternative therapies with examples

Social and psychological aspects of cancer

Psychological carcinogenic risk factors

There is a great deal of speculation and anecdotal evidence connecting psychological factors and both the risk of developing cancer and its prognosis. Much of the research on the relationship between stressful life experiences and the onset of cancer has been poorly designed. However, the few well-conducted trials have failed to establish a link. A large study of women with newly diagnosed breast cancer found that women who have a severely stressful life experience in the year before the diagnosis, or in the 5 years afterwards, do not seem to be at increased risk of developing a recurrence of the disease. Moreover, a meta-analysis addressed the influence of psychological coping strategies (including fighting spirit, helplessness/hopelessness, denial and avoidance) on cancer survival and recurrence. This meta-analysis found that there was little consistent evidence that psychological coping styles play an important part in survival from or recurrence of cancer.

Psychological distress in cancer patients

Psychological distress is frequent in patients with cancer and is often overlooked or even deliberately neglected by clinicians. However, over the last few decades, more oncologists have appreciated that psychological distress and psychiatric disorders such as anxiety, depression and delirium (in hospitalized patients) are frequent co-morbid conditions. Increasingly, the outcome measures in clinical trials of new therapies have included quality-of-life evaluation and not just assessed tumour response and survival endpoints. A number of factors have been found to be associated with an increased risk of psychological distress in patients with cancer (Table 4.1). Clinical features of anxiety include anorexia, fatigue, loss of libido, weight loss, anhedonia (the inability to experience pleasure from activities usually found enjoyable), insomnia and suicidal ideation. Many of these key symptoms are at times attributed to cancer and as few as one-third of cancer patients who might benefit from antidepressants are prescribed them.

As well as pharmacological treatments, psychological interventions are frequently employed in the care of people with cancer. These interventions have a positive effect on psychological morbidity and functional

Oncology: Lecture Notes, Third Edition. Mark Bower and Jonathan Waxman.
© 2015 by John Wiley & Sons, Ltd. Published 2015 by John Wiley & Sons, Ltd.
Companion Website: www.lecturenoteseries.com/oncology

Table 4.1 Factors increasing the risk of psychological morbidity in cancer patients

History of mood disorder
History of alcohol or drug misuse
Cancer or its treatment associated with visible deformity
Younger age
Poor social support
Low expectation of successful treatment outcome

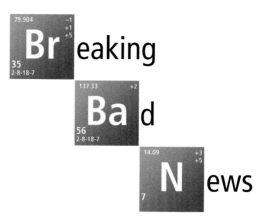

Figure 4.1 Breaking bad news.

adjustment and may ameliorate disease and treatment-related symptoms. The most useful psychological intervention appears to be a group of treatments termed cognitive-behavioural psychotherapy. These include behavioural therapy, behaviour modification and cognitive therapy in various combinations. In behavioural therapy, a formal analysis of the patient's problem leads to an individualized programme of techniques aimed at changing their behaviour. Cognitive therapies explore how thoughts influence feelings and behaviour and aim to modify thought processes directly. These therapies consist of identifying maladaptive thought patterns (such as hopelessness in depression) and teaching patients to recognize and challenge these. Probably the most widely employed psychosocial intervention for cancer patients is supportive counselling that along with information and patient education empowers patients.

Psychosocial problems in cancer survivors

Even after successful curative treatment of cancer, patients continue to suffer psychological morbidity. The psychological sequelae in cancer survivors may relate to the illness and its treatment as well as family and personal issues. The majority of children who survive cancer cope well with long-term adjustment although adults generally fare less well. Three well-recognized scenarios in this context are:

- The Lazarus syndrome (difficulty with returning to normal life)
- The Damocles syndrome (fear of recurrence and terror of minor symptoms)
- The Survivor syndrome (guilt about surviving where others have died)

Cancer survivors also suffer social problems including financial difficulties, particularly with insurance and mortgages. They have also been found to have greater problems in obtaining employment and keeping jobs and these may be compounded by frequent follow-up clinic visits.

Breaking bad news

Medical students have identified breaking bad news as their greatest fear in terms of communicating with patients and in the first half of the 20th century it was routine practice to hide the diagnosis from patients with cancer (Figure 4.1). It is uncertain whether this was a paternalistic policy to protect the patient or because physicians avoided a difficult task that many found unpleasant (and one that might lead them to question their own clinical practices). Although many students believe that good communication skills are innate, it is clear that like so many things the techniques can be taught and learnt (Table 4.2). The way in which the diagnosis is communicated to patients is an important determinant of subsequent psychological

Table 4.2 Top tips for communicating with patients

Clarify patient's statements

Use open questioning (not leading)

Note verbal and non-verbal clues

Enquire about patient's psychosocial problems (e.g. depression)

Keep patients to the point

Prevent needless repetition

Provide verbal and visual encouragement

Obtain precise information

Use brief questions

Avoid jargon

stress and, even if patients recall little of the conversation that followed, they state that the competence of the doctor at breaking bad news is critical to establishing trust. Why do doctors fear breaking bad news? Obviously the information causes pain and distress to patients and their relatives, making us feel uncomfortable. We fear being blamed and provoking an emotional reaction. Breaking bad news reminds us of our own mortality and fears of our own death. Finally, we often worry about being unable to answer a patient's difficult questions since we never know what the future holds for either our patients or ourselves. Breaking bad news to patients should not involve protecting them from the truth but rather imparting the information in a sensitive manner at the patient's own pace.

Breaking bad news to patients requires preparation and this aspect is very often overlooked. The setting for these discussions should be quiet, comfortable and confidential, so that the whole ward does not eavesdrop and so that your bleep and mobile phone do not constantly intrude. An adequate period of time (at least 30 minutes) should be set aside and the patient should be asked if she/he wants someone else present. The conversation should open with a question to find out how much the patient already knows. An open question such as "What have you already been told about your illness?" can reveal not only what has been said and how much has been understood but also the emotional state of the patient ("I'm so terrified it's cancer"). This opening gambit frequently takes care of much of the hard work for you ("I think it's cancer but the doctors do seem to want to say"). Under these circumstances the diagnosis can be confirmed in an empathetic fashion. If this initial question does not open up a useful avenue, a warning shot should be fired off ("I have the results of your biopsy and I'm afraid that the news is not good"). Following this warning shot, wait for the patient to respond and check if the patient wants to be told more. This cycle of warning shot, pause and checking should be repeated when elaborating on details of the diagnosis and treatment options. In this way the patient determines how much information is delivered. Certainly long monologues are overwhelming and confusing and it is hopeless and insensitive to use this opportunity to try and teach pathophysiology. Learning to identify and acknowledge a patient's reaction is essential to breaking bad news. In general, prognostication with respect to "how long have I got Doc?" and the quoting of 5-year-mortality statistics are rarely helpful. Few doctors can explain the implications of skewed distributions, medians and confidence intervals, let alone in a way that is accessible to patients. Many patients will ask for these predictions hoping

for reassurance. In these circumstances it is always easier to give false reassurance but the temptation must be resisted as you will not be doing your patient a favour in the long run. After answering the patient's enquiries, it should be possible to synthesize their concerns and medical issues into a concrete plan. Even in the bleakest of situations setting short-term achievable plans leaves the patient with a goal for the future and hope. The plan should include an explicit arrangement for following up the conversation and a method for the patient to contact you if something arises before the next planned visit.

The immense bravery and gallows humour of a few patients in the face of death can bring unexpected, almost guilty comfort to bad news breakers. Francois Truffaut, the French new wave film director died of brain cancer at the age of 52. In his last published letter, he wrote "film critics were 20 years ahead of conventional medicine, when my second film (Tirez sur le pianiste) came out they said it could only be made by someone whose brain was not functioning properly".

Coping strategies

Increased interaction and empathy with cancer patients has costs to health-care professionals that need to be appreciated and addressed. Improved communications bring health-care professionals closer to the patient and may increase feelings of inadequacy when faced with insoluble issues and of failure when patients die. Health-care professionals dealing with dying patients and their families risk burn-out, and although the medical profession is notoriously resistant to external help, a team spirit, adequate training through communication workshops and peer support are important elements in coping with these emotional stresses. Another technique that is frequently employed is distancing, which may protect the doctors from their feelings but often reduces their compassion and their capacity to care for patients. Although the burden of caring for people with cancer falls most heavily on doctors and nurses, other staff members may also be affected. Indeed, when patients are dying their distress and that of their caregivers trickle down to everyone in the clinic or ward.

Medical burn-out

The depletion of physical and mental resources induced by excessive striving to reach an often unrealistic work-related goal is termed burn-out. Burn-out of staff working in cancer care is common and victims often describe themselves as workaholics. The Maslach burn-out inventory is a tool that measures burn-out and a quarter of consultant oncologists in the United Kingdom have scores that denote this. The consequences of medical burn-out include emotional exhaustion, leading to psychological detachment from patients and the sensation that little is being achieved in terms of personal accomplishment. This may account for the high frequency of experienced oncologists changing roles in their 50s, taking on management positions or jobs with cancer charities or immersing themselves increasingly in research rather than patient contact.

Unconventional treatments

The unmet emotional needs of patients have been held responsible for the increasing use of unconventional treatments for cancer. The void that patients may feel at a vulnerable stage in their lives may be filled with complementary treatments, alternative therapies or quackery.

Complementary and alternative therapies

According to the Cochrane Project, complementary and alternative medicine (CAM) is a broad domain of healing resources that encompasses all health systems, modalities and practices and their accompanying theories and beliefs, other than those intrinsic to the politically dominant health system of a particular society or culture in a given historical period. Thus, whilst orthodox medicine is politically dominant, CAM practices outside this system are, for the most part, isolated from the universities and hospitals where health care is taught and delivered. As some CAM disciplines (e.g. acupuncture) become increasingly incorporated into conventional medicine they therefore lose their "alternative" status. Indeed, it is this co-operation of health systems that led to the introduction of the term "complementary medicine" rather than the title "alternative medicine".

Every year around 20% of the population in the United Kingdom use CAM and this is interpreted as a measure of disillusion with conventional medicine. In contrast, the prevalence of use in the United States is 40% and in Germany it is >60%. There is a prolonged history in Germany of CAM use and indeed Samuel Hahnemann (1755–1843), who first described homoeopathy (Box 4.1), was a German physician. The pantheon of complementary and alternative therapies includes alternative therapies

> **Box 4.1 Homoeopathy – does it work?**
>
> The underlying principle of homoeopathic medicine is the use of extremely low-dose preparations prescribed according to the belief that like should be cured with like (readers may wish to refer to the Mitchell and Webb sketch "Homeopathic A&E" on YouTube). Treatments are chosen according to the symptoms that they elicit when administered to healthy people. Since raw onions cause crying, stinging eyes and a runny nose, *Allium cepa* (derived from onions) is used as a homoeopathic remedy for hayfever. The most notorious experimental trial that attempted to explain the mechanism of action of homoeopathy was undertaken by Jacques Benveniste. He hypothesized that water had the ability to remember solutes that had been dissolved in it after finding that very dilute solutions of allergens could elicit basophil responses. In a show trial experiment, the then editor of *Nature*, Sir John Maddox brought a team of independent referees to observe the experiments in Benveniste's laboratory. The observers included James Randi, a magician and investigator of the paranormal, and under his scrutiny Benveniste's team was unable to repeat the findings. Since that failure, Benveniste has continued to pursue the storage of memory in water, claiming to be able to store an electronic record in water that can be transferred back into an email format. These claims have been met with even greater scepticism and have earned him an unprecedented second Ig Nobel Prize.
>
> Despite these claims the most widely believed theory of the mechanism of homoeopathy remains a placebo effect and more effort has been focused on establishing the efficacy of homoeopathy. A meta-analysis, published in the *Lancet*, examined over 100 randomized, placebo-controlled trials and found a significant odds ratio of 2.45 in favour of homoeopathy. Homoeopathic medicines can be purchased over the counter at chemists and health stores. In contrast to other forms of CAM, homoeopathy is supported by the NHS through both the National Homoeopathic Hospital in London and the fact that homoeopathic remedies may be prescribed on the NHS by any doctor registered with the General Medical Council.

with recognized professional bodies (e.g. acupuncture (Box 4.2), chiropractic, herbal medicine (Box 4.3), homoeopathy, osteopathy), complementary therapies (e.g. Alexander technique, aromatherapy, Bach and other flower extracts, body work therapies including massage, counselling stress therapy, hypnotherapy, meditation, reflexology, shiatsu, healing,

---

Box 4.2 Acupuncture

Acupuncture was originated over 2000 years ago in China. It was used by William Osler, the celebrated Canadian-born physician who was both Chief of Staff at The Johns Hopkins University and subsequently Regius Professor of Medicine at Oxford University at the start of the 20th century. The recent resurgence in popularity of acupuncture dates from President Nixon's visit to China in the 1970s. The stimulation of acupuncture points by fine needles is intended to control the Qi energy circulating between organs along channels or meridians. The 12 main meridians correspond to the 12 major functions or "organs" of the body and acupuncture points are located along these meridians. The analgesic actions of acupuncture may be explained by a conventional physiological gating model and acupuncture is known to release endogenous opioids. There is convincing evidence supporting the value of acupuncture in the management of both nausea and acute pain. The evidence base for the use of acupuncture in chronic pain is less secure and current evidence suggests that it is unlikely to be of benefit for obesity, smoking cessation and tinnitus. For most other conditions the available evidence is insufficient to guide clinical decisions. Acupuncture appears to be a relatively safe treatment in the hands of suitably qualified practitioners, with serious adverse events being extremely rare. It has been estimated that 1 million acupuncture treatments are given on the NHS in England each year, at an estimated cost of £26 million, equivalent to all other complementary therapies combined. A further 2 million acupuncture treatments are given in the private sector annually.

Box 4.3 Herbalism

The most widely used herbalism in the United Kingdom is Chinese and derives from the Daoist concepts of balancing the yin and yang elements of Qi energy. The revenue from herbal products in the United Kingdom exceeds £40 million per year. Perhaps the most familiar example of herbal medicine is the use of St John's wort (*Hypericum perforatum*) for treating mild to moderate depression. Systematic reviews of randomized controlled trials confirm its efficacy over placebo and its equivalence to amitryptilline with fewer side effects. St John's wort is, however, not free of side effects and has important drug interactions caused by inducing hepatic microsomal enzymes. Other more severe toxicities have been described with herbal medicines including rapidly progressive interstitial renal fibrosis in several women after taking Chinese herbs containing powdered extracts of *Stephania tetrandra* prescribed by a slimming clinic.

Maharishi Ayurvedic medicine, nutritional medicine, yoga), alternative therapies that lack professional organization but have established and traditional systems of health care (e.g. anthroposophical medicine, Ayurvedic medicine, Chinese herbal medicine, Eastern medicine (Tibb), naturopathy, traditional Chinese medicine) and, finally, there are other "new age" alternative disciplines (e.g. crystal therapy, dowsing, iridology, kinesiology, radionics).

Many doctors remain concerned about the use of CAMs. These concerns may be based on a number of factors including that patients may be seen by unqualified practitioners, may risk delayed or missed diagnosis, may decline or stop conventional therapies, may waste money on ineffective therapies and may experience dangerous adverse effects from treatment. Moreover, the scientific academic training in medicine leads many doctors to question the value of those therapies where a plausible mechanism of action is not available. At present practitioners of CAM in the United Kingdom are free to practice as they wish without clear regulation; greater co-operation and respect between conventional doctors and complementary therapists would improve patient care.

Quackery

The word quack is supposedly derived from "quacksalver", a 17th century variant spelling of quicksilver or mercury, which was used in certain remedies that the public came to recognize as harmful. Pseudoscience uses the language and authority of science without recognizing its methods. It produces claims that cannot be proven or refuted and often poses as the victim (scientists are suppressing the truth). A quack may reasonably be defined as a pseudoscientist who is selling something, and a charlatan as a cynical pseudoscientist who knows one is deceiving the public. It is a sorry monument to human greed and stupidity that more money is spent on health frauds every year than on medical research. Quacks are convincing because they tell people what they want to hear. Moreover, it is almost impossible for the cancer quack to fail. When a patient deteriorates, the cancer quack resorts to lines such as "if only you had come to me sooner". However, we should appreciate that quacks can teach us a great deal whilst we retain an honest and informed practice of medicine. Their popularity is attributed to

Box 4.4 The Luigi Di Bella cure

This treatment is named after its proponent, Professor Luigi Di Bella (1912–2003), a retired physiologist who lived in Modena. It is based on a combination of somatostatin, vitamins, retinoids, melatonin and bromocriptine. Adrenocorticotrophic hormone (ACTH) and low doses of the oral chemotherapeutic agents cyclophosphamide and hydroxyurea are sometimes also included. It was claimed that the treatment stimulated the body's self-healing properties without damaging healthy cells. No scientific rationale or supportive experimental evidence was provided and despite claims to have cured thousands of patients no clinical results were published in peer-reviewed scientific journals. In December 1997, a judge in the southern Italian city of Maglie ruled that the health authority should fund this treatment for a patient and this pattern was followed elsewhere. Although the initial child died of cancer, unprecedented public interest in the unconventional therapy led to public demonstrations with the right-wing media in Italy championing the cause. The socialist Italian government under considerable pressure decided to carry out phase II open-label studies in several cancer centres. Scrutiny of Di Bella's own clinical records of 3076 patients revealed that 50% lacked evidence that the patient had cancer and a further 30% had no follow-up data. Adequate data were available for just 248 patients of whom 244 had, in addition, received conventional treatments for their tumours. These findings rattled Di Bella's credibility and in October 1998 the findings of the first clinical trial were published in the *British Medical Journal*. Of 386 patients, just three had shown a partial response. The findings, however, failed to shake Di Bella's confidence. He accused drug companies of conspiring against him, and suggested that the results were sabotaged by mainstream doctors. Even in 2003, some 3000 patients received Di Bella-based cancer treatments paid for by three Italian regional health services.

Box 4.5 Shark cartilage

In 1993, William Lane a marine biologist and entrepreneur published a book entitled *Sharks Don't Get Cancer* following the discovery that some species of sharks have lower than predicted rates of cancer. This was followed by a prime-time television documentary focusing on a Cuban study of 29 cancer patients who received shark cartilage preparations. This resulted in patients clambering for sharks' cartilage and a consequent devastation of North American shark populations. According to the National Marine Fisheries Service "the Atlantic shark … is severely over-capitalized" and it is estimated that over 200,000 sharks are killed in American waters just for their cartilage every month. The powdered cartilage has modest anti-angiogenic activity *in vitro*; however, oral administration results in the digestion of these proteins prior to absorption. An open-label phase II clinical trial, which was in part funded by shark cartilage manufacturers, found not a single responder amongst 58 patients although both nausea and vomiting were reported. Cartilage Technologies subsequently announced that it would support no additional research on shark cartilage as a cancer remedy. It is, however, intriguing that squalamine, an aminosterol antibiotic isolated from shark livers, inhibits angiogenesis and suppresses the growth of tumour xenografts in animal models. Squalamine is easily synthesized without the need to fish for sharks and is under clinical trial investigation in age-related macular degeneration as well as solid tumours.

"The Zapper", a 9 V electrical device for zapping away cancers.

Euthanasia

Euthanasia is the intentional killing by act or omission of a dependent human being for his or her alleged benefit. The term "assisted suicide" is used when someone provides an individual with the information, guidance and means to take his or her own life with the intention that they will be used for this purpose. Although active euthanasia remains illegal in the United Kingdom, it was legalized in Australia's Northern Territory in 1995, but this bill was overturned by the Australian parliament in 1997. In 1998, Oregon State, USA, legalized assisted suicide following a ballot of the population. There were 129 deaths under Oregon's Physician Assisted Suicide Act between 1998 and 2002. Euthanasia was legalized in

their patience and ability to listen carefully and show both interest and affection (Box 4.4). As well as this, quacks encourage patients to take an active role in their health care, thus empowering them. The internet appears to have made cancer quackery even easier. Whilst much health information on the web is evidence based and of high quality, the open access has also been abused. Entrepreneurs have recognized the value of the web as a free-for-all market and have used it to promote fraudulent cancer treatments ranging from £100 a pound shark cartilage powder (Box 4.5) to

2000 in Holland and in 2002 in Belgium. A survey published in 1994 showed that half of a mixture of hospital consultants and general practitioners in England had been asked by a patient to take active steps to hasten death and that a third of those asked had complied with the patient's request. The reason people choose euthanasia is mostly out of fear of losing autonomy and/or bowel/bladder control, and an increasing proportion of the British public wishes to allow euthanasia for patients in certain incurable disease scenarios.

Ethics

Much of the teaching of contemporary ethics focuses on the "thought experiments" devised by Philippa Foot, a British philosopher and founder of modern virtue ethics, who lived in California. Her experiments centre around runaway trolleybuses in San Francisco with people tied to the rails. The individual is able to operate sets of railway points to divert the trolleybus onto another route … but what is this? … there is another body on that track too! The points operator is set ethical dilemmas around which track to divert the trolleybus down; should they kill five convicts or a pregnant mother (and similar scenarios). The strategies that we take to these ethical dilemmas have been divided into three: Aristotelian virtue ethics, Authoritarian and Formulaic. The Aristotelian approach emphasizes the role of the aristocratic character in evaluating ethical behaviour, the wisdom of the privileged nobility, a role often adopted by judges in contemporary society. The authoritarian attitude is based upon the written rules or rights published either as religious text or laws. These historical texts (Koran, Bible, Talmud, etc.) often do not directly address modern ethical dilemmas, such as genetic testing or surrogacy and hence require interpretation, which is often itself contested. The formulaic approaches to ethics include the deontological moral philosophy of Immanuel Kant and the utilitarianism of Jeremy Bentham, whose skeleton is preserved in a dressed auto-icon that is displayed at University College, London. In the simplest terms, the deontological argument is that you should only do actions to others that you would be willing to have done to yourself. The utilitarian view is that you should take the action that provides the greatest benefit to the maximum number of people.

Four principles underpin medical ethics: respect for autonomy, non-maleficence, beneficence and justice. In health-care decisions, respect for autonomy means that the patient is allowed to act intentionally, with understanding and without controlling influences. This is the basis of informed consent. The principle of non-maleficence requires that we do not intentionally cause harm or injury to a patient, either through acts of commission or omission. In common language this is avoiding negligence and is based on Hippocrates' (460–377 BC) original decree "primum non nocere". The principle of beneficence is the duty of health-care professionals to provide benefit to patients and prevent harm befalling them. These duties apply not only to the individual patient but to the society as a whole and therein frequently lies the problem. In practice, double effect reasoning, first attributed to Thomas Aquinas (1224–1274), may apply when an action has two outcomes – one good and one bad – and allows a lesser harm for a greater good.

Justice in health-care terms is defined as fairness in distribution of care particularly when allocating scarce resources. A number of political doctrines interpret this differently. Karl Marx (1818–1883), of course, believed in egalitarianism "from each according to his abilities, to each according to his needs". Modern health care is rarely provided on this basis but rather on a system that distributes care according to a number of factors including need, effort, contribution, merit and free-market exchanges. Utilitarian philosophers, on the other hand, advocate a system that balances benefit between the collective public and the individual.

Perhaps the most interesting example of the rationing of health care is the Oregon health plan. The Oregon health plan was set up in 1987 with the aim of serving more low-income people using federal funds through a system that prioritizes heath care. An extensive list of more than 700 physical health, dental, drug dependency and mental health services was drawn up and their priority publicly debated in order to reflect a consensus of social values of Oregonians. The list of 587 approved procedures went into operation in 1994. The innovation that most sharply and controversially characterizes this systematic approach is its commitment to providing a standard health benefit based on ranking the effectiveness and value of all medical treatments. To determine which conditions are to be covered, Oregon's Health Services Commission ranks diagnoses from the most important (treatment has the greatest impact on health status) to the least important. This prioritization introduces a transparent approach to health-care rationing and was originally designed to use the savings achieved to extend coverage to more people. Moreover, it requires public involvement in health policies and incorporates public values into the rankings. The top five ranked items were the diagnosis and treatment of head injury, insulin-dependent diabetes mellitus, peritonitis, acute glomerulonephritis (including dialysis) and pneumothorax. At the cut-off cusp, medical treatment of contact and atopic dermatitis and symptomatic urticaria are covered, as is repair of damaged knee ligaments, but the treatment of sexual dysfunction with psychotherapy or medical and surgical approaches does not make the cut, nor does the medical treatment of chronic anal fissure nor complex dental prostheses. The Oregon Health Services Commission also excluded treatment for hepatocellular cancer and widely disseminated cancer.

Sociology of oncology

Inequalities in health are not confined to the marked differences between wealthy and poor nations but are recapitulated within countries, such as the United Kingdom. Eight tube stations on the Jubilee tube line separate Westminster from Canning Town in Newham and the life expectancy of a child born in Westminster exceeds that of a child born in Newham by 6 years – almost 1 year lost for each stop travelled. How much of this disparity is attributable to differences in health care is uncertain, even in a state health monopoly that is free at the point of delivery. Certainly, Marxist health analysts such as Howard Waitzkin propose that doctor–patient encounters reproduce the dominant ideologies of wider society and that medicine is a tool for social control. Modern medicine stands accused of serving the interests of capital and of ensuring that people adhere to the norms of behaviour. Many oncological health inequalities are behavioural and medicine has branded these as self-inflicted; for example, tobacco use and diet. Similar arguments have accused medicine of gender discrimination. Women are greater users of health care because they live longer and because of the medicalization of reproductive health. It is also worth noting that the only national cancer screening programmes are for women (mammogram and cervical smears). Medicine has a long history of reinforcing a subordinate role for women in society, leading to both radical and reformist responses from the feminist movement. Equivalent oncological responses would be the alternative medicine movement, which wishes to overthrow the current practice of oncology, and complementary medicine, which wishes to change cancer medicine from within, encouraging the adoption of a wider vision and a more holistic approach.

The use of metaphors in cancer medicine has been attacked by both Susan Sontag and John Diamond, who use their personal experiences of cancer to describe the negative implications of these metaphors. Many of these metaphors are bellicose, "the fight against cancer" belittles the patient as "a victim". The use of these figures of speech may render cancer socially as well as physically devastating and "losing the battle against cancer" denigrates a patient's role in the society.

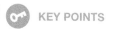 KEY POINTS

- Psychological problems affect most cancer patients including long-term issues in cancer survivors
- Breaking bad news is a learnt skill that requires practice but is rewarding if done well
- Coping strategies are required to insulate clinicians from burn-out
- The use of unconventional therapies by cancer patients is the norm not the exception and in part reflects the desire to have some control over their lives and illness

Part 2

Types of cancer

5

Breast cancer

Learning objectives

✓ Explain the epidemiology and pathogenesis of breast cancer

✓ Recognize the common presentation and clinical features of breast cancer

✓ Describe the treatment strategies and outcomes of breast cancer

Diseases of the breast, including tumours, have been attracting medical interest for more than 5000 years. The earliest written records of breast cancer are in the Edwin Smith papyrus, from ancient Egyptian civilizations of 3000–2500 BC. Hard and cold lumps were recognized as tumours, whilst abscesses were hot. The next major advances in the management of breast cancer occurred during the golden age of surgery at the end of the 19th century, following advances in antisepsis and anaesthesia. William Halsted in Baltimore described radical mastectomy in 1894. Moreover, in an early example of surgical audit, he reported a local recurrence rate in 50 women of only 6%. The next major advance in the management of breast cancer occurred in 1896 with the development of surgical oophorectomy as a treatment strategy for advanced breast cancer, which was pioneered by George Beatson in Glasgow (the Beatson Institute for Cancer Research in that city is named after him). Geoffrey Keynes, the brother of macroeconomist John Maynard Keynes and an expert in the watercolours of William Blake, developed lumpectomy and radiotherapy as a breast conservation measure in the 1930s whilst appointed as surgeon at St Bartholomew's Hospital in London. In the 1960s and 1970s the second-wave feminism movement in Europe and America took breast cancer as a campaigning point and their efforts led to increased focus on breast cancer treatment and research. Copying the AIDS awareness red ribbons, breast cancer activists adopted pink ribbons and now there is a rainbow of different cancer ribbons. These campaigns directly led to improvements in screening access, and screening programmes were introduced without a significant evidence base for efficacy and against the views of the medical establishment. As a consequence of increased screening, the survival rates of breast cancer have risen steadily over the last 30 years. A list of 5-year survival of breast cancer patients by stage of disease can be found in Table 5.2. Breast cancer patients were largely viewed as the property of the surgeons. In the United Kingdom in the last few years central governmental directives have led to multidisciplinary working. This has directly led to a decrease in the use of mutilating surgery and an increase in the use of adjuvant treatments. As a result of early detection and adjuvant therapies survival in breast cancer has increased significantly from around 65% in the 1980s to 85% in current times.

Epidemiology

Breast cancer is a common disease (Table 5.1 and Table 1.1). According to the most recent figures, 49,936 women are affected annually and 11,684 die in the United Kingdom as a result of this condition. The risk of breast cancer is influenced by family history, age, diet, social class and nulliparity. The risk of breast cancer rises with duration of exposure to oestrogens, so that early menarche, late menopause, low parity and hormone replacement therapy (HRT) all increase the risk. There is a protective effect of a full-term

Oncology: Lecture Notes, Third Edition. Mark Bower and Jonathan Waxman.
© 2015 by John Wiley & Sons, Ltd. Published 2015 by John Wiley & Sons, Ltd.
Companion Website: www.lecturenoteseries.com/oncology

Table 5.1 UK registrations for (female) breast cancer 2010

	Percentage of all cancer registrations	Rank of registration	Lifetime risk of cancer	Change in ASR (2000–2010)	5 year overall survival
	Female	Female	Female	Female	Female
Breast cancer	31	1st	1 in 8	+6%	85%

pregnancy, provided the pregnancy is achieved prior to the woman's 30th birthday. There is a minor protective effect of having more than five pregnancies, but probably no protective effect from breastfeeding. Oestrogen-only HRT, as well as combined oestrogen and progestogen HRT, increases the risk of breast cancer in proportion to the duration of HRT administration. Both the oral contraceptive pill and alcohol and coffee consumption have been linked to breast cancer, but the associations are controversial. Breast cancer risk increases with age, plateauing during the menopausal years of 45–55. Women are at increased risk from breast cancer from non-vegetarian diets; it is not clear what the reason for this should be. Women who are more than two standard deviations above average height and weight are at a greater risk from breast cancer, as are women of social classes I and II.

A family history of breast cancer is a very important risk factor for breast cancer. If more than two first-degree relatives are affected, the risk to other female family members increases by a factor of 2. There are clear links between breast cancer and other cancers, with associations between ovarian and endometrial cancer and colonic tumours. There are four relatively common genes that lead to an increased risk of breast cancer and these are: BRCA1 and 2, CHEK2 and FGFR2. The prevalence and penetrance (percentage of people with the mutation that have the cancer) of mutations in these genes vary but lead to a lifetime risk of breast cancer of greater than 80% and up to 60% of ovarian cancer. BRCA1 gene is located on chromosome 17q21 and is a tumour suppressor gene, the product of which is involved in cell cycle regulation. The BRCA1 product binds with Rad51, a major protein of 3418 amino acids, which is involved in sensing and directing the molecular response to double-stranded DNA damage. Thus mutations of BRCA allow damage to DNA to go unrepaired and an accumulation of DNA mutations leads to cancers. BRCA2 gene is located on chromosome 13q12 and also has a role in DNA repair. To commemorate its discovery in 1994, a cycle path in Cambridge was painted with 10,257 stripes of colour, representing the nucleotide base sequence of the BRCA2 gene.

The detected incidence of breast cancer is increasing in England and Wales. Similarly, death rates have fallen by nearly 30% over the last 15 years and survival chance has increased from 65% to 85%. These rises in incidence and survival are almost certainly due to the successes of the screening programme, which has led to the earlier detection of tumours at an earlier stage, with the resultant better prognosis. There are also contributions to this fall in mortality rate from an increased use of adjuvant chemotherapy and hormonal therapy.

Presentation and screening

Women with breast cancer generally present to their clinicians with a lump in their breast. On average,

Table 5.2 Five-year survival of women with breast cancer by stage of disease

Tumour stage	Percentage of patients at diagnosis	Stage definition	5-year survival
Stage I	41	Tumour <2 cm, no nodes	88%
Stage II	45	Tumour 2–5 cm and/or moveable axillary nodes	69%
Stage III	9	Chest wall or skin fixation and/or fixed axillary nodes	43%
Stage IV	5	Metastases	12%

there is a delay of approximately 3 months between the woman first noting the mass in her breast and her seeing a hospital clinician. As a result of concerns over the care of women with breast cancer, the investigation and treatment of this disease has been prioritized. Women in whom breast cancer is suspected must be seen in "outpatients" within 2 weeks of receipt of the referral letter.

Alternative sources of referral are from breast screening programmes. In the United Kingdom the breast cancer screening program was introduced as a political initiative during an election campaign. It was alleged that more money was spent on advertising the initiative than in the provision of screening facilities. The NHS Breast Screening Programme (NHSBSP) offers mammographic screening to all women aged 50–70 at 3 yearly intervals and currently over 2.7 million women are screened per year. A large proportion of screen-detected breast cancers are smaller than 2 cm without spread to the axillary lymph nodes or are *in situ* tumours only. Tumours are usually identified as a soft-tissue density or microcalcification within the breast. Large population-based randomized trials have suggested that mammographic screening reduces the mortality from breast cancer by 25% as a consequence of earlier diagnosis. However, breast screening is not without harm; radiation exposure, pain, psychological stress and perhaps most importantly overdiagnosis. Overdiagnosis remains the most controversial issue in breast cancer screening and refers to the detection and subsequent treatment of breast cancers that would never have caused any harm to the patient in her natural lifetime (see Box 3.5). In 2013, a Cochrane review of screening trials involving 600,000 women concluded that for those trials where there was adequate randomization, there was no survival advantage to screening. Total 10-year breast cancer mortality was the same in screened and unscreened groups.

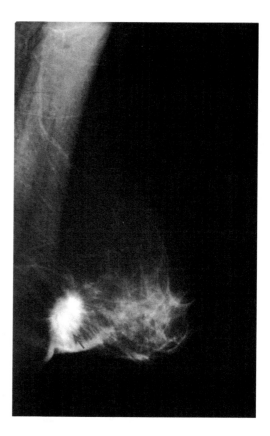

Figure 5.1 Lateral view of a breast mammogram showing a large, dense, speculated mass highly suggestive of breast cancer.

Diagnosis

The current standard is for women to be seen in a multidisciplinary setting that offers a "one-stop shop" for diagnosis. Surgeons, with a special interest in breast cancer work in a clinic with oncologists, with access to same-day cytology and imaging services. A careful history should be obtained from the patient prior to examination when seen in outpatients. The mass may be thought to be benign or malignant. Benign lumps are more likely in younger women and tend to be painful and enlarge before menstruation.

Malignant lumps tend to be more common in older women and are generally painless: only 30% of malignant breast lumps are painful and just 10% of lumps seen in new patients are malignant. Occasionally, women present with features of locally advanced (Figures 5.3 and 5.5) or metastatic disease (Figure 5.6).

Diagnosis is carried out by clinical, mammographic (Figure 5.1), ultrasonographic, cytological and histological means. After clinical examination, mammography (a soft-tissue X-ray of the breast), aspiration cytology (removal of cells by means of a needle and syringe) and core biopsy (removal of a solid piece of breast tissue) should be performed to further assess the significance of the breast lump. In younger women, ultrasonography rather than mammography is the radiological investigation of choice. If there is confirmed malignancy, all women should then proceed to surgery within 2 weeks of diagnosis, as recommended by national guidelines.

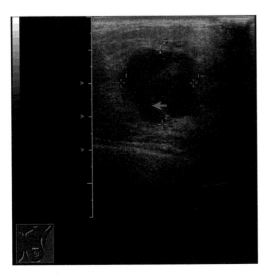

Figure 5.2 Breast ultrasound showing large, echo-dense, irregular, primary breast cancer lesion.

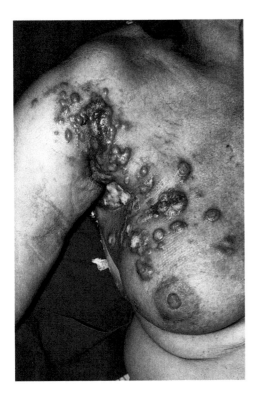

Figure 5.3 Local recurrence of breast cancer showing multiple ulcerating skin nodules.

Staging and grading

There are two main pathological variants of breast cancer: ductal (70%) and lobular, and these may be *in situ* or invasive (or a mixture of both) (see Figure 1.9). Tumour grading was first described by Bloom and Richardson and bears their eponyms. This grading scheme depends upon the degree of tumour tubule formation, the mitotic activity and the nuclear pleomorphism of the tumour (see Box 1.3). As one might expect, poorly differentiated tumours have a worse prognosis than moderately differentiated ones, which in turn have a worse prognosis than well-differentiated breast cancer (Table 5.3). There may be pre-invasive changes and these are described as either ductal (DCIS) or lobular carcinoma *in situ* (LCIS). LCIS are additionally graded according to their microscopic features (see Figure 1.9).

Stage is defined according to the TNM classification, which is updated every 10 years or so (Table 5.4; see also Box 3.1). The subscript "P" denotes a pathological staging following surgery. The Nottingham prognostic index based upon the tumour size, N stage and tumour grade is used to predict 10-year survival in early breast cancer.

Treatment

Surgery

Surgery for breast cancer depends upon the clinical stage of the disease. If the mass is less than 5 cm in size and not fixed, the preferred treatment is removal of the lump, which is termed "lumpectomy" or by the rather more elegant term "wide local excision". Axillary lymph node dissection was conventionally performed, but now this has largely been replaced by sentinel lymph node biopsy which, if positive, may then be followed by an axillary clearance. The sentinel node is the hypothetical first node draining a cancer. The reason for sampling the axillary nodes is that if the nodes are affected, there is a significant advantage in this group of women to adjuvant chemotherapy. In the "node-negative" woman there is a very much smaller advantage to adjuvant chemotherapy. In an older woman there may be an argument against routine axillary dissection. The reason for this is that adjuvant treatment with chemotherapy within this group of women is not dictated by lymph node status, because the advantage is much smaller than in younger women and the toxicity of the treatment outweighs these modest gains. It is clear, however, that

Table 5.3 Breast cancer grading and prognosis

Grade	5-year survival
G1: Well differentiated	95%
G2: Moderately differentiated	75%
G3: Poorly differentiated	50%

knowledge of the axillary nodal status does provide prognostic information.

For a woman whose tumour measures >5 cm in size, the preferred surgical option is mastectomy, which is removal of the breast with axillary dissection. This is to reduce the chance of local recurrence. For more advanced breast cancer, the value of surgical treatment is much more contentious and elderly women may be treated with hormonal therapy alone if the breast cancer expresses oestrogen receptors and/or progesterone receptors (see Figure 1.14). In a younger woman, neoadjuvant chemotherapy may be given in the first instance, to reduce the size of the tumour and this may then be followed by surgery and radiotherapy. There is a major role for reconstructive surgery and this may be carried out at the time of primary surgery or at a later date upon completion of adjuvant radiotherapy or chemotherapy. The psychological gain is tremendous and needs to be considered in older as well as younger women, for breasts are considered valued personal property in older just as much as in younger women.

Adjuvant radiotherapy

After lumpectomy, radiotherapy is given to the breast. This is done in order to reduce the risk of local recurrence of the tumour. Without radiation this risk is between 40% and 60%; whereas with radiation, the risk is reduced to approximately 4–6%, which is the same as that for more radical surgical procedures. Radiotherapy is generally given over a 6-week period and requires daily attendance at hospital. The side effects of radiation include tiredness and burning of the skin, which is generally mild. More serious consequences of radiation are seen only rarely and include damage to the brachial nerve plexus and, with more old-fashioned treatment machines and plans, damage to the coronary blood vessels. Rarely, a second cancer, such as an angiosarcoma, may follow at the site of radiotherapy treatment.

Adjuvant hormonal therapy

Treatment with tamoxifen has been shown to have an advantage in terms of disease-free and overall survival in both pre- and postmenopausal women and is now given routinely to this group of patients. It is usually recommended that treatment should extend for 5 years. There is no advantage to adjuvant tamoxifen in oestrogen receptor-negative tumours. There have been changes in our understanding of the oestrogen receptor. Two different classes of oestrogen receptor (ER), described as α and β, have been identified. Tamoxifen is a selective ERα-antagonist, which, in turn, has effects on the progesterone receptor. In postmenopausal women, recent studies suggest that a newer group of drugs, the aromatase inhibitors, may be even more effective than tamoxifen as adjuvant therapy. The current standard is to give sequential therapy with tamoxifen and then an aromatase inhibitor. Treatment is given for a total of 5 years. Approximately 10% of circulating oestrogens derive from adrenal precursors, such as androstenedione, through the action of aromatase enzymes. The aromatase inhibitors block this action, limiting the synthesis of oestrone and oestrone sulphate produced by a second series of enzymes – the sulphatase system (Figure 5.4). Use of aromatase inhibitors is associated with osteoporosis. There have been reports of cases of endometrial carcinoma associated with the use of tamoxifen. The estimated risk is one case per 20,000

Table 5.4 TNM staging of breast cancer

T stage (primary tumour)	N stage (nodal status)	M stage (metastatic status)
T0: No detectable primary tumour	N0: No nodes involved	M0: No metastases
T1: Tumour less than 2 cm	N1: Mobile axillary nodes	M1: Spread to distant organs
T2: Tumour measuring between 2 and 5 cm	N2: Fixed axillary nodes	
T3: Tumour measuring greater than 5 cm	N3: Involved supra- or infraclavicular nodes	
T4: Tumour of any size extending into skin or chest wall		

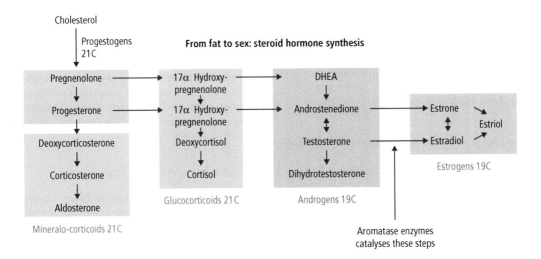

Cholesterol

Progestogens 21C

From fat to sex: steroid hormone synthesis

Pregnenolone → 17α Hydroxy-pregnenolone → DHEA

Progesterone → 17α Hydroxy-pregnenolone → Androstenedione → Estrone

Deoxycorticosterone · Deoxycortisol · Testosterone · Estradiol · Estriol

Corticosterone · Cortisol · Dihydrotestosterone

Aldosterone

Estrogens 19C

Mineralo-corticoids 21C · Glucocorticoids 21C · Androgens 19C

Aromatase enzymes catalyses these steps

Figure 5.4 Sex hormone synthesis pathway (21C, 21 carbon compound 19C, 19 carbon compound). DHEA, dehydroepiandrosterone.

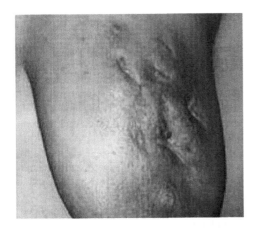

Medical metaphors:
Breast Cancer: Peau d'orange

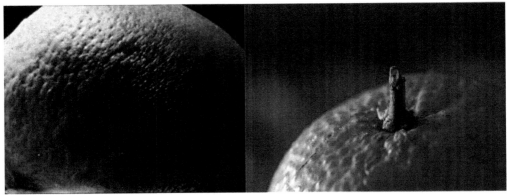

Figure 5.5 Peau d'orange is caused by lymphoedema of the skin with tethering of the sweat ducts giving a dimpled appearance to the swollen skin resembling the skin of an orange.

women per year of use. Selective oestrogen receptor modulators (SERMS) targeting tumour, and not normal tissues, may avoid the risk of uterine malignancy. However, there may be advantages to non-selective oestrogen inhibitors in terms of the prevention of osteoporosis.

Adjuvant chemotherapy and receptor targeting therapy

Adjuvant chemotherapy has a significant place in the management of breast cancer. Adjuvant chemotherapy using the cyclophosphamide, methotrexate, fluorouracil (5FU) (CMF) programme was the first shown to be of benefit. A large international study showed that more intensive therapy using the FEC (5FU, epirubicin, cyclophosphamide) regimen is more effective than CMF. The addition of taxanes (paclitaxel, docetaxel) chemotherapy given in the adjuvant setting confers further benefits. Third generation adjuvant chemotherapy (FEC-T), combining FEC and docetaxel, is now considered to be the standard. There is no evidence that intensifying adjuvant therapy any further using, for example, high-dose treatments with bone marrow or peripheral blood stem cell support, improves the disease-free interval or the overall survival. About a quarter of breast cancers express the epidermal growth factor receptor 2 (EGFR2), also known as Her-2/neu and c-erbB-2 (see Figure 1.14). This is the target for the monoclonal antibody trastuzumab (Herceptin). For patients with Her-2 receptor-positive tumours, treatment with adjuvant trastuzumab may be considered. Treatment is conventionally given for periods of 12–18 months. The advantage to treatment with trastuzumab is small, but is recommended because of the poorer survival of women with tumours that strongly express Her-2. The toxicity of treatment with trastuzumab is significant, and particularly of note are the direct cardiac effects that may manifest as heart failure.

Treatment of metastatic breast cancer

The treatment of metastatic breast cancer depends very much upon the age of the patient and the sites of metastasis. It is only rarely curable and so life quality issues are immediately important. When we described this point to one patient, she replied: "my dear, it's the quality of death that bothers me".

In older women whose metastases are in the skin or bone, the preferred treatment option is hormonal

therapy (see Figure 3.26), provided that the tumour expresses oestrogen and/or progestogen receptor positivity. The agent of first choice is tamoxifen because of its lack of toxicity and efficacy. Approximately 70% of women aged 70 respond to this therapy.

In a younger woman the growth of breast cancer is frequently dependent upon oestrogens derived chiefly from the ovaries. In a premenopausal woman, hormonal therapy is generally less effective than in postmenopausal women, and at the age of 30, just 10% of patients overall will respond to treatment at all. But regardless of this statistic oophorectomy, that is, removal of the ovaries by either radiotherapeutic, surgical or medical means, is generally the first therapeutic stratagem. Surgical oophorectomy is unnecessary, given that an equivalence of effect is provided by the use of medical treatment with a luteinizing hormone receptor hormone (LHRH) agonist. How much easier is it to provide a simple 3-monthly depot injection than to expose a woman to laparoscopy and surgical oophorectomy. Radiotherapy is not a particularly successful way of causing gonadal failure. Ovaries are relatively radiotherapy resistant and the conventional dosages of radiotherapy given to sterilize may not sterilize a younger woman and certainly will not lead to an instant reduction in circulating ovarian steroid hormones. So for a premenopausal woman, treatment with an LHRH agonist is generally recommended as the first therapeutic hormonal manoeuvre.

Other sources of hormones are from the adrenal glands, diet and peripheral tissues. As a result of our knowledge of the steroid biosynthetic pathways, inhibitors of these pathways have been developed. In recent years we have seen the introduction of aromatase inhibitors into clinical practice. These drugs inhibit the enzymes that convert androgens manufactured in the adrenals into oestrogens (Figure 5.6). Further hormonal therapies are also likely to become available because of Pharma interest in the development of oestrogen sulfatase inhibitors. The sulfatases are enzymes involved in the final steps of oestrogenic steroid synthesis and sulfatase inhibitors are in clinical development currently.

Triple negative breast cancers lack expression of ER, PR and HER2; they constitute about 15% of all breast cancers and have an aggressive natural history. These triple negative tumours resemble BRCA1-associated breast cancers and are highly sensitive to chemotherapy with DNA-damaging agents such as cisplatin, and the effects of these drugs can be potentiated by the use of poly-ADP ribose polymerase (PARP) inhibitors which disable DNA base excision repair. PARP inhibitors (postfix: -parib) are also

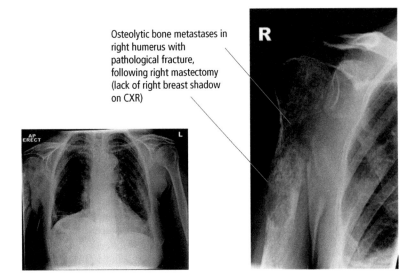

Osteolytic bone metastases in right humerus with pathological fracture, following right mastectomy (lack of right breast shadow on CXR)

Figure 5.6 Metastatic breast cancer.

effective in BRCA1-associated breast and ovary cancers. Angiogenesis inhibitors, such as the monoclonal antibody bevacizumab, have also been shown to have a modest beneficial effect in breast cancer. The erythroblastic leukaemia oncogene (ErbB) family of receptor tyrosine kinases includes four members: epidermal growth factor receptor (EGFR), HER 2, HER3 and HER4. A significant proportion of breast cancers express HER2 which may be targeted with the monoclonal antibody trastuzumab or the oral kinase inhibitor lapatinib that inhibits both HER2 and EGFR. Breast cancer therapy is rapidly evolving into a form of personalized medicine where treatment is based on decisions made from tumour array comparative genome hybridization (CGH) and next generation sequencing techniques (see Figure 1.13).

In both pre- and postmenopausal women, radiation treatment is very effective in controlling bone pain. The addition of regular bisphosphonate therapy both relieve bone pain and reduce skeletal events such as fractures and spinal cord compression. If lungs or liver are affected, then chemotherapy is required. Overall, between 40% and 60% of patients respond to chemotherapy and this response is for a median duration of 1 year. The median survival of women with metastatic breast cancer ranges between 18 and 24 months, with 5–10% alive after 5 years. It should be noted that there are patients with very prolonged survival, and these include those women who have, for example, single sites of metastatic disease.

High-dose chemotherapy

Breast cancer responds to chemotherapy, but often after responding, patients relapse and die. There have been attempts to maximize response rates by intensifying chemotherapy. High-dose treatments were popular in the early 1980s. Response rates were found to be higher than for conventional treatment; toxicity, however, was significantly worse, and death rates reached 20% as a result of the side effects of treatment. Even more significantly, patients who responded and survived the toxicity later relapsed, and the median duration of response was no better than that expected with conventional treatment.

In the 1990s, there was an increase in the numbers of patients receiving high-dose therapy for breast cancer. This was possible as a result of the improvement in supportive therapy, principally bone marrow rescue, either with stem cells or with marrow. Mortality has decreased and now is 5% in the best centres. Overall, there has been no significant improvement in the expectation for survival for patients with metastatic breast cancer, and only 20% of patients are alive 2 years after the transplantation. It has been recently argued that the relatively good results of intensive therapy reported in early studies are entirely the result of the selection of good-prognosis patients for treatment with high-dose therapy, and that the same effects could be achieved with less intensive, conventional therapy. It may be the case that early intensive therapy given as adjuvant treatment to patients with

poor-risk tumours will lead to improved survival, but this has not been shown in any randomized study.

Carcinoma *in situ*

The introduction of universal mammography has led to an enormous increase in the diagnosis of relatively benign breast conditions such as DCIS and LCIS. The latest ONS statistics describe 5765 men and women diagnosed with carcinoma *in situ* in 2011. DCIS, diagnosed by excision biopsy and untreated will progress to invasive cancer in 40% of patients over 5 years. Treatment with adjuvant radiotherapy will limit this progression rate to 1–4% per annum. Mastectomy is an alternative to radiation therapy. Both radiotherapy and mastectomy are equally effective in local disease control. In randomized control studies tamoxifen has been shown to prevent local recurrence in women who have DCIS. LCIS is associated with a high incidence of bilaterality reaching up to 40% and mirror biopsy is recommended of the contralateral breast. Adjuvant treatment with radiotherapy is not helpful in preventing LCIS recurrence. The mortality rate from carcinoma *in situ* is less than 1%.

Paget's disease of the nipple

This is an eczematous condition of the nipple, associated in 80% of cases with an underlying ductal carcinoma and in about 20% of cases with underlying DCIS. It was named after Sir James Paget, who also bagged Paget's disease (of bone) and extramammary Paget's disease as eponyms. He was a friend of Charles Darwin and Thomas Huxley as well as father to Stephen Paget who first proposed the "seed and soil" hypothesis of tumour metastasis.

Male breast cancer

Breast cancer in men is rare accounting for <1% breast cancer (349 cases in the United Kingdom in 2011). At presentation, men with breast cancer are on average 10 years older than women with breast cancer and >40% are stage III or IV. Initial treatment combines mastectomy and tamoxifen as most tumours express ER. Mastectomy is required in order to obtain "good" tumour margins which minimizes the risk of local recurrence. The overall survival is worse than in women and relates to the advanced stage at diagnosis with overall 5-year survivals of 40–60%.

 ONLINE RESOURCE

Case Study: A TV producer with a breast lump.

 KEY POINTS

- Breast cancer is the most common cancer in women accounting for almost one-third of all cancers in women
- A family history of breast cancer and the overall duration of oestrogen exposure are the main risk factors for breast cancer
- Most women with breast cancer present through the NHS Breast Screening Programme (NHSBSP), with a breast lump or less commonly with manifestations of metastatic disease
- The clinical management of breast cancer is truly multi-disciplinary, including surgery, radiotherapy, chemotherapy, novel agents and palliative care
- Eighty-five per cent of women diagnosed with breast cancer in the United Kingdom survive 5 years

6

Central nervous system cancers

Learning objectives

✓ Explain the epidemiology and pathogenesis of central nervous system (CNS) cancers

✓ Recognize the common presentation and clinical features of CNS cancers

✓ Describe the treatment strategies and outcomes of CNS cancers

The first recognized resection of a primary brain tumour was performed in 1884 by Rickman Godlee in collaboration with the Westminster Hospital neurologist Alexander Bennett. It should be remembered that the removal of the cerebral cortex tumour was performed before any diagnostic imaging was available (X-rays were discovered in 1895 by Wilhelm Röntgen), but even then the surgeon knew to operate on the contralateral side to the clinical signs!

Scientists use animal models to study genetics, development and oncogenesis, and the most common models are mice (see onco-mice in Box 1.1), fruit flies (*Drosophila melanogaster*) and nematode worms (*Caenorhabditis elegans*) (Figure 6.1). However, fish have also turned out to be useful subjects – in particular zebrafish (*Danio rerio*), which are tropical freshwater minnows with five horizontal stripes running from their mouth to the caudal fin. Zebrafish are the vertebrate model for studying the genetics of embryonic development because the embryos are transparent and the genome sequence is known and can readily be modified by knockouts. A less well-known fish model of cancer is the damselfish (*Pomacentrus partitus*) that lives on coral reefs and has several vertical stripes. Deb and Flo in *Finding Nemo* are damselfish, so here is an excuse to watch that masterpiece of subtlety and metaphor again.

Damselfish neurofibromatosis is a naturally occurring, neoplastic disease of these fish that consists of multiple neurofibromata and neurofibrosarcomas. It has been proposed as an animal model for neurofibromatosis type 1 in humans. However, whilst von Recklinghausen's neurofibromatosis type 1 is vertically transmitted as an autosomal dominant trait, damselfish neurofibromatosis is transmitted horizontally between fish and is thought to be due to an oncogenic retrovirus named damselfish neurofibromatosis virus (DNFV).

Epidemiology

There were 9365 people diagnosed with a brain tumour in 2011 in the United Kingdom and 4975 deaths from brain tumours. Brain tumours are slightly more common in men than in women. Fifteen per cent of adults diagnosed with brain tumours survive for 5 years. A further 400 children are diagnosed with central nervous system (CNS) tumours in the United Kingdom each year. CNS tumours are the second most common cancer in childhood after leukaemia and account for 27% of all cancers in children. Metastases

Oncology: Lecture Notes, Third Edition. Mark Bower and Jonathan Waxman.
© 2015 by John Wiley & Sons, Ltd. Published 2015 by John Wiley & Sons, Ltd.
Companion Website: www.lecturenoteseries.com/oncology

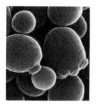
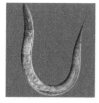

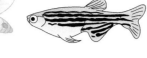
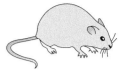

Saccharomyces cerevisiae (yeast)

Caenorhabditis elegans (nematode – roundworm)

Drosophila melanogaster (fruitfly)

Danio rerio (zebrafish)

Mus musculus (mouse)

Figure 6.1 The oncologist's menagerie. The five most common animal models used in laboratory studies of cancer.

to the brain are about 10 times more common than primary brain tumours. The most common primary tumour sites amongst patients with brain metastases are lung, breast, melanoma and kidney. In addition, nasopharyngeal cancers may directly extend through the skull foramina. Meningeal metastases occur with leukaemia and lymphoma, breast and small-cell lung cancers, and from medulloblastoma and ependymal glioma as a route of spread. Primary tumours of the CNS account for 1.5% of all cancers and 3% of cancer deaths (Table 6.1). About 58% of CNS tumours arise in the brain, 23% in the meninges, 11% in the pituitary and 8% in the spinal cord. Similarly, astrocytomas account for 34% of CNS tumours, meningiomas for 21% and pituitary adenomas for 8%. The World Health Organization (WHO) International Classification of Diseases (ICD) attributes a code to all diseases and the current version is ICD-10, the first version of the ICD that has removed homosexuality from its ridiculous classification as a mental illness! CNS tumours are broadly grouped into malignant or benign tumours and the grade of the tumours in the WHO classification can be loosely translated into aggressive (generally grades II–IV) and indolent (generally grade I) tumours. Most (95%) astrocytomas are aggressive, but only 8% of meningiomas and 1–2% pituitary tumours are aggressive.

Aetiology

Although the cause of most adult brain tumours is not established, a number of inherited phakomatoses are associated with brain tumours. Phakomatoses are a group of familial conditions with unique cutaneous and neurological manifestations and dysplasias of a number of organ systems. Phakomatoses include:

- Neurofibromatosis (von Recklinghausen's disease)
- Tuberous sclerosis (Bourneville's disease)
- von Hippel–Lindau disease (cerebroretinal angiomatosis)
- Sturge–Weber syndrome (encephalotrigeminal angiomatosis)
- Osler–Rendu–Weber syndrome
- Fabry's disease (angiokeratoma corporis diffusum)

The first three of these are associated with brain tumours; von Recklinghausen's neurofibromatosis with cranial and root schwannomas, meningiomas, ependymomas and optic gliomas (see Figure 2.15); tuberous sclerosis with gliomas and ependymomas; and von Hippel–Lindau disease with cerebellar and retinal haemangioblastoma (Table 6.2). In addition, an increased incidence of brain tumours is a feature

Table 6.1 UK registrations for primary brain cancer 2010										
	Percentage of all cancer registrations		Rank of registration		Lifetime risk of cancer		Change in ASR (2000–2010)		5-year overall survival	
	Female	Male	Female	Male	Female	Male	Female	Male	Female	Male
Brain cancer	3	3	8th	10th	1 in 77	1 in 77	0%	+10%	16%	15%

Table 6.2 Phakomatoses associated with brain tumours

Condition	Inheritance and genetics	Cutaneous manifestations	Eye	Nervous system	Brain tumours
Von Reckling-hausen's neuro-fibromatosis (NF-1)	Autosomal dominant NF-1 gene (encodes neurofibromin that regulates GTPases in signal transduction)	Café au lait macules, axillary freckles	Lisch nodules (pigmented iris hamartomas)	Neurofibromata	Schwann cell tumours of spinal and cranial nerves, meningiomas, ependymomas, optic gliomas
Acoustic neurofi-bromatosis (NF-2)	Autosomal dominant NF-2 gene (encodes Merlin protein involved in cell adhesion)	Café au lait macules less common than in NF-1	Presenile cataracts	Bilateral acoustic neuromas Neurofibromata	Schwann cell tumours of spinal and cranial nerves, meningiomas, astrocytomas, ependymomas, optic gliomas
Tuberous sclerosis	Autosomal dominant TSC1 gene (encodes hamartin protein) and TSC2 gene (encodes tuberin protein)	Adenoma sebaceum, Shagreen patches, subungual fibromata, café au lait spots		Seizures, mental retardation	Giant cell astrocytoma of the foramen of Munro, gliomas, ependymomas
Von Hippel–Lindau	Autosomal dominant VHL gene (encodes VHL protein involved in ubiquitination)	Skin hamartomas	Retinal angiomas		Cerebellar haemangioblas-tomas, ependymomas, pheochromocy-toma

of Gorlin's basal nevus syndrome (medulloblastoma), Turcot syndrome (gliomas) and Li–Fraumeni syndrome (glioma) (see Table 2.3).

High-dose ionizing radiation to the head region administered in the past for benign conditions such as scalp tinea capitis fungal infection (ringworm) increases the risk of nerve sheath tumours, gliomas and meningiomas. There is much public concern that low-frequency non-ionizing electromagnetic fields such as those emitted by 60 Hz power cables may increase the risk of brain tumours, but there is no consistent evidence to support this hypothesis. Similarly, despite scares, there is no evidence to support an association with wireless radiofrequency devices such as mobile phones. This joins the long list of things that cause cancer according to the *Daily Mail*. It includes Facebook, deodorant, hair dye, talcum powder, mouthwash, tooth whitener, oral sex, chips and chocolate.

Pathology

Primary nervous system tumours may be glial tumours, non-glial tumours or primary cerebral non-Hodgkin's lymphoma (Table 6.3). As you may recall from embryology lectures, the early embryo has three distinct germ layers of cells:

- Endoderm, the innermost layer that gives rise to the digestive organs, lungs and bladder
- Mesoderm, the middle layer that gives rise to the muscles, skeleton and blood system
- Ectoderm, the outer layer that gives rise to the skin and nervous system

Neuroectodermal tumours are classified on the basis of the predominant cell type and include tumours of both central and peripheral nervous system derived

Table 6.3 Central nervous system tumours

Gliomas	Non-glial brain tumours
Astrocytomas Grade I (non-infiltrating pilocytic astrocytoma) Grade II (well-to-moderately differentiated astrocytoma) Grade III (anaplastic astrocytoma) Grade IV (glioblastoma multiforme)	Meningioma Pituitary adenoma Craniopharyngioma Extragonadal germ cell tumour Primary cerebral lymphoma Choroid plexus tumours
Other glial tumours Ependymoma Oligodendroglioma Medulloblastoma	**Primary spinal cord tumours** Schwannoma Extradural meningioma Intramedullary ependymoma Astrocytoma

cells. After embryonic development ceases, neurons do not divide, but glial cells retain the ability to proliferate throughout life and thus most adult neurological tumours are derived from glial cells and are named gliomas. Glial cells (from the Greek term for glue) surround the neurons holding them in place, supplying them with nutrients and insulating them from one another; glia also remove pathogens and dead neurons.

Gliomas account for 50% of brain tumours and are divided into grade I (non-infiltrating pilocytic astrocytoma), grade II (well-to-moderately differentiated astrocytoma), grade III (anaplastic astrocytoma) and grade IV (glioblastoma multiforme). The prognosis deteriorates with rising tumour grade. In addition to these astrocytomas, there are other glial tumours including ependymomas that arise from ependymal cells (the epithelial like cells that line the ventricles of the brain and spinal cord), and oligodendrogliomas that arise from oligodendrocytes (the cells that make myelin sheaths). In the peripheral nervous system, neurofibromata (derived from non-myelin forming Schwann cells) and schwannomas (derived from Schwann cells that make myelin) are the most frequent glial tumours.

Medulloblastoma is a glial tumour of childhood usually arising in the cerebellum, which may be related to primitive neuroectodermal tumours elsewhere in the CNS. Non-glial brain tumours include pineal parenchymal tumours, extragonadal germ cell tumours, craniopharyngiomas, meningiomas and choroid plexus tumours. Meningioma is the commonest non-glial tumour and constitutes 21% of brain tumours. The majority of spinal axis tumours in adults are extradural, metastatic carcinoma, lymphoma or sarcoma. Primary spinal cord tumours include extradural meningiomas (26%), schwannomas (29%),

intramedullary ependymomas (13%) and astrocytomas (13%).

Seventy per cent of primary brain tumours in adults are supratentorial, situated above the tentorium cerebelli, the tent of dura mater that lies between the cerebellum and the inferior portion of the occipital lobes. In contrast, primary brain tumours in children are usually located below the tentorium (Table 6.4).

Presentation

Glial tumours

Glial tumours may produce both generalized and focal effects, and these will reflect the site of the tumour and the speed of its growth. General symptoms from the mass effect, increased intracranial pressure, oedema, midline shift and herniation

Table 6.4 Brain tumours by age and site

Adult	Child
Supratentorial Metastases Glioma Meningioma Pituitary tumour	**Supratentorial** Craniopharyngioma Pinealoma Optic glioma
Infratentorial Metastases Acoustic neuroma Cerebellar haemangioblastoma	**Infratentorial** Medulloblastoma Cerebellar astrocytoma Ependymoma of fourth ventricle

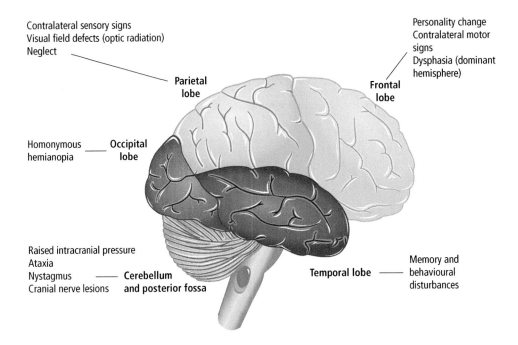

Contralateral sensory signs
Visual field defects (optic radiation)
Neglect

Personality change
Contralateral motor signs
Dysphasia (dominant hemisphere)

Parietal lobe

Frontal lobe

Homonymous hemianopia — Occipital lobe

Raised intracranial pressure
Ataxia
Nystagmus — Cerebellum
Cranial nerve lesions and posterior fossa

Temporal lobe — Memory and behavioural disturbances

Figure 6.2 Common presentation of brain tumour by site.

syndromes are all seen, including progressive altered mental state and personality, headaches, seizures and papilloedema. Focal symptoms depend upon the location of the tumour (Figure 6.2). Although seizures are a feature of up to half of all glial tumours, fewer than 10% of first fits are due to tumours and only 20% of supratentorial tumours present with fits.

Meningioma

These tumours, which are more common in women, present as slowly growing masses producing headaches, seizures, motor and sensory symptoms and cranial neuropathies, depending on their site (Table 6.5 and Figure 6.3). Meningiomas are some of the few tumours that produce characteristic changes on plain skull X-rays with bone erosion, calcification and hyperostosis (excess growth of bone) (Figure 6.4).

Spinal axis tumours

The sites of spinal axis tumours are 50% thoracic, 30% lumbosacral and 20% cervical or foramen magnum. These tumours present with radicular symptoms due to nerve root infiltration, syringomyelic disturbance (dissociated sensory loss of pain and temperature sensation) due to central destruction by

intramedullary tumours, or sensorimotor dysfunction (limb weakness and a sensory level) due to cord compression.

Investigation and staging

Neuroradiology has developed into the most important investigation in patients with suspected brain tumours, following the introduction of computed tomography (CT) in the mid-1970s by Geoffrey Hounsfield and magnetic resonance imaging (MRI) in the 1980s. Newer techniques, such as positron emission tomography (PET), single photon emission computerized tomography (SPECT) and functional MRI have also found roles in the diagnosis and management of patients with brain tumours. MRI with gadolinium enhancement is the imaging technique of choice with advantages over CT particularly for posterior fossa tumours and non-enhancing low-grade gliomas (see figures in Chapter 1). PET with fluorodeoxyglucose-18, which accumulates in metabolically active tissues, may help to differentiate tumour recurrence from radiation necrosis (Figure 6.4). Stereotactic biopsy is required to confirm

Table 6.5 Clinical features of meningiomas by site

Tumour site	Clinical features
Parasagittal falx	Progressive spastic weakness Numbness of legs
Olfactory groove	Anosmia Visual loss Papilloedema (Foster–Kennedy syndrome) Frontal lobe syndrome
Sella turcica	Visual field loss
Sphenoid ridge	Cavernous sinus syndrome (medial) Exophthalmos and visual loss (middle) Temporal bone swelling and skull deformity (lateral)
Posterior fossa (foramen magnum, tentorium)	Hydrocephalus (tentorium) Gait ataxia and cranial neuropathies V, VII, VIII, IX and X (cerebellopontine angle) Suboccipital pain, ipsilateral arm and leg weakness (foramen magnum)

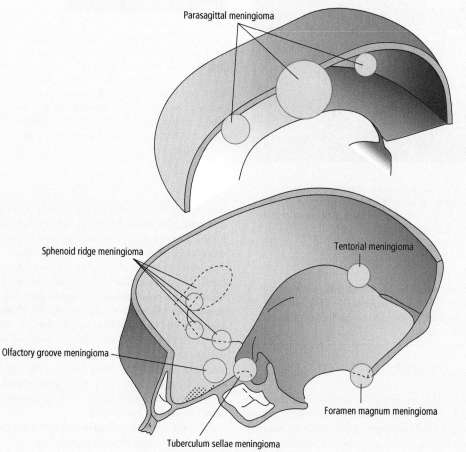

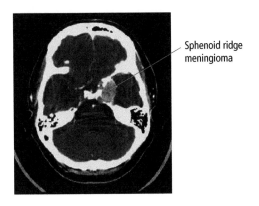

Sphenoid ridge
meningioma

Figure 6.3 CT scan image of meningioma.

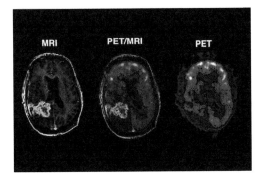

Figure 6.4 Co-registered and separate MRI and
18-fluorodeoxyglucose PET scan images from a patient
with a paraventricular high-grade glioma, demonstrating
high glucose utilization by the tumour.

the diagnosis, although occasionally tumours are diagnosed on clinical evidence, because biopsy might
be hazardous, for example, in brain stem gliomas.

Treatment

Some gliomas are curable by surgery alone and some
by surgery and radiotherapy; the remainder require
surgery, radiotherapy and chemotherapy, and these
tumours are rarely curable. Surgical removal should
be as complete as possible within the constraints of
preserving neurological function. Radiation can increase the cure rate or prolonged disease-free survival
in high-grade gliomas and may also be useful symptomatic therapy in patients with low-grade glioma,
who relapse after initial therapy with surgery alone

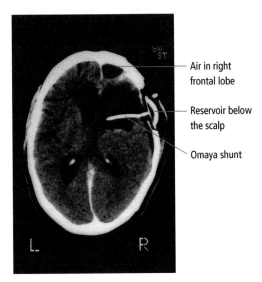

Air in right
frontal lobe

Reservoir below
the scalp

Omaya shunt

Figure 6.5 CT scan from a patient showing an Omaya
shunt (a closed cerebrospinal fluid (CSF) shunt joining the
lateral ventricle with a reservoir below the scalp) in place that
is leaking, resulting in air seen in the right anterior brain and
fluid accumulating around the shunt site. Omaya shunts
may be placed to relieve non-communicating
hydrocephalus caused by obstruction to CSF flow within
the ventricular system, or to administer intrathecal
chemotherapy.

(Figure 6.5). Newer radiotherapy delivery techniques
that have been pioneered in the treatment of brain
tumours include both Gamma Knife and CyberKnife
treatments, which have caught the attention and
interest of the gently dozing neurosurgeon in the multidisciplinary team. Gamma Knife radiotherapy is delivered by 201 cobalt-60 sources arranged in a ring in a
helmet that is bolted to the patient's skull. CyberKnife
radiotherapy uses a linear accelerator to deliver
radiotherapy via a robotic arm that is linked to an
image guidance system. CyberKnife radiotherapy
does not need a skull frame because the real-time
image linking means that if the patient moves, the
robotic arm also moves so that the radiotherapy dose
is delivered to the correct site.

Chemotherapy with lipid-soluble nitrosoureas or
temozolomide may prolong disease-free survival in
patients with oligodendrogliomas and high-grade
gliomas, although its high toxicity may not always
merit this approach. One recent advance is the
use of biodegradable wafers implanted with BCNU
chemotherapy that may be inserted at the time of
surgery. Gene therapy has been adopted for trials in

gliomas with viral vectors being administered either into the blood or directly into the tumour by surgeons. The genetically modified viral vectors may be non-replicating viruses that deliver a transgene that causes an anticancer effect, or replicating oncolytic viruses that directly lyse cancer cells by replicating. Gliomas are a good model to try these methods because they are pretty much the only cells dividing in the brain (apart from microglia and endothelial cells). Similarly, anti-angiogenic therapies chiefly targeting vascular endothelial growth factor (VEGF) are used in clinical trials in high-grade glioma. Another line of research in gliomas has focussed on the development of immunotherapy targeting HER2 expression and autologous dendritic cell therapies. Similarly, some gliomas have activation of the AKT intracellular signalling pathway and this can be targeted by a number of drugs in development. The name AKT originates from the inbred strain of mouse that developed spontaneous lymphomas from which the AKT protein kinase was identified.

Therapy of meningiomas is surgical resection, which may be repeated at relapse. Radiotherapy reduces relapse rates and should be considered for high-grade meningiomas or incompletely resected tumours. Relapse rates are 7% at 5 years if completely resected and 35–60% if incompletely resected.

Unlike with other brain tumours, surgical resection does not have a useful role in primary cerebral lymphomas. In immunocompetent patients, the combination of chemotherapy and radiotherapy produces median survivals of 40 months. In contrast, in the immunocompromised patients, especially those with HIV infection, the prognosis is far worse, with a median survival of under 3 months. Palliative radiotherapy or best supportive care is the appropriate treatment options here.

Complications of treatment

Early complications of cranial radiotherapy which occur in the first 3–4 months are due to reversible damage to myelin-producing oligodendrocytes. This recovers spontaneously after 3–6 months. It causes somnolence or exacerbation of existing symptoms in the brain and Lhermitte's sign (shooting numbness or paraesthesia down the back and limbs precipitated by neck flexion) in the cord. Late complications include radiation necrosis, causing irreversible neu-

Table 6.6 Five-year survival rates of adult patients with brain tumours

Tumour	5-year survival
Grade I glioma (cerebellar)	90–100%
Grade I glioma (other sites)	50–60%
Grade II (astrocytoma)	16–46%
Grade III (anaplastic astrocytoma)	10–30%
Grade IV (glioblastoma multiforme)	1–10%
Oligodendroglioma	50–80%
Meningioma	70–80%

rological deficits due to damage to blood vessels. This may mimic disease recurrence; it is radiation dose related and occurs in up to 15% of patients, with the highest frequency in children who have also received chemotherapy. PET scanning may differentiate radionecrosis and relapse.

Prognosis

The prognosis of glial tumours depends upon the histology, the grade and size of the tumour, on the age and performance status of the patient and on the duration of the symptoms (Table 6.6). The median survival for anaplastic astrocytoma is 2–5 years, and for glioblastoma multiforme is 10–14 months. Meningiomas, if completely resected, are usually cured and the median survival is over 10 years.

 ONLINE RESOURCE

Case Study: The consultant's mother.

 KEY POINTS

- Metastases to the brain are more common than primary brain tumours
- Most CNS cancers in adults are gliomas or meningiomas and are supratentorial
- CNS tumours usually present with fits, signs of raised intracranial pressure or disrupted function related to the location of the tumour

7

Oesophageal cancer

Learning objectives

✓ Explain the epidemiology and pathogenesis of oesophageal cancer
✓ Recognize the common presentation and clinical features of oesophageal cancer
✓ Describe the treatment strategies and outcomes of oesophageal cancer

---

The British playwright Harold Pinter was diagnosed with cancer of the oesophagus and wrote the eloquent poem 'Cancer Cells', whilst undergoing chemoradiotherapy, which illustrates his understanding of the molecular basis of cancer. The poem can be read at: http://www.theguardian.com/books/2002/mar/14/poetry.haroldpinter.

Epidemiology and pathogenesis

Cancer of the oesophagus is a relatively uncommon cancer in the United Kingdom with 8332 diagnoses and 7603 deaths in 2011, but the incidence is rising, at least in men (Table 7.1) and causes awful suffering. Oesophageal cancer is rare under the age of 45 and the incidence rises steeply with age. It is two to three times more frequent in men. Worldwide, oesophageal cancer is the sixth most common cause of death from cancer and it is 20–30 times more common in China than in the United States.

Two-thirds of cases of oesophageal cancer are adenocarcinomas, typically of the lowest third of the oesophagus, whilst one-third of cases are squamous cell cancers occurring usually in the upper two-thirds of the oesophagus. The incidence of adenocarcinoma relative to squamous cancer is rising. Tobacco is a major risk factor for both histological types of oesophageal cancer, but the two types otherwise vary not only in their histology and anatomical distribution but also in their risk factors. Chronic irritation appears to be a major precipitant of squamous cell cancer and may be caused by alcohol, caustic injury, radiotherapy or untreated achalasia. The Plummer–Vinson syndrome (also known as Patterson–Kelly–Brown syndrome) of chronic iron deficiency anaemia, dysphagia and oesophageal web is associated with squamous cell cancer of the oesophagus, particularly in impoverished populations. Tylosis is an autosomal dominant abnormality, characterized by hyperkeratosis (skin thickening) of the palms and soles. It carries a 95% risk of squamous cell cancer of the oesophagus by the age of 70. Chewing betel quid or paan, a mixture of betel leaf, areca nut and slaked lime causes mild euphoria and stains your teeth red. It also

---

Oncology: Lecture Notes, Third Edition. Mark Bower and Jonathan Waxman.
© 2015 by John Wiley & Sons, Ltd. Published 2015 by John Wiley & Sons, Ltd.
Companion Website: www.lecturenoteseries.com/oncology

Table 7.1 UK registrations for oesophageal cancer 2010

	Percentage of all cancer registrations		Rank of registration		Lifetime risk of cancer		Change in ASR (2000–2010)		5-year overall survival	
	Female	Male	Female	Male	Female	Male	Female	Male	Female	Male
Oesophageal cancer	2	3	13th	8th	1 in 110	1 in 56	–9%	+7%	12%	13%

increases the risk of both cancers of the oral cavity and squamous cell cancer of the oesophagus.

In contrast, the major precipitant of oesophageal adenocarcinoma appears to be gastro-oesophageal reflux disease (GORD). Related markers of reflux, such as hiatus hernia, obesity, frequent antacid and histamine H2 blockers, are also associated with an increased risk. Barrett's oesophagus (named after Norman Barrett, a thoracic surgeon at St Thomas' Hospital, London) is an acquired premalignant condition that develops in 5–8% of adults with reflux leading to metaplasia of the normal squamous epithelium of the lower oesophagus to columnar epithelium, which may become dysplastic, see Box 1.2. Other causes of distal oesophageal irritation such as hiatus hernia, achalasia and scleroderma can also lead to Barrett's oesophagus and overall it affects 0.5–2% of the adult population. The annual rate of transformation from Barrett's oesophagus to oesophageal adenocarcinoma is 0.12%, which is 11 times greater than the normal risk. The risk is highest for obese white men over 45 years old who smoke. Over the last three decades, there has been a radical shift in the histology of oesophageal cancer in the industrialized world, with a marked decline in squamous cell cancers and a rise in adenocarcinomas. This may reflect alterations in the number of smokers and in the obesity and nutrition of patients.

Prevention

Half of all cases of oesophageal cancer could be prevented by giving up smoking, drinking less alcohol and improving diet, substituting fresh fruit and vegetables for poorly preserved, high salt foods contaminated with nitrosamine carcinogens or microbial toxins. Endoscopic surveillance is recommended every 2–5 years for patients with Barrett's oesophagus, but the evidence that screening is effective is absent. Low-grade dysplasia requires aggressive anti-reflux

management, whilst multifocal or high-grade dysplasia should be treated by surgical resection.

Presentation

Patients present with dysphagia or odynophagia (pain on swallowing), weight loss and, less frequently, with haematemesis. At the time of diagnosis, more than half of the patients will have locally advanced, unresectable disease or metastases present. Left supraclavicular lymphadenopathy (Virchow's node), hepatomegaly and pleural effusion are common features of metastatic dissemination. Rudolf Virchow is said to have described the association after diagnosing it in himself. He also challenged Bismarck to a duel with sausages but that is another story. The diagnosis is usually confirmed by upper gastrointestinal endoscopy (Figure 7.1) and barium studies (Figure 7.2).

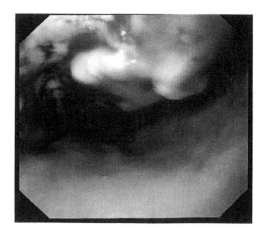

Figure 7.1 Endoscopic view of cancer of the mid-oesophagus.

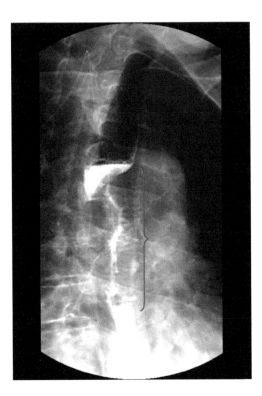

Figure 7.2 Oesophageal cancer. Gastrografin swallow image showing a long tight stricture of the distal third of the oesophagus with shouldering that encroaches on the gastro-oesophageal junction. This malignant stricture was due to adenocarcinoma of the oesophagus.

Staging and grading

Although CT or PET-CT staging is most helpful in defining operability and presence of nodal involvement (Figure 7.3), additional information can be obtained from using endoscopic ultrasound which is able to evaluate the depth of invasion. This allows the surgeon to have a better view as to the extent of the resection that is required.

Treatment

Only 40% of patients will have localized disease at presentation and are candidates for oesophagectomy with or without neoadjuvant or postoperative adjuvant chemoradiation. Oesophagectomy shortens the oesophagus so a section of the stomach is pulled up into the chest cavity (Figure 7.4). Adjuvant chemoradiotherapy, either prior to surgery (neoadjuvant), or following resection, appears to improve survival but the gain is likely to be modest. Surgery has a 5–10% mortality rate and may be complicated early by anastomotic leaks, and later by strictures, reflux and motility disorders. At diagnosis, 25% of patients will have local extension and are treated with palliative radiotherapy, which may cause oesophageal perforation and haemorrhage, pneumonitis and pulmonary fibrosis, as well as transverse myelitis (inflammation of the spinal cord leading to sensory, motor and sphincter deficits). The remaining 35% of patients will have metastases at presentation and are usually treated symptomatically or with palliative chemotherapy if they are fit. Although cancer of the oesophagus is sensitive to chemotherapy, the duration of response is typically short and may be measured in weeks. Cisplatin-based combination regimens have higher response rates, but this may be offset by their greater toxicity. Symptomatic relief from dysphagia in patients unsuitable for surgery may be achieved by endoscopically placed oesophageal self-expandable metallic stents or plastic stents (see Figure 3.5).

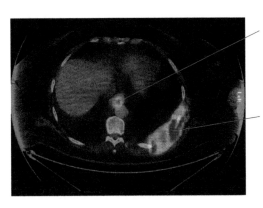

FDG uptake within mid-to-distal oesophagus associated with concentric mural thickening

FDG uptake in left posterior rib destructive metastasis

Figure 7.3 PET-CT scan of metastatic squamous cell cancer of the oesophagus.

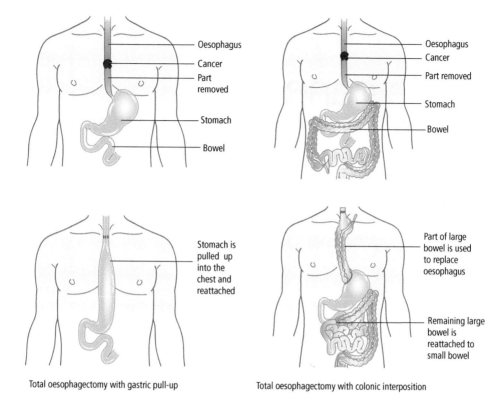

Total oesophagectomy with gastric pull-up   Total oesophagectomy with colonic interposition

Figure 7.4 Types of total oesophagectomy. Reproduced with permission of CancerHelp UK.

Table 7.2 Five-year survival rates of patients with oesophageal cancer, according to stage at presentation

Stage	T stage (local tumour)	N stage (nodal status)	M stage (metastatic status)	5-year survival
0	Tis	N0	M0	>95%
I	T1	N0	M0	50–80%
IIA	T2–3	N0	M0	30–40%
IIB	T1–2	N1	M0	10–30%
III	T3–4	N0–1	M0	10–15%
IV	Any T	Any N	M1	<2%

Tis, carcinoma *in situ*; T1, invasion of lamina propria; T2, invasion of muscularis propria; T3, invasion of adventitia; T4, invasion of adjacent structures.

 ONLINE RESOURCE

Case Study: An actuary with a leak.

 KEY POINTS

- Two-thirds of cancers of the oesophagus are adenocarcinomas of the lower one-third and smoking and gastro-oesophageal reflux disease (GORD) are the main risk factors
- One-third of cancers of the oesophagus are squamous cell cancers of the upper two-thirds and smoking and chronic irritation including alcohol are the main risk factors
- Patients present with dysphagia, odynophagia and weight loss
- Only a minority of patients present with potentially curable disease

Prognosis

The 5-year survival rates of patients with oesophageal cancer according to stage at presentation are detailed in Table 7.2.

8

Gastric cancer

Learning objectives

✓ Explain the epidemiology and pathogenesis of gastric cancer
✓ Recognize the common presentation and clinical features of gastric cancer
✓ Describe the treatment strategies and outcomes of gastric cancer

Epidemiology and pathogenesis

Gastric cancer is the 13th most common malignancy in the United Kingdom and constitutes approximately 2% of all cancers. The male-to-female ratio is 1.5:1. In 2010, nearly 7266 people were diagnosed with stomach cancer in the United Kingdom and 4830 died of stomach cancer. The average age at presentation is 65 years. The survival for gastric cancer has tripled over the last 25 years but currently only 18% of patients are alive 5 years after diagnosis (Table 8.1). Surprisingly, gastric cancer is the second most common cause of cancer deaths worldwide with 988,000 new diagnoses in 2008. There are extreme geographical variations, with the incidence being five times higher in Japan than in the United States.

The incidence of gastric cancer has fallen in the industrialized world over the last few decades. This is particularly the case for distal tumours of the stomach. It had been thought that one of the reasons for the decrease in the West is better food refrigeration and decline in the use of salt as a food preservative. Whilst smoking increases the risk of stomach cancer, diet also has an important role. Higher consumption of citrus fruit, allium vegetables (the onion family) and brassicas (the cabbage family) all reduce the risk; so eat fresh fruit and vegetables. In contrast, a high salt intake (>6 g/day) and Asian pickled vegetables increase the risk of stomach cancer.

In 1926, the Nobel Prize for medicine was awarded to a Dane, Dr Johannes Fibiger, who had described a nematode worm that he called *Spiroptera carcinoma*, which caused stomach cancers in rats that he caught in an infested sugar refinery. It was subsequently shown that the cancers were in fact only metaplasia and that the cause was vitamin A deficiency. Although Fibiger has been branded a fibber, it turns out that chronic infection is the cause of most human gastric cancers. The single most common cause of gastric cancer is infection with *Helicobacter pylori*: probably the most common chronic bacterial infection in man. This bacterium colonizes over half of the world's population. Infection is usually acquired in childhood and, in the absence of antibiotic therapy, persists for the life of the host. How *H. pylori* causes gastric cancer remains unclear. Strains that have cytotoxin-associated gene (CagA) are more oncogenic and the products of these genes regulate protein secretion by epithelial cells. In addition, chronic *H. pylori* infection leads to the local production of inflammatory cytokines that are also thought to be involved in oncogenesis. Infection by *H. pylori* explains the aetiology of cancers developing in patients with atrophic gastritis. *Helicobacter* infection is more common in patients with gastric cancer than in "controls", particularly in younger patients.

Oncology: Lecture Notes, Third Edition. Mark Bower and Jonathan Waxman.
© 2015 by John Wiley & Sons, Ltd. Published 2015 by John Wiley & Sons, Ltd.
Companion Website: www.lecturenoteseries.com/oncology

Table 8.1 UK registrations for gastric cancer 2010

	Percentage of all cancer registrations		Rank of registration		Lifetime risk of cancer		Change in ASR (2000–2010)		5-year overall survival	
	Female	Male	Female	Male	Female	Male	Female	Male	Female	Male
Gastric cancer	2	3	14th	10th	1 in 120	1 in 64	−28%	−32%	17%	18%

Presentation

Patients with gastric cancer generally present to their general practitioner with symptoms of abdominal pain. Classically, the pain is epigastric and worse with meals. The differential diagnosis includes benign peptic ulceration. The routine prescription of protein pump inhibitors, without investigation by endoscopy, may lead to late diagnosis and the presence of advanced disease at diagnosis. Because the symptoms of gastric cancer are very similar to those of peptic ulceration and because peptic ulceration is very common and not necessarily routinely investigated, early diagnosis of gastric cancer in the West presents a difficult problem. Fewer than 2% of patients with first-time dyspepsia will have gastric cancer but the risk is greater in people over 55 years and those with dysphagia, vomiting, weight loss, anorexia or symptoms of gastrointestinal bleeding. Walk-in endoscopy clinics, however, are becoming much more widely available in the United Kingdom, and it is hoped that they will impact upon survival figures for gastric cancer.

After initial assessment, which should include a full blood count, liver function tests and chest X-ray, more specialized investigations should be undertaken. These should include endoscopy with biopsy, ultrasonography and CT imaging of the abdomen and chest. There have been advances in endoscopic ultrasound that have allowed improvements in local staging of gastric tumours. These improvements are such that mucosal invasion can be distinguished from submucosal invasion. The majority of patients with gastric cancer present with inoperable disease; only 20% of patients have disease that is potentially curable.

Staging and pathology

The TNM staging system is widely used for staging gastric cancer, as with all TNM staging it may be modified by a prefix and a suffix (Table 8.2).

Table 8.2 Prefixes used to qualify TNM staging

Prefix	Means staging is based on:
c	Clinical examination
p	Pathological examination of a surgical specimen
y	Assessment after neoadjuvant therapy
r	Assessment of recurrence
a	Assessment at autopsy
Suffix	
G (1–4)	Grade of tumour
R (0–2)	Completeness of resection margins (none, microscopic, macroscopic)
L (0–1)	Invasion into lymphatic vessels (none, present)
V (0–2)	Invasion into veins (none, microscopic, macroscopic)

Ninety-five per cent of all gastric tumours are adenocarcinomas. The remainder are squamous cell cancers and lymphomas. Small cell cancers are reported only rarely. In around 5% of the cases, the stomach wall is diffusely involved by cancer resulting in a rigid thick stomach wall called linitis plastica or leather bottle stomach.

Treatment

Surgery

The only significant chance for a cure rests with surgery. Laparoscopic staging is carried out prior to definitive laparotomy. There is considerable debate concerning the operative procedures of first choice. Older retrospective data suggested that survival was improved with total gastrectomy compared with subtotal gastrectomy. Current practice is total

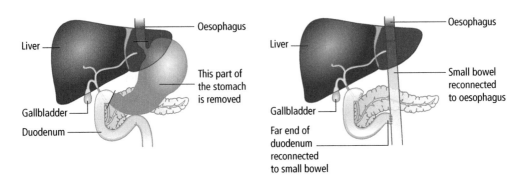

Figure 8.1 Total gastrectomy with Roux-en-Y anastomosis. (Roux-en-Y anastomosis is named after a Swiss surgeon, César Roux rather than the restaurateur brothers of the same surname.) Reproduced with permission of CancerHelp UK.

gastrectomy for proximal tumours in the upper third of the stomach and subtotal gastrectomy with resection of adjacent lymph nodes for distal lower two-thirds cancers (Figures 8.1 and 8.2). The operative mortality in the United Kingdom varies from 5% to 14% and is directly related to the number of these operations performed by the surgeon.

Surgical developments have been led by the Japanese, who have to deal with the highest incidence of carcinoma of the stomach in the world. The current recommendation by the Japanese Society for Research in Gastric Cancer is for extensive lymphadenectomy, which involves the removal of the lymphatic chains along the coeliac axis and hepatic and splenic arteries. This sort of dissection also has the advantage of allowing more accurate staging for gastric cancer and has been associated with improved survival. Tumours of the gastro-oesophageal junction are increasing in the West and are treated surgically by subtotal resection of the oesophagus, along with the cardia and gastric fundus.

A few patients are diagnosed with early-stage disease where the cancer is confined to the mucosa and submucosa, most commonly in patients who are on an endoscopic surveillance programme in East Asian countries with high incidences of gastric cancer. These early-stage-localized gastric cancers may be treated with curative endoscopic mucosal resection and survival is in excess of 90%. Advances in endoscopy, endoscopic ultrasonography and endoscopic surgery thus have produced great improvements in limiting the morbidity of interventional therapies. Significant improvements have been seen in Japan as a result of the wide-scale implementation of screening endoscopy. In Japan, up to 40% of patients are found to have early-stage tumours, which contrasts with the situation in the West.

Adjuvant treatment

A large randomized trial showed that perioperative chemotherapy (before and after surgery) increased

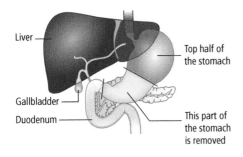

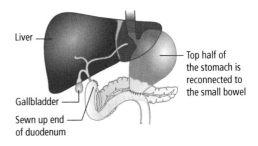

Figure 8.2 Partial gastrectomy. Reproduced with permission of CancerHelp UK.

rates of surgery, progression-free survival and overall survival in gastric cancer. The most widely used chemotherapy regimens are epirubicin, cisplatin and infusional 5-fluorouracil (5FU) (ECF) or epirubicin, cisplatin and capecitabine (ECX).

Treatment of metastatic or locally inoperable gastric cancer

Patients with inoperable local disease or metastases may be treated with palliative chemotherapy. Over the years, many treatment programmes have been introduced and the majority have contained 5FU. There is uncertainty as to whether or not combination therapy offers benefit. The response rates are higher but the overall survival is similar for combination chemotherapy compared with single-agent 5FU treatment. In the 1970s, there was considerable enthusiasm following the introduction of a combination therapy containing 5FU, adriamycin (doxorubicin) and mitomycin C. This treatment schedule, known as the "FAM regimen", was initially reported as leading to responses in 40% of patients, with a median duration of response of approximately 9 months. Randomized trials have since shown that the same order of response can be obtained with single-agent 5FU, with the same expectations of survival. In recent times, there has been considerable support for combination chemotherapy using epirubicin and cisplatin with either continuous infusion 5FU (ECF) or its oral prodrug capecitabine (ECX) or a combination of epirubicin, oxaliplatin and capecitabine (EOX). A surprising recent discovery is that about 20% of gastric cancers overexpress the epidermal growth factor receptor HER-2 and are thus potentially amenable to treatment with the monoclonal antibody trastuzumab or the small molecule lapatinib that targets this receptor in breast cancer too. Currently, NICE approves the use of trastuzumab for patients with metastatic gastric cancers that strongly overexpress HER-2. Occasionally, bleeding from inoperable tumours may be alleviated by embolization (Figure 8.3) or radiotherapy.

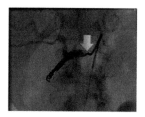 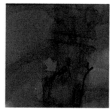

Figure 8.3 Coil embolization, using a detachable platinum coil inserted by interventional radiologist. To reduce haemorrhage from a primary gastric tumour, selective catheterisation of the gastroduodenal artery () was followed by coil embolisation ().

Survival

In the West, more than two-thirds of patients present with advanced tumours. The median survival of patients with advanced local disease or metastatic tumour is approximately 6 months.

ONLINE RESOURCE

Case Study: The belly of an emperor.

KEY POINTS

- The most common cause of gastric cancer is infection with *Helicobacter pylori* and in the United Kingdom the incidence of gastric cancer is falling whilst the survival is rising
- Patients with gastric cancer present with epigastric pain indistinguishable from peptic ulcer disease but dysphagia, vomiting, weight loss, anorexia or symptoms of gastrointestinal bleeding all make the diagnosis of cancer more likely

9

Hepatobiliary cancer

Learning objectives

✓ Explain the epidemiology and pathogenesis of liver cancer

✓ Recognize the common presentation and clinical features of liver cancer

✓ Describe the treatment strategies and outcomes of liver cancer

Epidemiology

Hepatobiliary cancer is the sixth most common malignant tumour in the world. The highest incidences are seen in South East Asia. In the United Kingdom, hepatobiliary cancer is relatively uncommon. In 2011, 4348 men and women were registered with liver cancer and sadly 4106 died. The male to female ratio for liver cancers is 1.7:1 and the risk rises with increasing age with 90% diagnosed in people over 55 years of age. In the United Kingdom the 5-year survival for patients with this cancer is just 5% (see Table 9.1).

Pathogenesis

Primary liver cancers are divided into four main groups of tumour:

- Hepatocellular cancer (HCC), also called hepatoma, is derived from hepatocyte cells (75%)
- Biliary tree cancers, also known as cholangiocarcinomas, are derived from cells lining the bile ducts (25%)
- Angiosarcoma derived from cells of the blood vessel of the liver (1–2%)
- Hepatoblastomas derived from immature liver cells chiefly affects children (80% liver tumours in those <15 years old)

The aetiology and clinical management of these different tumours varies. HCC is associated with chronic infection with hepatitis B virus (HBV) and hepatitis C virus (HCV). Around 2 billion people worldwide are infected with HBV and 10% of people infected with HBV develop chronic HBV, whilst 170 million people are infected with HCV and >80% develop chronic HCV infection if left untreated (see Table 2.10).

Table 9.1 UK registrations for hepatobiliary cancer 2010

	Percentage of all cancer registrations		Rank of registration		Lifetime risk of cancer		Change in ASR (2000–2010)		5-year overall survival	
	Female	Male	Female	Male	Female	Male	Female	Male	Female	Male
Liver cancer	1	2	19th	14th	1 in 215	1 in 120	+31%	+44%	5.7%	5.1%

Chronic HBV infection is prevalent in up to 15% of males in certain populations and the lifetime risk of developing HCC is 40% in this group of men. An epidemiological study of 22,707 Taiwanese male government employees followed over 10 years found that the relative risk of liver cancer was 98 for men with HBV. To put this risk into context, the relative risk for lung cancer amongst smokers is around 17. In a study from the National Cancer Centre in Korea, 74.6% of the patients with HCC were HBV positive. The HBV genome encodes four proteins: C (core protein), P (a DNA polymerase), S (surface antigen) and X (whose function is not clear but acts as a weak oncogene) (see Chapter 2). How chronic HBV causes cancer is unclear, but it is thought that the constant proliferation of hepatocytes caused by the need to replace virus-damaged cells and the chronic inflammatory response in the liver are the main culprits. Support for this hypothesis comes from HCV-induced liver cancer. HBV and HCV are very different viruses genetically, but both cause similar chronic infection and inflammation of the liver and both are associated with a high risk of liver cancer.

In terms of the model for chemical carcinogenesis, these viruses appear to act as tumour promoters rather than initiators. This is supported by synergism in risk between chronic HBV infection and mutagens such as aflatoxin B1. Aflatoxin B1 is derived from the fungus *Aspergillus fumigatus* which commonly infects foods such as peanuts that are stored in damp conditions and which causes mutation of p53. In one study from China, the relative risk of liver cancer in people with chronic HBV was 7, in those exposed to aflatoxin was 3, but in those exposed to both chronic HBV and aflatoxin was 60.

HCC are associated with other causes of chronic liver damage including alcoholism and other hepatitides causing cirrhosis such as primary biliary cirrhosis, haemochromatosis and acute and chronic hepatic porphyrias (acute intermittent porphyria, porphyria cutanea tarda, hereditary coproporphyria and variegate porphyria).

Tumours of the biliary tree are divided into (Figures 9.1 and 9.2):

- intrahepatic bile duct cancers (which are treated in the same way as HCCs).
- perihilar cholangiocarcinomas (also known as Klatskin tumours) occurring at bifurcation of hepatic ducts.
- extrahepatic cholangiocarcinomas.
- gallbladder cancers.

Biliary tree tumours occur at increased frequency in primary sclerosing cholangitis with a lifetime risk of developing cholangiocarcinoma of 10–20%. Congenital conditions that cause dilatation of the biliary tract such as choledochal cysts and Caroli's disease also transform into cholangiocarcinoma in 25% of patients. Gallstones and cholecystectomy do not influence the risk of biliary tree cancer. In South East Asia, where these tumours are common, they are seen in association with biliary infestation with liver flukes (*Clonorchis sinensis* and *Opisthorchis viverrini*) that affect 30 million people worldwide (see Table 2.12).

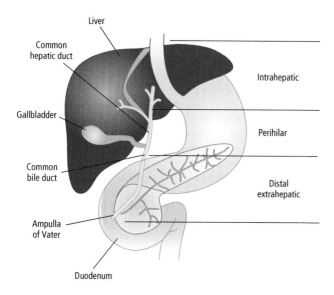

Figure 9.1 Anatomy of biliary tract cancers.

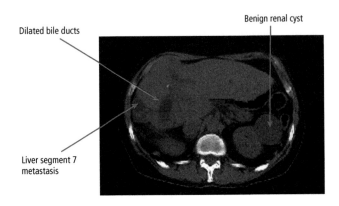

Benign renal cyst

Dilated bile ducts

Liver segment 7 metastasis

Figure 9.2 CT scan demonstrating intrahepatic dilated bile ducts that were due to cholangiocarcinoma. There is also a low attenuation metastasis in segment 7 of the liver and an incidental (benign) renal cyst.

The aetiology of hepatoblastoma is not known. Hepatic angiosarcoma is associated with exposure to the vinyl chloride monomer (VCM), choloroethene (C_2H_3Cl) that is polymerized to the plastic polyvinyl chloride (PVC), that is used to make everything from vinyl records and PVC trousers to guttering and catheters. The mechanism for this is not clear, and the development of this tumour does not always occur in those men and women who have the heaviest exposure to VCM, as for example, in those workers involved in autoclave cleaning in chemical works. When workers exposed to VCM are examined for their lifetime risk of developing angiosarcoma this is overall clearly four times higher than in the general population. Where there is a coincident HBV infection, the risk increases 25-fold compared with the general population.

Prevention

The central role of hepatitis viruses in the aetiology of HCC offers opportunities for primary prevention, eradication and screening as strategies to prevent cancer. A vaccine based on the surface antigen envelope protein of HBV (HBVsAg) protects against the acquisition of HBV. The widespread introduction of this vaccine in Taiwan has been shown to reduce the risk of HCC in children and a similar protection in adults is likely. Second, antiviral therapy against hepatitis B that is effective at lowering HBV titres may reduce the risk of liver cancer amongst people with chronic HBV. Similarly, therapy for chronic HCV may also reduce the risk of HCC in chronically infected individuals and recent advances have led to combination treatments that have high rates of clearing HCV without the use of interferons. Finally, screening people with

chronic HCV and HBV may reduce the mortality of liver cancer by diagnosing patients earlier with surgically resectable HCC. Liver ultrasound and serum α-fetoprotein (AFP) screening should be performed every 6 months in patients with chronic HBV or HCV. There are significant concerns with regard to the increasing infection rates with hepatitis C in Europe. It is thought that the risk of developing hepatobiliary cancer in the presence of chronic hepatitis C infection is even greater than that associated with hepatitis B infection.

Presentation

Patients with hepatobiliary cancer generally present with advanced disease. Typical presentations are with jaundice, liver pain and weight loss. A patient with a suspected diagnosis of hepatobiliary cancer should be referred to the appropriate surgical unit for investigation. The management of these conditions is very complex and should only be in centres of excellence with highly specialized surgical units, who achieve significantly better results.

Standard investigations for patients with HCC should include blood counts, liver function tests, renal function tests, chest X-rays, ultrasound assessment and CT imaging. Ultrasonography has developed considerably over the last decade, and these technical improvements have been matched by improved standards in endoscopic assessment of the patient. Hepatobiliary cancers are associated with raised serum levels of AFP, which is characteristically raised to many thousands of ng/mL. In patients with cirrhosis, who may have AFP levels raised to a few hundreds of ng/mL, increasing levels point to the development of hepatobiliary cancer. Surprisingly, those

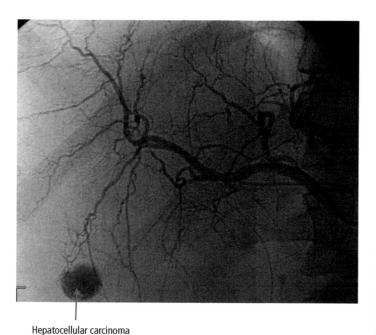

Hepatocellular carcinoma

Figure 9.3 Selective angiography of the right hepatic artery showing a small area of hypervascularity due to hepatocellular carcinoma. As this was inoperable (there were four other lesions in different segments of the liver), it was treated by transcatheter arterial chemoembolization (TACE).

patients whose tumours do not secrete AFP are more likely to have favourable outcomes. Hepatobiliary tumours produce other serum markers such as carcinoembryonic antigen (CEA) and carbohydrate antigen 19-9 (CA19-9) which may also be useful in the monitoring progress. The diagnosis of HCC may often be established non-invasively using dynamic imaging modalities (CT, MRI or contrast-enhanced ultrasound) and this avoids the risk of tumour spread at biopsy.

Characteristically, patients with cholangiocarcinoma present with obstructive jaundice and usually require biliary drainage. This can be achieved either by a radiologist placing a percutaneous transhepatic biliary drain (PTBD) or by endoscopic retrograde cholangiopancreatogram (ERCP) and placement of a biliary stent. Histological confirmation of the diagnosis of cholangiocarcinoma is usually made at ERCP with needle aspiration or brush cytology or by radiological guided percutaneous biopsy.

Staging and grading

Hepatobiliary tumours are described as well, moderately or poorly differentiated. Staging for hepatic and biliary tract tumours is according to the TNM classification.

Treatment

Liver resection is the only treatment that offers a chance for cure for liver cancer. Surgery is limited by the degree of spread of the tumour and the presence or absence of background cirrhosis. The aim of surgery generally is to remove the lobe of the liver containing the tumour. Liver transplantation is potentially curative for patients with solitary HCC <5 cm or up to 3 nodules all <3 cm yielding 5-year survival rates above 70%; however, just 10% of patients with liver cancers have operable tumours. When curative surgery is not possible, hepatic transarterial chemoembolization (TACE), percutaneous tumour ablation including radiofrequency ablation sclerotherapy (see Figure 3.12) and systemic anticancer therapy may be appropriate (Figure 9.3). Sorafenib, an oral receptor tyrosine kinase inhibitor that inhibits angiogenesis, has emerged as a valuable palliative treatment for unresectable HCC that prolongs median overall survival from 5.5 to 9.2 months. Unfortunately, treatment with this agent is not allowed in England as a result of an inappropriate, in the view of most oncologists and their patients, decision by NICE.

Table 9.2 Five-year survival rates of patients with hepatic and biliary tract cancers

Tumour	5-year survival
Hepatocellular cancer	5%
Gallbladder cancer	5%
Cholangiocarcinoma	5%
Periampullary cholangiocarcinoma	50%

Cholangiocarcinomas are chemosensitive but rarely operable. A combination of gemcitabine and cisplatin chemotherapy is currently the gold standard treatment for inoperable cholangiocarcinoma.

Prognosis

Five-year survival for patients with operable liver cancer is in the order of 33% when management involves partial liver resection. The 5-year survival of patients transplanted is 80%. The median survival of patients who are not treated with curative intent is 6–7 months (Table 9.2). The median survival of patients in the Far East is much poorer, and the vast majority die within 2–3 months of diagnosis.

 ONLINE RESOURCE

Case Study: The co-infected Côte d'Ivorian.

 KEY POINTS

- Liver cancer is the sixth most common cancer globally due mainly to infection with hepatitis B and C viruses but is much less frequent in the United Kingdom
- Screening people with chronic hepatitis virus infection and cirrhosis using ultrasound and blood tests of α-fetoprotein can detect tumours at an earlier stage when they are potentially curable by surgery
- Patients with liver cancer present with jaundice, pain and weight loss

10

Pancreatic cancer

Learning objectives

✓ Explain the epidemiology and pathogenesis of pancreatic cancer

✓ Recognize the common presentation and clinical features of pancreatic cancer

✓ Describe the treatment strategies and outcomes of pancreatic cancer

---

The list of celebrities who have died from cancer of the pancreas is lengthy, from the Dirty Dancing actor Patrick Swayze to the Apple founder Steve Jobs; amongst the casualties is Roger (Syd) Barrett the former singer and founder of the psychedelic progressive rock band Pink Floyd. Syd left the band in 1968 after 3 years and became a troubled recluse in Cambridge bothered by the paparazzi. In 1975 his former band mates released the album "Wish you were here" including the tribute track "Shine on you crazy diamond". We recommend that all students listen to a version of this song on YouTube.

Epidemiology

Cancer of the pancreas is the tenth most common cancer, and is now the fifth most frequent cause of cancer deaths. There is an equal incidence between the sexes. In 2011, there were 8733 new diagnoses and 8320 deaths attributed to cancer of the pancreas. It is very sad to note that registration figures virtually equal mortality rates. The 5-year survival is just 3% (Table 10.1).

Pathogenesis

Family history contributes to 5–10% pancreatic cancers and includes familial cancer predisposition syndromes as well as hereditary chronic pancreatitis (Table 10.2).

In addition to genetic predisposition, environmental causes have been associated with an increased risk of pancreatic cancer. Smoking increases the risk 1.5–3-fold; similarly, obesity and lack of physical exercise are risk factors. Chronic pancreatitis increases the risk three times and diabetes (both type 1 and type 2) doubles the risk.

Well over 90% of all pancreatic malignancies are exocrine adenocarcinomas, usually arising from ductal cells (85%) but cancers arising from acinar cells and stem cells are also included. You may recall that exocrine glands secrete their products into a duct whilst endocrine glands secrete directly into the bloodstream. Pancreatic exocrine cancers develop from ductal epithelial cells through a sequence of epithelial premalignant lesions known as pancreatic intraepithelial neoplasia, with the sequential accumulation of somatic mutations in genes including the oncogene K-RAS and the tumour suppressor genes: P53, P16/CDKN2A and SMAD4/DPC4. Pancreatic adenocarcinoma cells express a wide variety of receptors that are potential therapeutic targets including epidermal growth factor (EGF) receptors, vascular endothelial growth factor (VEGF) receptors and insulin-like growth factor (IGF) receptors. Pancreatic adenocarcinoma also expresses a wide variety of hormone receptors and these include receptors for somatostatin, gonadotropin-releasing hormone, steroid hormones, IGFs and VEGFs. It should be emphasized

---

Oncology: Lecture Notes, Third Edition. Mark Bower and Jonathan Waxman.
© 2015 by John Wiley & Sons, Ltd. Published 2015 by John Wiley & Sons, Ltd.
Companion Website: www.lecturenoteseries.com/oncology

Table 10.1 UK registrations for pancreatic cancer 2010

	Percentage of all cancer registrations		Rank of registration		Lifetime risk of cancer		Change in ASR (2000–2010)		5-year overall survival	
	Female	Male	Female	Male	Female	Male	Female	Male	Female	Male
Pancreatic cancer	3.8	3.6	8th	12th	1 in 74	1 in 73	+7%	+0%	3.8%	3.6%

that these receptors are present in exocrine pancreatic cancers but are rarely present in the uncommon secretory endocrine pancreatic tumours. The rare endocrine tumours of the pancreas are known as islet cell tumours or nesidioblastomas and include gastrinomas, insulinomas and pancreatic carcinoids. These tumours may be functional or non-secretory.

Presentation

Patients with cancer of the pancreas present with many different symptoms. These include abdominal and back pain, weight loss, anorexia and fatigue. In many patients the disease is asymptomatic, until they present with obstructive jaundice. Other, less common presentations include superficial venous thrombosis (Trousseau's sign), a palpable gallbladder in the presence of obstructive jaundice (Courvoisier's law states that this combination is unlikely to be due to gall stones) and diabetes. Because of the anatomical position of the tumour, late presentation is very common. The patient with a suspected diagnosis of pancreatic cancer should be referred by his or her GP to a general surgeon or a gastroenterologist and be seen in outpatients within 2 weeks of receipt of the GP's letter of referral. The clinician should organize a number of tests, which include full blood count, renal and liver function tests, a chest X-ray and a CT scan of the abdomen (Figure 10.1). Abdominal ultrasonography is also helpful but endoscopic ultrasound (EUS) is probably the most valuable diagnostic test when coupled with percutaneous needle biopsy. The measurement of serum levels of the carbohydrate antigen tumour marker CA19-9 is less helpful in the diagnosis of cancer of the pancreas as it may be elevated in most causes of obstructive jaundice (false positive) and may be normal in patients with pancreatic cancer (false negative). CA19-9 is, however, useful in monitoring cancer of the pancreas in patients with raised levels at diagnosis.

Table 10.2 Familial cancer predisposition syndromes that increase the risk of pancreatic cancer

Syndrome	Gene affected	Lifetime risk of cancer of pancreas
Hereditary pancreatitis	PRSS1	25–40%
Peutz–Jeghers syndrome	STK11	11–36%
Familial atypical multiple mole melanoma syndrome (FAMMM)	CDKN2A	10–19%
Hereditary breast ovary cancer syndrome	BRCA-2	3–5%
Lynch syndrome (hereditary non-polyposis colon cancer)	DNA mismatch repair genes	4%

Pancreatic cancer

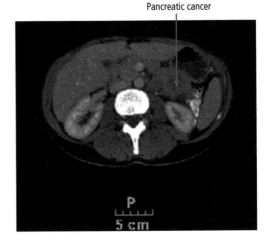

Figure 10.1 CT scan of a mass in the tail and body of the pancreas showing a low attenuation centre, suggesting central necrosis of an adenocarcinoma of the pancreas.

Investigation of the patient with pancreatic cancer is aimed at establishing the diagnosis and defining operability. After the initial tests have been carried out, the patient should proceed to EUS or, if not available, endoscopic retrograde cholangiopancreatography (ERCP). At ERCP, cytology specimens may be obtained from brushings, suction of the pancreatic duct or biopsy. ERCP is more invasive than other diagnostic imaging modalities and carries a significant complication rate so it is usually reserved for patients with biliary obstruction who require stenting. A failure to obtain a diagnosis by endoscopy should be followed by further investigation. Fine needle aspiration cytology under CT scan is usually successful at obtaining a tissue diagnosis.

Staging and grading

As with other cancers, numerous different staging systems are used including the TNM classification. The group staging system is summarized below:

- Stage I: cancer confined to the pancreas (T1N0M0 if <2 cm, T2N0M0 if >2 cm).
- Stage II: cancer has grown into the adjacent duodenum or bile duct but not spread to the lymph nodes (T3N0M0).
- Stage III: cancer has spread to the lymph nodes with (T3N1M0) or without (T1–2N1M0) direct tumour extension.
- Stage IV A: cancer has invaded into the stomach, spleen, colon or nearby large blood vessels and lymph nodes may (T4N1M0) or may not (T4N0M0) be involved.
- Stage IV B: there is spread to distant organs by metastases (T1–4N0–1M1).

The vast majority of pancreatic cancers are exocrine adenocarcinomas of ductal origin and they are graded as either well, moderately or poorly differentiated tumours. The tiny minority of endocrine tumours are classified according to the products that they secrete.

Treatment

There is considerable nihilism attached, quite reasonably, to the treatment of a patient with pancreatic cancer. The initial management consists of relieving symptoms of pain and obstructive jaundice. For less than 20% of patients is there any hope for operability, as defined by imaging. No attempt should be made to proceed to surgery until jaundice has completely resolved. Jaundice is dealt with by relief of biliary obstruction, either by endoscopic stenting or by percutaneous transhepatic stenting of the biliary system (Figure 10.2). Pain may be relieved by the use of opiates or may resolve with the relief of biliary obstruction. At laparotomy, only a third of the 20% of patients with radiologically operable disease turn out to have surgically operable tumours.

Pancreatic surgery requires a considerable degree of specialization and should not be carried out outside of the setting of a specialist treatment centre. The reason for this is simple: specialist centres achieve better survival rates and lower morbidity and mortality rates. The operation of choice is Whipple's procedure, and this involves removal of the distal half of the stomach (antrectomy), gallbladder (cholecystectomy), distal common bile duct (choledochectomy), head of the pancreas, duodenum and proximal jejunum (pancreatoduodenectomy), and regional lymph nodes. Reconstruction consists of attaching the pancreas to the jejunum (pancreaticojejunostomy), the common bile duct to the jejunum (choledochojejunostomy), and the stomach to the jejunum (gastrojejunostomy), to allow bile, digestive juices and food to flow! There are modifications of this procedure, such as the pylorus-conserving pancreaticoduodenectomy, that are associated with less postoperative morbidity and equivalent efficacy.

Thirty years ago, surgery for pancreatic cancer was associated with a very high morbidity of approximately 25%. This has fallen in specialist centres to 5%, with the expectation that 20% of patients with operable disease will survive 5 years. Post-operative adjuvant chemotherapy with 5-fluorouracil and folinic acid, or gemcitabine modestly improves survival. Trials of chemoradiation, as an adjunct to surgery, marginally improve survival but at a cost of considerable toxicity. Ampullary carcinomas of the pancreas generally present with early-stage disease because of their anatomical position. These tumours are associated with better prognoses than cancers of the rest of the pancreas.

Treatment of inoperable disease

Patients with inoperable pancreatic cancer have a poor prognosis and the treatment of this condition is palliative. The median survival is 4–6 months. Active treatment with chemotherapy may be advised. The most successful chemotherapy programmes have response rates of up to 40%, but the median

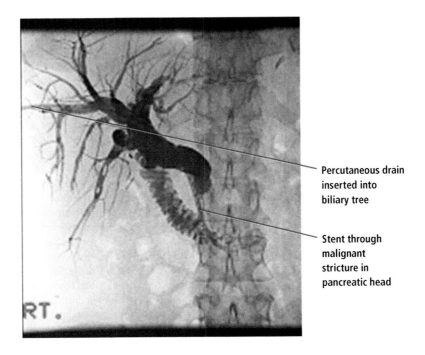

Percutaneous drain inserted into biliary tree

Stent through malignant stricture in pancreatic head

RT.

Figure 10.2 Two stents: bilirary obstruction due to malignant stricture in head of pancreas.

duration of survival of these responding patients is just 1 month longer than might be expected without active treatment. Because pancreatic cancer is relatively common, a number of chemotherapy agents have been tried for this condition. Combination therapy using the more toxic agents, such as anthracyclines and taxanes, offers little benefit. The current consensus view is that gemcitabine with either capecitabine or carboplatin or cisplatin probably offers as good an opportunity for disease palliation as any other combination. Quality-of-life issues are paramount in this condition because of the poor prognosis for inoperable disease.

The expression by pancreatic exocrine cancer cells of numerous receptors and the poor results with systemic chemotherapy have led to strategies targeting these receptors. EGF receptor inhibitors including the protein kinase inhibitor erlotinib and the monoclonal antibody cetuximab have been studied with limited success. The VEGF pathway has also been targeted with the anti-VEGF monoclonal antibody bevacizumab and receptor tyrosine kinase inhibitors of VEGF receptors including sorafenib. Again the results are disappointing. The IGF pathway that is activated in pancreatic and other cancers is a novel target for therapeutic strategies and monoclonal antibodies targeting both the ligand (IGF1 and IGF2) and the receptor (IGF receptor 1, IGFR1) are under

investigation along with receptor tyrosine kinase inhibitors of IGFR1.

The transfer of suicide genes to tumour cells by retroviral vectors has also been applied in pancreatic cancer cell lines. This approach is known as gene-directed enzyme prodrug therapy (GDEPT). The adenovirus vector that was used carried the herpes simplex virus thymidine kinase gene that phosphorylates the prodrug ganciclovir into deoxyGTP that is incorporated into replicating DNA, causing strand termination. This GDEPT strategy inhibited gene expression and cell growth of pancreatic cancer cell lines. This strategy is being investigated in clinical trials.

An alternative approach to the management of pancreatic cancer is to focus only on treating the symptoms: stenting to relieve jaundice and coeliac axis nerve block to relieve pain. This procedure blocks the pain fibres originating from the pancreas and ensures good quality of life. The technique requires skill and is relatively well tolerated.

Prognosis

The outlook even for patients with operable pancreatic cancer is unfortunately not particularly good, with

Table 10.3 Clinical manifestations of secretory endocrine tumours

Tumour	Major feature	Minor feature	Common sites	Percentage malignant	MEN associated
Insulinoma	Neuroglycopenia (confusion, fits)	Permanent neurological deficits	Pancreas (β-cells)	10	10%
Gastrinoma (Zollinger–Ellison syndrome)	Peptic ulceration	Diarrhoea, weight loss, malabsorption, dumping	Pancreas Duodenum	40–60	25%
VIPoma (Werner–Morrison syndrome)	Watery diarrhoea, hypokalaemia, achlorhydria	Hypercalcaemia, hyperglycaemia, hypomagnesaemia	Pancreas, neuroblastoma, SCLC, phaeochromocytoma	40	<5%
Glucagonoma	Migratory necrolyic erythema, mild diabetes mellitus, muscle wasting, anaemia	Diarrhoea, thromboembolism stomatitis, hypoaminoacidaemia, encephalitis	Pancreas (α-cells)	60	<5%
Somatostatinoma	Diabetes mellitus, cholelithiasis, steatorrhoea, malabsorption	Anaemia, diarrhoea, weight loss, hypoglycaemia	Pancreas (β-cells)	66	Case reports only

MEN, multiple endocrine neoplasia; SCLC, small cell lung cancer; VIP, vasoactive intestinal polypeptide.

a 20% chance of 5-year survival. The outlook for those patients with locally advanced or metastatic disease is very poor, with a median survival of 3–4 months. It is for this reason that there is such an emphasis upon quality of life in pancreatic cancer, rather than on the prospects for cure.

Pancreatic endocrine tumours

This is a fascinating group of tumours, interesting not only because of their biology, but also because patients with these tumours are expected to do well. Pancreatic endocrine tumours include tumours arising from islet cells (insulinomas, glucagonomas, gastrinomas and VIPomas) and neuroendocrine tumours originating from enterochromaffin cells (carcinoids). The bizarre constellation of symptoms produced by carcinoids are interesting even to medical students, as are the gastrointestinal symptoms resulting from gastrinomas and VIPomas, and the hypo- and hyperglycaemia from insulinomas and glucagonomas, respectively (Table 10.3). Old school general physicians will expect every medical student reading this book to be able to recount the umpteen skin conditions associated with carcinoid tumours, as well as describe the reasons for the effects of this tumour on the heart. They will take delight in quizzing you on their ward rounds, so we suggest that you google these symptoms and signs if there is an inpatient with carcinoid on your ward. These endocrine malignancies can be associated with enormously long natural histories, which may date back over decades.

The major treatment options for pancreatic endocrine tumours include octreotide to decrease hormonal secretion, and chemoembolization to reduce the symptoms that result from tumour bulk. Octreotide is an octapeptide mimic of somatostatin that inhibits the secretion of a whole host of peptide hormones including gastrin, glucagon, growth hormone, insulin, pancreatic polypeptide (PP) and vasoactive intestinal polypeptide (VIP). Octreotide also reduces pancreatic and intestinal fluid secretion, hence it is used in the management of malignant bowel obstruction. Octreotide has a median period of effect of 1 year in carcinoids, but leads to no clinical evidence of disease regression. Interferon may also lead to a reduction in secretory symptoms of carcinoid tumours. Where symptoms are significant and octreotide has failed, embolization is considered, both to the primary site and to hepatic metastases. Embolization is a significant enterprise and is associated with mortality rates of 3–5% in even the best centres. It should therefore be considered with great care before it is undertaken. The mTOR inhibitor everolimus and sunitinib both have been found to have activity in neuroendocrine pancreatic cancers. Everolimus used in combination with octreotide should be considered the current treatment standard, near trebling progression free survival in a "landmark" clinical trial. The authors of Lecture Notes like landmarks.

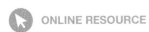

ONLINE RESOURCE

Case Study: Once a surgeon, always a surgeon.

KEY POINTS

- Pancreatic cancer is the 10th most common cancer in the United Kingdom and hereditary syndromes account for 5–10% cases
- Most patients present with advanced disease, causing pain, weight loss and obstructive jaundice and only 3% survive 5 years
- Fewer than one in five have operable disease and most patients are treated palliatively with or without systemic chemotherapy
- Pancreatic endocrine tumours have a more indolent course and may secrete a number of peptide hormones causing a variety of different syndromes that may be alleviated by octreotide

11

Colorectal cancer

Learning objectives

✓ Explain the epidemiology and pathogenesis of colorectal cancer

✓ Recognize the common presentation and clinical features of colorectal cancer

✓ Describe the treatment strategies and outcomes of colorectal cancer

---

One of England's greatest sportsmen, Bobby Moore died of metastatic bowel cancer in 1993 at the age of 51. He had an orchiectomy and radiotherapy for testicular cancer in 1964, two years before captaining England to World Cup victory, so although his radiotherapist may have helped win the World Cup, he may also have led ultimately to a radiation-induced secondary cancer that killed our sporting hero. This is another example of why it is better to be a medical oncologist than a radiotherapist.

Epidemiology

Colorectal cancer is a major cause of morbidity in the West. In 2011, 41,581 people were diagnosed with colorectal cancer and 15,609 died of the disease. The incidence has risen modestly over the last quarter of a century and the 5-year overall survival has doubled over the same time interval to around 50% (Table 11.1). The introduction of screening by one-off flexible colonoscopy or faecal occult blood (FOB) testing is likely to alter the incidence and mortality over the next decade. Colorectal cancers evolve over a 10-year period from polyp to invasive cancer. It is likely that a single colonoscopy every 10 years provides effective screening and prevention, but the cost of all those endoscopies for the entire population is unaffordable and so cannot be used as a screening tool.

Pathogenesis

Although family history, including hereditary colorectal cancer syndromes, contributes to a third of cases of colorectal cancer, in the 1960s and 1970s, there was increasing recognition of the possibility of a dietary basis to colorectal cancer. The disease was thought to be uncommon in the developing world, whilst the high red meat/low fibre diet and obesity in the more developed market economies were seen to be responsible for a higher incidence of colorectal cancer. Much of the data on the link between diet and colorectal cancer comes from the European Prospective Investigation into Cancer and Nutrition (EPIC) study.

Consumption of both red meat and processed meat (ham, bacon, sausages, pate, tinned meat) are associated with an increased risk (Table 11.2). High fibre diets increase the transit time of the stool and decrease the colorectal epithelial exposure to carcinogens within the stool. Higher consumption of dietary fibre especially cereal fibre reduces mainly left-sided colon cancers. Overall vegetable consumption also reduces the risk, but the benefit of fruit has not been confirmed in meta-analyses despite the constant advise to eat five fruits (or vegetables) a day. This advice is not based on facts and has been conjured up by some committee, in a similar way to the alcohol consumption advisory figures. Nevertheless, the authors suggest that you do not tell young children this

---

Oncology: Lecture Notes, Third Edition. Mark Bower and Jonathan Waxman.
© 2015 by John Wiley & Sons, Ltd. Published 2015 by John Wiley & Sons, Ltd.
Companion Website: www.lecturenoteseries.com/oncology

Table 11.1 UK cancer registration for colorectal cancer 2010

	Percentage all cancer registrations		Rank of registration		Lifetime risk of cancer		Change in ASR (2000–2010)		5-year overall survival	
	Female	Male	Female	Male	Female	Male	Female	Male	Female	Male
Colorectal cancer	11	14	3rd	3rd	1 in 19	1 in 14	+6%	+5%	56%	54%

information as the reaction of their mothers is wholly unpredictable.

Aspirin has been shown to have a protective effect against colorectal cancer, and epidemiological studies of prolonged aspirin use have shown a consistent reduction of up to 50% in the risk of colorectal cancers. This decrease in risk is thought to be due to the inhibitory effect of aspirin on cyclooxygenase-2, which is an enzyme found in high concentrations in colorectal tissue and promotes the growth of polyps. In randomized studies, aspirin has been shown to reduce the incidence of adenomatous polyps in patients screened after the excision of a primary colorectal tumour. There has, however, only been a single randomized trial of aspirin prophylaxis, which has shown no evidence for a reduction in colorectal cancer incidence and the toxicity; especially the risk of gastrointestinal haemorrhage means that it is premature to recommend aspirin as chemoprevention. Patients with both Crohn's disease and ulcerative colitis are at risk from developing colonic tumours, and this risk rises to over 10% after 20 years follow-up. The risk factors for colorectal cancer in patients with inflammatory bowel disease include the duration of colitis and the extent of colonic involvement.

Up to 20% of patients with colorectal cancer have a family history of colorectal cancer. There are two significant familial causes for colorectal cancer: familial adenomatous polyposis (FAP) and hereditary non-polyposis colorectal cancer (HNPCC). FAP is an autosomal dominant condition that accounts for 1% of all colorectal cancer. The gene for FAP was mapped to chromosome 5q21 in 1987 and the responsible gene APC was cloned in 1991. All patients with FAP develop colorectal cancer by the age of 40 years, so prophylactic colectomy is offered to teenagers with FAP. HNPCC, or Lynch syndrome, is responsible for 2–5% of colorectal cancers. HNPCC is characterized by colorectal cancers occurring at an early age, and they are often sited on the right side of the colon. In addition, HNPCC is associated with endometrial carcinoma, and gastric, renal, ureteric and central nervous system malignancies. In this condition, the genetic abnormalities include microsatellite instability and mutated mismatch-repair genes (most frequently hMSH2 and hMLH1).

In the vast majority of non-inherited colorectal malignancy, the molecular changes consist of a sequential accumulation of mutations in genes including p53 and deletion of the colorectal gene (DCC), K-Ras and APC. Indeed, it was the identification by polymerase chain reaction (PCR) of a K-Ras mutation that led pathologists to confirm the cause of death of King Ferdinand I of Aragon, the King of Naples. After his death, his body was mummified and embalmed in 1494 and placed in a wooden sarcophagus at the Abbey of San Domenico Maggiore, Naples. In 2006, an autopsy was performed revealing a large pelvic

Table 11.2 The effect of dietry intake on risk of colorectal cancer

Dietary factor	Effect on CRC incidence	Quantification
Meat		
Red meat	Increased risk	17–30% increase in risk per 100–120 g/d
Processed meat	Increased risk	9–50% increase in risk per 25–50 g/d
Fibre		
Cereal fibre	Decreased risk	10% decrease in risk per 10 g/d
Vegetables	Decreased risk	2% decrease in risk per 100 g/d
Dairy products	Decreased risk	16% decrease risk per 400 g/d

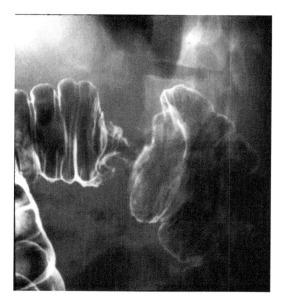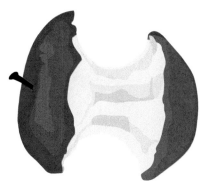

Figure 11.1 Medical metaphors: colon cancer: apple core lesion.

mass and the molecular analysis was consistent with a primary bowel cancer. Three-quarters of colorectal cancers are adenocarcinomas arising via an accumulation of genetic changes from benign adenomatous polyps (see Figure 2.8). Adenomas are usually slow growing and the risk of malignant transformation increases with their size and how long they have been present.

Presentation

Patients with colorectal tumours present to their general practitioners with a history of altered bowel habit and rectal bleeding. This may also be accompanied by weight loss and abdominal pains. These symptoms are suggestive of malignancy, and accordingly an urgent referral should be made to a specialist bowel surgeon. The patient should be seen within 2 weeks of receipt of the general practitioner's referral letter. It is unfortunate that sometimes these symptoms are disregarded by GPs and dismissed as due to piles or irritable bowel syndrome, and IBS of course, does not cause rectal bleeding.

Diagnosis

In outpatients, the surgeon should take a full history from the patient and examine him or her. This should include a rectal examination, which may show the patient to have melaena. Proctoscopy and sigmoidoscopy should be performed in the outpatient setting. Blood tests should be organized, which should include a full blood count, renal function and liver function tests. A chest X-ray should be carried out and a barium enema or colonoscopy arranged as an outpatient procedure. The barium enema may show narrowing of the colon. In malignancy, this narrowing is typical and has the appearance of an apple core (Figures 11.1 and 11.2). Endoscopy may show a stenosing lesion or a polyp. Biopsies should be taken of the suspicious area.

Staging and grading

The tumour should be examined histologically. It is described as being either well, moderately or poorly differentiated. The original staging system for colorectal cancer was reported by Cuthbert Esquire Dukes, a British pathologist, in 1932. With various modifications this system is still in use today. Dukes' stage reflects the degree of invasion of the tumour. Dukes' stage A is specified when a tumour is confined to the mucosa. Dukes' stage B is a tumour that perforates the serosa, and Dukes' stage C is given when lymph nodes are affected. Tumours of the colon are, furthermore, divided according to their anatomical sub-sites. These are the appendix, caecum, ascending colon, hepatic

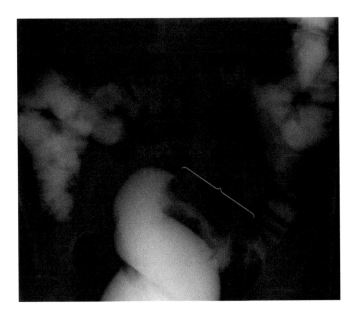

Figure 11.2 Barium enema investigation showing irregular stricture of the sigmoid colon with shouldering giving an apple core appearance typical of sigmoid colon cancer.

flexure, transverse colon, splenic flexure, descending colon and sigmoid colon. Finally, the tumour can be staged according to the TNM clinical classification system (Table 11.3).

Treatment

The suspicion of malignancy having been raised, the patient should be worked up for surgery including an assessment of operability by CT scanning and by MRI. The CT scan will show whether or not there are enlarged lymph nodes within the abdomen and will define the possibility of further spread involving the liver. The MRI is more accurate than a CT scan in defining operability and in the staging of a rectal primary. If there is no gross evidence of dissemination, the patient with a colonic tumour should be admitted to hospital for colectomy. Removal of the primary is still considered in the presence of metastatic disease to reduce the risk of perforation or obstruction. However, the use of endoscopically placed stents has developed for those unfit for surgery or as a bridge to surgery in patients presenting with bowel obstruction (Figures 11.3 and 40.13).

The surgical plan depends upon the experience and practice of the clinician. There have been considerable developments in the area of laparoscopic surgery. If the patient is therefore considered to be an appropriate candidate, a laparoscopic colectomy might be performed. The results of rectal surgery are

Table 11.3 TNM staging of colorectal cancer

T stage (primary tumour)	N stage (nodal status)	M stage (metastatic status)
T0: No evidence of primary tumour	N0: No nodes	M0: No distant metastases
T1: Tumour invades submucosa	N1: Metastasis in one to three pericolic nodes	M1: Distant metastases
T2: Tumour invades muscularis	N2: Metastasis in four or more pericolic nodes	
T3: Tumour invades through the muscularis	N3: Metastasis in any lymph node	
T4: Tumour perforates the peritoneum		

Small bowel

Centrally placed loops of dilated bowel
Valvulae conniventes (extend across
whole bowel wall)

Large bowel

Peripheral loops of dilated bowel
Haustrae (do not cross whole diameter of colon)

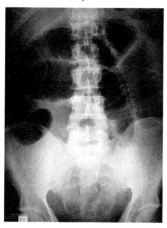
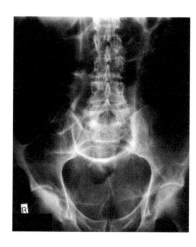

Figure 11.3 How to tell
small bowel obstruction from
large bowel obstruction on an
X-ray.

critically surgeon dependent, and much better results are obtained in centres where the surgeon specializes in this procedure.

Surgery for colonic cancer

At operation, a midline incision should be performed and the abdominal contents inspected. The tumour should be mobilized and removed together with a good margin of normal tissue. The tumour should be inspected and frozen sections performed to ensure that the resection edges of the apparently normal gut contain no tumour. An end-to-end anastomosis is then made. If the patient is found to have three to five liver metastases at operation, these should be resected at an appropriate time, as successful resection is associated with a good prognosis and the possibility of cure. If there are more than three to five metastases, no operative action should be taken. Extensive resection of the lymph nodes should be performed, providing histopathological information which affects the patient's management.

Surgery for rectal cancers

The surgery that is performed depends upon the site of the carcinoma and a preoperative assessment of operability. Tumours of the upper and middle third of the rectum are treated by anterior resection. In this procedure, the rectum is mobilized from the sacral hollow, and the tumour is removed together with an adequate margin of normal tissue. This normal margin ranges between 2 and 5 cm. The mesorectum and lateral pararectal tissue should be removed. Lesions of the lower third of the rectum are treated by abdominoperineal resection, which requires a permanent colostomy. The rectum is mobilized, and the peritoneum at the base of the bladder or posterior vagina is incised. The lateral ligaments are divided and the anus excised. The quality of surgery in rectal cancer is critically important. Extensive lymphadenectomy is associated with significantly improved chances for survival.

Complications of surgery

A neurogenic bladder is very common after pelvic surgery but will usually recover within 10 days. Ureteric tears or transections may complicate surgery, but only rarely so. Sexual dysfunction in males is inevitable after rectal surgery, and the most common problems are retrograde ejaculation and erectile impotence. Change in sexual function in women has not been assessed because of the sexist bias of surgeons who have not thought it necessary to investigate this aspect of life. Surgery is complicated by a mortality rate of 1–2%.

Adjuvant treatment for colonic cancer

Following recovery from surgery, no additional treatment is recommended for patients with Dukes' stage

A disease. The value of adjuvant chemotherapy for Dukes' B disease remains controversial. This is because no major advantage has been shown for adjuvant chemotherapy within this group of patients. Patients with Dukes' C (node positive) tumours, however, should receive adjuvant chemotherapy. The reason for this is that there is a survival advantage in this group of patients. An online web-based tool (Adjuvant! Online) to estimate the recurrence rates, survival and benefits of adjuvant chemotherapy is available that can help patients and doctors with these decisions. The currently advocated adjuvant chemotherapy regime is FOLFOX, a combination of short-term infusional 5-fluorouracil, folinic acid and oxaliplatin administered every fortnight for 6 months.

Adjuvant treatment for rectal cancer

Patients with rectal cancer may receive preoperative neoadjuvant radiotherapy. This has been shown to limit pelvic recurrence for low rectal tumours. It is disputed whether neoadjuvant radiotherapy improves survival. Alternatively, after the patient has recovered from surgery, he or she may receive pelvic radiotherapy. This has been shown in randomized studies to decrease the risk of pelvic recurrence by 5–10%. Patients with more advanced tumours (T3 and T4) may be treated with neoadjuvant chemoradiotherapy prior to surgery. There is increased postoperative morbidity with chemotherapy given in conjunction with radiotherapy. Trial results show that neoadjuvant chemoradiotherapy improves disease-free survival and possible overall survival. Neoadjuvant chemoradiotherapy may lead to a complete remission in up to 70% of patients. There have been studies reported where patients achieving a complete tumour response with neoadjuvant chemoradiation have not proceeded to rectal surgery. In one of these studies just 20% of patients achieving a complete response progressed. There is a school of thought that is emerging that considers that in those patients achieving a complete response with chemoradiation observation is reasonable, reserving rectal surgery for those patients who relapse.

Management of metastatic disease

In the situation where there are limited metastases from colorectal cancer, consideration is given to the possibility of curative surgical treatment. If the patient is fit, and there are three to five hepatic metastases or less than three pulmonary metastases, resection may be considered to be appropriate. If surgery is successful, then the prognosis is relatively good, with survival chances ranging up to 40% at 5 years.

Generally, however, metastatic colorectal carcinoma has a poor prognosis, and the current recommendation for appropriate treatment is with 5FU-based regimens and radiotherapy. There is debate as to whether or not the addition of folinic acid is of an advantage to the patient. The current consensus is that there is a benefit at least in terms of remission rates, although no consensus has been reached regarding survival. The treatment regimen of first choice was called the "De Gramont regimen" and includes fortnightly 5FU and folinic acid given for 6 months. A host of new treatments have recently become available for patients with colorectal cancer. The most commonly used chemotherapy regimens are FOLFOX and FOLFIRI. The addition of irinotecan and oxaliplatin to 5FU in these regimens has improved median survival from 9 to 18 months. Recently the addition of bevacizumab, a humanized monoclonal antibody against vascular endothelial growth factor (VEGF), to both the FOLFOX and FOLFIRI regimens has led to a further modest improvement in survival. Cetuximab, a partially humanized monoclonal antibody against the epidermal growth factor receptor (EGFR), and panitumumab, a fully humanized antibody against EGFR, have both been shown to prolong survival in patients with metastatic colon cancer that lack mutations in K-Ras. Tumours are now evaluated for mutations of the Ras gene in order to define suitability for treatment. As a result of the use of these agents, survival in metastatic colorectal cancer has been extended from 18 months to almost 2 years. In this context, the cost of treatment becomes a significant political issue but, amongst the discussion on the politics of cancer care, little attention seems to be paid to the cost of not treating the patient. Dying from metastatic colorectal cancer without drug treatment is an expensive process, and the authors of this chapter are not merely considering financial cost when we make this statement.

Screening

As with other cancer screening programmes, the identification of high-risk groups for screening is important. Early colonoscopic screening studies focused on

Table 11.4 Screening scheme for colorectal cancer

Risk	Action	Age
Low risk 1 relative >45 years *or* 2 relatives >70 years	Reassure: no colonoscopy	
Low–moderate risk 2 first-degree relatives, average age 60–70 years	Single colonoscopy	Aged 55 years
Moderate risk 2 first-degree relatives, average age 50–60 years	5-yearly colonoscopy	Aged 35–65 years or starting
1 first-degree relative <45 years		Start screening 5 years before the age when cancer was diagnosed in the youngest relative
Moderate–high risk 2 first-degree relatives, average age <50 years	3–5-yearly colonoscopy	Begin age 30–35; refer to genetics
3 close relatives (not AC)		
High risk 3 close relatives AC +ve (HNPCC) (FAP)	2-yearly colonoscopy Annual sigmoidoscopy from teens	Age 25–65; refer to genetics And counselling

AC, Amsterdam criteria; FAP, familial adenomatous polyposis; HNPCC, hereditary non-polyposis colorectal cancer.

very high risk groups such as those with hereditary colon cancer syndromes and those with extensive inflammatory bowel disease. It is estimated that there may be a genetic predisposition to colorectal cancer in more than 20% of patients with these tumours. In the vast majority of colorectal cases there is, however, at present no direct evidence of there being a genetic risk. Patients with a risk of developing colorectal tumours can be stratified as having low, low–moderate, moderate, moderate–high or high risk of developing malignancy. The criteria for proceeding to screening for these patients are defined as in Table 11.4. Randomized controlled studies of whole population screening with FOB have shown that screening every 2 years those aged 45–74 reduces colorectal cancer mortality by 15–18%. Conversely, a screening one-off flexible sigmoidoscopy at the age of 55–64 reduces colorectal cancer incidence by 33% and mortality by 43%.

In 2006, the NHS bowel cancer screening programme introduced FOB tests for people aged 60–69 years every 2 years (Figure 11.4). It is estimated that if the uptake of FOB testing reaches 60% by the year 2026, 20,000 deaths from bowel cancer will be prevented in the United Kingdom. For every 1000 FOB tests completed, 20 (2%) will be abnormal and 16

(1.6%) patients will proceed to a colonoscopy, 6 (0.6%) of these will have polyps, 2 (0.2%) will have cancer and 8 (0.8%) a normal colonoscopy. The cost estimate equation for FOB testing is £1000 for each life-year saved. FOB testing will miss tumours and lead to a number of false positive findings. Colonoscopy is a more accurate means of detecting cancers but

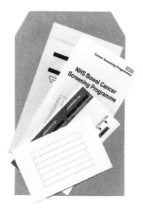

Kit contains:
Full instructions
Six cardboard sticks to collect the samples
A red and white test card
A prepaid hygienic envelope to return the sample

Figure 11.4 NHS faecal occult blood (FOB) screening kit.

requires full bowel preparation and sedation and carries a risk of perforation (around 1 in 1500). Although the costs of colonoscopy for screening normal populations is, unfortunately, not economic, it is the investigation of choice for high-risk populations (Table 11.4). Because of studies showing the benefits and safety of one-off sigmoidoscopy, NHS England is planning to supplement FOB screening with flexible sigmoidoscopy screening of the population at 55 years of age.

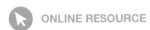 ONLINE RESOURCE

Case Study: A bunged up copper.

 KEY POINTS

- Colorectal cancer is the third most common cancer in the United Kingdom, and both family history and diet are implicated in causation
- Screening with faecal occult blood testing or one-off sigmoidoscopy reduces colorectal cancer mortality
- Patients with colorectal cancer present with altered bowel habit, rectal bleeding, weight loss or abdominal pain
- The clinical management of colorectal cancer involves a combination of surgery, chemotherapy and radiotherapy with increasing use of novel targeted therapies

12

Kidney cancer

Learning objectives

✓ Explain the epidemiology and pathogenesis of kidney cancer
✓ Recognize the common presentation and clinical features of kidney cancer
✓ Describe the treatment strategies and outcomes of kidney cancer

---

Epidemiology

In 2010, 10,144 people were diagnosed with kidney cancer and 4189 died of the disease in the United Kingdom. The incidence of kidney cancer is rising faster than almost any other cancer. Around 54% of all kidney cancer patients survive 5 years from diagnosis (Table 12.1). We are at a point where we now understand many of the molecular changes in kidney cancer. Treatments for kidney cancer have been designed targeting these changes and can be given in England and Wales subject to the sometimes draconian decisions and whimsy of the National Institutes for Health and Care Excellence.

Over 90% of kidney cancers arise from the renal cortex and are thought to originate chiefly from cells of the proximal convoluted tubules of the nephrons. These tumours are known variously as renal cell cancer, renal adenocarcinoma, clear cell renal cancer, hypernephroma or if you are a really old clinician, Grawitz tumour. About 10% of kidney cancers arise in the renal pelvis and are urothelial transitional cell tumours derived from the transitional cell epithelium of the collecting system.

Pathogenesis

A number of factors have been found to increase the risk of kidney cancer including smoking that also increases the risk of urothelial cancers of the ureters and bladder presumably because of urinary excretion of tobacco-related carcinogens. Obesity and hypertension also increase the risk of kidney cancers. Much recent attention has focused on the molecular biology of kidney cancers including genetic predispositions.

The molecular basis of some of the familial syndromes associated with an increased risk of kidney cancer is recapitulated in spontaneous kidney cancer (see Table 12.2). For example, the mTOR pathway, angiogenesis and the MET receptor have all been found to be disrupted in spontaneous kidney cancers and provide potential therapeutic targets. In clear cell renal cancer, loss of heterozygosity at chromosome 3p (the site of the VHL gene locus) leads to inactivation of hypoxia-inducible factors. This in turn leads to activation of vascular endothelial growth factor receptor (VEGFR) and epidermal growth factor receptor (EGFR), with resultant new vessel formation and tumour development. VEGFR and EGFR upregulation

---

Oncology: Lecture Notes, Third Edition. Mark Bower and Jonathan Waxman.
© 2015 by John Wiley & Sons, Ltd. Published 2015 by John Wiley & Sons, Ltd.
Companion Website: www.lecturenoteseries.com/oncology

Table 12.1 UK registrations for kidney cancer 2010

	Percentage of all cancer registrations		Rank of registration		Lifetime risk of cancer		Change in ASR (2000–2010)		5-year overall survival	
	Female	Male	Female	Male	Female	Male	Female	Male	Female	Male
Kidney cancer	2	4	10th	7th	1 in 90	1 in 56	+38%	+27%	55%	53%

are features of renal cell cancer that have been exploited for treatment.

Presentation

Patients with renal cancers commonly present with pain in the loins or blood in the urine. The classic triad of flank pain, haematuria and fever is only found in 10%. Kidney cancers can produce non-metastatic systemic effects including erythropoietin production causing polycythaemia, rennin secretion causing hypertension, parathyroid-hormone-related peptide (PTHrP) production yielding hypercalcaemia and interleukin-6 secretion causing paraneoplastic pyrexia. Less common presentations in males include varicocoeles due to occlusion of the testicular veins. The left testicular vein drains into the left renal vein, whilst the right testicular vein drains directly into the inferior vena cava (IVC). About a quarter of patients present with metastatic disease and the most common sites for secondary spread in kidney cancer are lung, liver, bone and brain. Increasingly kidney cancers are detected as incidental findings during imaging investigations for other indications and this may account in part for the rising incidence in recent years and the improved survival as these tumours are often surgically curable. The Bosniak classification of CT-detected renal cysts predicts the chance that the cyst is malignant based on features such as multi-septation, rim enhancement and presence of soft tissue elements.

Outpatient diagnosis

The urologist will assess the patient in the outpatient clinic, taking a full medical history and examining the patient. Investigations to be organized will include full blood count, liver and renal function tests and a chest X-ray. Further investigation will also include a CT scan of the abdomen (Figure 12.1) and the thorax to define operability. Angiography and an intravenous urogram (IVU) (Figure 12.2) may also have to be performed.

Table 12.2 Familial cancer predisposition syndromes and kidney cancers

Syndrome	Kidney cancer risk	Other manifestations	Gene affected
von Hippel–Lindau disease (VHL)	70% develop clear cell RCC by age 60 years	Phaeochromocytoma (Type 1 VHL) Haemangioblastoma CNS or retinal (Type 2 VHL)	VHL 3p regulates hypoxia inducible factor 1α (HIF)
Hereditary papillary renal cell cancer (HPRCC)	Type 1 papillary RCC	None	MET (receptor for hepatocyte growth factor)
Hereditary leiomyomatosis renal cell cancer (HLRCC)	10% develop type 2 papillary RCC (10%)	Leiomyomata of skin and uterus	Fumerate hydratase (FH)
Birt–Hogg–Dubé syndrome (BHD)	15–30% develop RCC	Skin fibrofolliculomas, lung cysts	Folliculin (FLCN)

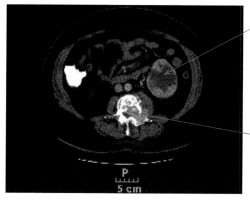

Renal cancer primary

Bone metastasis eroding vertebra and extending into the spinal canal and through the neural foramen

Figure 12.1 Metastatic renal cancer. This CT scan shows a left renal inferior pole mass. In addition, there is erosion of the vertebral body and posterior elements of the third lumbar vertebra. This is associated with extension into the spinal canal causing cauda equina compression and through the neural foramen into the psoas muscle.

Staging and grading

Kidney cancers are either renal cell cancers (90%) (Figure 12.3) or transitional cell urothelial cancers of the renal pelvis (10%). The main subtypes of renal cell cancer are: clear cell (85%), papillary (10%) and chromophobe (<5%). Clear cell cancers are graded into four Fuhrman categories that are strongly correlated with prognosis. Occasionally primary kidney cancers are oncocytomas that behave relatively benignly and rarely metastasize. In addition, the kidney may be involved by a primary lymphoma or metastases from other sites. The patient with renal cell carcinoma is staged according to the spread of the disease, using the TNM staging criteria.

Treatment

Surgery

If the patient has no evidence of spread of the disease, then the urological surgeon will arrange for the patient to be admitted for nephrectomy. At operation, the kidney and vascular pedicle and associated lymph nodes are removed, together with the ureter

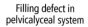

Filling defect in pelvicalyceal system

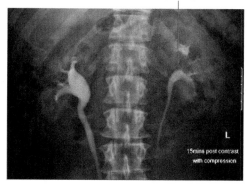

Figure 12.2 An intravenous urogram image demonstrating obstruction of the left pelvicalyceal system at the level of the pelviureteric junction with a filling defect. These appearances were due to a transitional cell carcinoma of the renal pelvis. Transitional cell cancer (TCC) of the renal pelvis arises in the collecting system and may be associated with TCC of the bladder and ureter. The biology, prognosis and treatment are similar to those of bladder cancer.

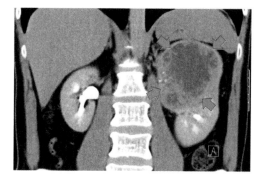

Figure 12.3 CT scan image of large left upper pole kidney mass. This is a Bosniak 4 renal cystic mass with a large necrotic component, multiple thick seprations and solid enhancing elements. At nephrectomy the pathological diagnosis was renal cell cancer.

and adrenal. Renal tumours have a propensity to invade along the renal vein. This invasion may extend into the IVC and right atrium. This does not represent a true invasion but is a tumour thrombus. If this is suspected, then a combined approach involving a urologist and a vascular surgeon is advised in an attempt to fully resect the tumour. For smaller and peripheral tumours, nephron-sparing surgery is performed (a fancy way of saying partial nephrectomy). Laparoscopic surgery for smaller tumours is also favoured as the surgical recovery is faster and the blood loss reduced.

Management of an inoperable primary tumour

Locally advanced, inoperable kidney cancer may cause significant symptoms, which may be poorly controlled by systemic palliative measures. These local symptoms can include haematuria, which may be so profound that regular blood transfusion is required, as well as loin pain, which may not respond to opiate analgesia. These symptoms can be treated by radiofrequency ablation, cryoablation, embolization or high-intensity frequency ultrasound. Radical nephrectomy in the presence of metastatic disease may relieve haematuria and pain but has minimal effect on the metastases despite earlier reports, although it may improve response to cytokine therapies. Two trials have shown that patients with metastatic disease who had nephrectomies lived longer. However, the survival benefit is measured in months and has to be weighed against the morbidity associated with surgery.

Adjuvant treatment

Adjuvant therapy, whether it is radiotherapy to the renal bed, chemotherapy, chemo-immunotherapy, cytokine therapy or anything else, is of no benefit after surgery.

Management of metastatic kidney cancer

Where there are single sites or limited numbers of metastases, there is a surgical option that needs to be considered. The removal of limited numbers of pulmonary metastases, or brain or bone metastases, leads to a chance for cure. Where there are multiple metastases the situation is different. There have been significant changes in the management of metastatic disease as a result of our understanding of the molecular biology of this group of tumours and access to novel therapies. Unfortunately, the rarer kidney cancers such as those associated with fumarate hydratase deficiency do not respond to systemic therapy and for these patients surgery is the only successful treatment option.

Chemotherapy

Chemotherapy is generally ineffective in the treatment of adenocarcinoma of the kidney with response rates below 10%. However, chemotherapy is given in the treatment of urothelial transitional cell tumours that resemble bladder cancers. The response rate of 60–70% is similar to that seen in patients with cancer of the bladder. Unfortunately, these responses are transient and last for a median time of 6–7 months.

Immunotherapy

Until recently, the most important therapy used for metastatic adenocarcinoma of the kidney was immunotherapy. The first agents used were bacillus Calmette–Guerin (BCG) and *Corynebacterium parvum*, but these have now been replaced by interleukin 2 (IL-2). Initial cytokine therapy for kidney cancer used interferon with modest response rates of 15%. In 1985, the results of treatment with IL-2 were first published, and 60% of patients with kidney cancer were reported to respond to treatment. This high response rate was not confirmed in subsequent studies, which were nevertheless encouraging in that, overall, approximately 20% of patients were seen to respond to treatment. The most significant aspect to IL-2 treatment is that responses are durable. Those few lucky patients who achieve a complete response may be cured of their malignancy. In the original dosage regimen, treatment had significant toxicities and even with current schedules the toxicity is high. It is with some surprise that the authors of this book have observed a resurgence of treatment with interleukin 2.

Anti-angiogenic therapy

The central role of angiogenesis in the biology of kidney cancer has led to drug treatments that inhibit the VEGF pathway. These include oral small molecule receptor tyrosine kinase inhibitors, "-nibs" and monoclonal antibodies, "-mabs". The former include sunitinib, sorafenib, pazopanib and axitinib, the latter include bevacizumab. These agents are the most widely used first-line therapies for advanced kidney cancer in the United Kingdom and have been shown to confer an overall survival benefit. In a recent randomized controlled trial pazopanib was compared to sunitinib in metastatic renal cell cancer. Both were equally effective, but pazopanib came out on top in terms of safety and quality of life.

Targeted therapy

The mammalian target of rapamycin (mTOR) pathway is downstream of the phosphoinositide 3 kinase and AKT (known as protein kinase B) pathway that is regulated by the phosphatase and tensin homologue (PTEN) tumour suppressor gene. This provides a valuable target in advanced kidney cancer. Temsirolimus and everolimus are mTOR inhibitors that are used as first-line therapy especially in advanced poor prognosis kidney cancer.

The optimal first-line treatment for advanced kidney cancer depends upon the organ function and performance status as well as the risk of progression of the malignancy. Many current trials aim to establish the gold standard first-line therapy as well as the most appropriate sequencing of lines of treatment.

Prognosis

The prognosis for localized adenocarcinoma of the kidney is variable. The survival rate for patients with good prognosis tumours is 60–80%, but if there is vascular or capsular invasion, only 40% survive 1 year. The median survival for patients with metastatic disease was 9 months. These statistics have significantly changed as a result of the development of new treatments for kidney cancer; with systemic treatment the median survival for patients with metastatic disease has been extended to 2 years. Kidney cancer survival is significantly longer for those who live in the least deprived areas of the United Kingdom compared to those who live in areas of greater material deprivation. Overall, 10% of patients with metastatic renal cell cancer survive 5 years from diagnosis and this group represents a curious feature of the malignancy. Even in the absence of metastases at presentation, the outlook for patients with transitional cell tumours is very poor, with 10% surviving for 1 year and 5% for 2 years.

 ONLINE RESOURCE

Case Study: A heart of gold and an oncocytoma.

 KEY POINTS

- The incidence of kidney cancer is rising, as is the survival as more tumours are detected at an earlier stage
- The molecular biology of kidney cancer has been unravelled and several targeted therapies have been developed
- The classic presentation of kidney cancer is with the triad of flank pain, haematuria and fever
- Paraneoplastic manifestations are relatively common in renal cancer including pyrexia, polycythaemia, hypercalcaemia and hypertension

13

Bladder cancer

Learning objectives

✓ Explain the epidemiology and pathogenesis of bladder cancer

✓ Recognize the common presentation and clinical features of bladder cancer

✓ Describe the treatment strategies and outcomes of bladder cancer

---

Epidemiology

In 2011, 10,399 people were diagnosed with bladder cancer and 5081 died of the disease in the United Kingdom (Table 13.1).

Worldwide more than one-third of a million people are diagnosed each year with bladder cancer and the global prevalence is estimated at 1.2 million. The highest incidence of bladder cancer is in industrialized nations of North America and Europe and in areas of endemic schistosomiasis in Africa and the Middle East. It is more than twice as common in men as in women.

Pathogenesis

The most important cause of bladder cancer is cigarette smoking, which accounts for over a third of all cases in the United Kingdom. The relative risk of bladder cancer in smokers is four and is attributed to tobacco-derived carcinogenic aromatic amines. Genetic polymorphisms modify this risk. "Slow acetylators" have a polymorphism of the N-acetyltransferase 2 (NAT2) gene that reduces the enzymes activity, which includes the detoxification of aromatic amines. Thus, people with the slow acetylator phenotype are more susceptible to smoking-induced bladder cancer, an intriguing example of the interaction between nature and nurture (or genetic and environmental factors) in the pathogenesis of cancer. Workers in the dye, paint and rubber industries are also at increased risk of bladder cancer through a similar mechanism as these industries use aromatic amines (such as aniline, benzidine and naphthylamine). Worldwide, 210 million people are infected with *Schistosoma haematobium* and 700 million people live in endemic areas. After malaria, it is the second most important parasitic disease and may be eradicated by a single oral dose of praziquantel, costing about 50p. Chronic bladder infection by *S. haematobium* increases the risk of bladder cancer (Figure 13.1), especially the less common squamous cell cancer of the bladder, and is estimated to cause over 10,000 cases per year globally. This is thought to be due to chronic irritation and long-term urinary catheters have also been shown to increase the risk for similar reasons.

There have been many developments in our understanding of the molecular biology of bladder cancer, and although these developments have not translated directly into treatment advances, they do provide significant prognostic information. Bladder tumours are thought to progress from a localized, superficial tumour to invasive and then metastatic disease. They are often multifocal. In an attempt to define the molecular events categorizing progression, it was originally noted that there was identical loss of heterozygosity in

Oncology: Lecture Notes, Third Edition. Mark Bower and Jonathan Waxman.
© 2015 by John Wiley & Sons, Ltd. Published 2015 by John Wiley & Sons, Ltd.
Companion Website: www.lecturenoteseries.com/oncology

Table 13.1 UK registrations for bladder cancer 2010

	Percentage of all cancer registrations		Rank of registration		Lifetime risk of cancer		Change in ASR (2000–2010)		5-year overall survival	
	Female	Male	Female	Male	Female	Male	Female	Male	Female	Male
Bladder cancer	2	5	11th	4th	1 in 110	1 in 40	–21%	–23%	50%	58%

multifocal bladder tumours. This original description, however, of what was thought to be a primary genetic event in this cancer, has not been confirmed. Multiple loss of genetic material has been described, with the most common losses centred on chromosome 9q22, which is the site of a gene called *patched* (PTC). This is thought to be a tumour suppressor gene in basal cell carcinoma and medulloblastoma. The PTC protein is a transmembrane receptor that downregulates the Hedgehog signalling pathway that plays a central role in embryonic development in insects and vertebrates (see Chapter 32, p. 259). There are other sites of chromosomal loss, particularly within chromosomes 3, 7 and 17. This loss of material can be used to follow up patients with bladder cancer, using fluorescence *in situ* hybridization (FISH) methodologies on urine cytology.

By far the most important of the recent findings in bladder cancer, however, has been the observation of overexpression of the human epidermal growth factor receptor (EGFR). This is reported in around 40% of the tumours of patients with bladder cancer. Overexpression correlates with a poor prognosis and treatments directed against EGFR may well have some future role as therapies for this malignancy.

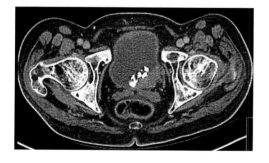

Figure 13.1 CT scan showing posterior wall bladder mass and calcification. The patient was from Egypt and had chronic schistosomiasis with an associated squamous cell cancer of the bladder.

Presentation

The initial symptoms include haematuria, dysuria and frequency of micturition. These symptoms are, unfortunately, sometimes treated with antibiotics by GPs for a period of time, prior to referral to a specialist. New urinary tract infections in older women should always be investigated actively, and symptoms occurring in a man should always be considered to be pathological and a referral made. Treating haematuria in a man with antibiotics without further investigation is negligent. There is of course a differential diagnosis, but one should have a very high index of suspicion of malignancy. Referral should be promptly organized to a specialist urological surgeon. The patient will be seen in an outpatient clinic. A careful history should be taken and an examination made. The patient's symptoms should be investigated further by performing a blood count, renal function tests, liver function tests and bacteriological and cytological examination of urine, to examine for the presence of infection and malignancy. An intravenous pyelogram (IVP) or increasingly a CT urogram may be ordered to examine the urothelial tract radiologically or an ultrasound investigation carried out.

These investigations should be organized promptly and the patient reviewed with the result within 2 weeks. A flexible cystoscopy is then generally organized and this takes place in the initial outpatient setting. If there is any suspicious appearance to the bladder, arrangements should then be made for a formal cystoscopy. The patient is anaesthetized for this procedure and the urethra and bladder carefully examined using a fibreoptic cystoscope. Any abnormal areas within the bladder should be biopsied together with areas of surrounding, apparently normal-looking bladder. The urologists at cystoscopy may describe a normal-looking bladder or the presence of a papilloma or solid tumour. The suspicious areas are treated by diathermy and the pelvis carefully examined in order to describe the clinical staging of the tumour.

Staging and grading

The tumour should then be examined pathologically and be given a grade according to differentiation. These grades are as follows:

- G1: well-differentiated tumour
- G2: moderately differentiated tumour
- G3: poorly differentiated tumour

Lesions are further characterized pathologically by their microscopic appearance as either transitional cell carcinoma or squamous carcinoma. Approximately 90% of patients in the United Kingdom have transitional cell carcinomas. The remainder are squamous carcinomas, adenocarcinomas, or rarely lymphoma or small cell tumours. There may be squamous metaplasia present within a transitional cell carcinoma and this is thought to be indicative of a poor prognosis. Adenocarcinomas may arise in a urachal remnant or result from direct invasion from a colorectal primary tumour. The urachus, you will recall from embryology lectures, is the canal that drains the bladder *in utero* into the umbilical cord that subsequently becomes the median umbilical ligament.

The tumour should also be staged according to the T (tumour), N (node) and M (metastatic categories) system (Table 13.2; see Figures 1.12 and 3.1).

Treatment

Treatment of superficial bladder cancer

The majority of transitional cell carcinoma of the bladder present as superficial tumours. The first step in the diagnosis and management of non-muscle invasive bladder cancer is cystoscopic transurethral resection of the bladder tumour (TURBT). After resection by diathermy at cystoscopy, approximately 60% of tumours will recur. The recurrence rate is greater where there are multiple tumours, associated carcinoma *in situ* or poorly differentiated tumours. For patients at low risk of recurrence, a single dose of intravesical mitomycin C may be administered following TURBT, whilst for those at high risk a course of intravesical bacillus Calmette–Guerin (BCG) is given to reduce the recurrence rate. Maintenance therapy with BCG, given for up to 2 years, has been shown to prevent recurrence, but the side effects mean that only 30% patients complete the course of maintenance therapy. Cystoscopic surveillance following TURBT is advocated. The recommendation for follow-up is slightly controversial, but in most practices cystoscopy is performed 3-monthly until the patient is tumour-free and thereafter 6-monthly for 2 years and yearly for 3 years. Practice varies throughout the

Table 13.2 TNM staging of bladder cancer

T (primary tumour)	N (nodal status)	M (metastatic status)
Tis: Carcinoma *in situ*	N0: No lymph node involvement	M0: No evidence of metastases
Ta: Papillary non-invasive tumour	N1: Single regional lymph node involvement	M1: Distant metastases
T1: Superficial tumour, not invading	N2: Bilateral regional lymph node beyond the lamina propria involvement	
T2: Tumour invading superficial	N3: Fixed regional lymph nodes muscle	
T2a: Tumour invading superficial muscle	N4: Juxtaregional lymph node involvement	
T2b: Tumour penetrating through superficial muscle		
T3a: Invasion of deep muscle		
T3b: Invasion through bladder wall		
T4a: Tumour invading prostate, uterus or vagina		
T4b: Tumour fixed to the pelvic wall		

A prefix "p" is given to describe the pathological staging of the tumour (e.g. pT3a).

United Kingdom. The requirement for lifelong routine monitoring and treatment in bladder cancer made it the most expensive cancer in terms of total medical care expenditure at least in 2001 when this cost was estimated at US$ 100,000 from diagnosis to death.

The authors of this book are impressed by the alacrity with which surgeons thrust out with knives advanced to excise bladders in patients with superficial bladder cancer. Many surgeons would view a recurrence-free survival of over 80% following cystectomy as a triumph of their surgical skills, but the truth (from several clinical trials) is that this recurrence-free survival is achieved by conservative treatment with intravesical BGC alone.

Treatment of invasive bladder cancer

The treatment of muscle-invasive carcinoma of the bladder is by surgery or radiation in those unfit for surgery. Radical cystectomy with urinary diversion is the preferred treatment for localized muscle-invasive bladder cancer and may in some cases be performed laparoscopically. Neoadjuvant cisplatin-containing chemotherapy before surgery has been shown to improve overall survival in two randomized controlled trials, whilst the use of post-operative adjuvant chemotherapy remains controversial. After cystectomy, patients must be nursed either in intensive care or in high-dependency beds. Continent bladders may be fashioned by the surgeon so that the patient does not require an ileostomy. Men are invariably rendered impotent by cystectomy. Little is known of the effects of cystectomy on female sexual function. There are well-known electrolyte disorders associated with ileostomies (chiefly dehydration and loss of sodium and potassium).

Radical radiotherapy is generally given to a total dose of 6500 cGy over a 6-week period. Treatment should be given to the whole pelvis, focusing down upon the bladder towards the end of treatment, or may be given to the bladder alone. Some radiotherapists insist on treating pelvic nodes in addition to the bladder primary. This leads to added toxicity and is illogical. If there are metastases present in pelvic nodes, there is a very high chance that they will also be present in intra-abdominal nodes so irradiating pelvic nodes had no logical benefit. Radiotherapy can also be used to reduce haematuria in advanced disease if TURBT is unable to control this. During radiotherapy, the patient may get cystitis or proctitis. At the end of treatment, he or she may suffer from a small, shrunken bladder as a consequence of radiation fibrosis. Both cystitis and proctitis are common after radiotherapy to the bladder, occurring in up to 30% of patients.

Adenocarcinoma of the bladder is thought to be relatively resistant to chemotherapy and radiotherapy, and as a consequence surgery is the main treatment option. Small cell bladder cancer and bladder lymphoma are managed with treatment regimens for small cell lung cancer and disseminated lymphoma, respectively.

Treatment of metastatic bladder cancer

When bladder cancer has spread beyond the bladder, it is conventionally treated with chemotherapy. Recent advances in the treatment of this disease mean that new hope is now offered to patients with metastatic cancer. A number of different treatment schedules have been used for treatment. The standard treatment currently is combination therapy with gemcitabine and cisplatin, chosen for efficacy and comparative lack of toxicity (Figure 13.2).

Bladder wall thickening

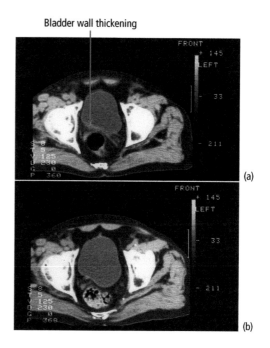

Figure 13.2 (a) CT scan demonstrating thickening of the posterior bladder wall due to invasive bladder cancer and (b) the same image after four cycles of platinum-based combination chemotherapy showing a reduction in bladder wall thickening.

Table 13.3 Bladder cancer survival

Stage	TNM	5-year survival
0	Ta/Tis N0 M0	98%
1	T1 N0 M0	88%
2	T2 N0 M0	63%
3	T3 or T4a N0 M0	46%
4	T4b or N1-3 or M1	15%

Prognosis

The consensus view is that TURBT and intravesical therapy prevent the progression of superficial to locally advanced or metastatic disease in 40% of cases. Overall, however, approximately 30% of patients with superficial tumours develop invasive disease. The prognosis for bladder cancer declines steeply with stage of disease (Table 13.3 and Figure 3.1). During the terminal phases of illness, patients require specialist care for symptom palliation. The disease may spread to bone, lung or liver, and opiate analgesia or local radiotherapy may be helpful in easing symptoms (Figure 13.3).

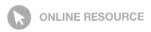 ONLINE RESOURCE

Case Study: The Albanian barber.

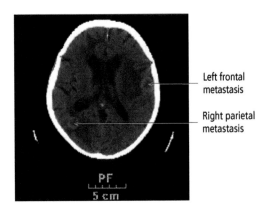

Left frontal metastasis

Right parietal metastasis

Figure 13.3 A man with a 3-year history of invasive bladder cancer treated with radical radiotherapy developed morning headaches and numbness of his right arm. His CT scan shown here shows two ring-enhancing metastases in the left frontal and right parietal regions with marked surrounding oedema.

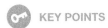 KEY POINTS

- Over a million people in the world are living with bladder cancer and cigarette smoking accounts for one-third of cases
- The initial symptoms include haematuria, dysuria and frequency of micturition and these should not be ignored by patients or their doctors

14

Prostate cancer

Learning objectives

✓ Explain the epidemiology and pathogenesis of prostate cancer
✓ Recognize the common presentation and clinical features of prostate cancer
✓ Describe the treatment strategies and outcomes of prostate cancer

---

Francois Mitterand was France's longest serving president. He was elected in May 1981 and left office after completing two whole 7-year terms in 1995. In November 1981, at the age of 65 and just 6 months into his first term, he was diagnosed with metastatic prostate cancer and commenced endocrine therapy. Eleven years into his presidency in 1992 he had developed hormone refractory disease, requiring radiotherapy. Throughout his presidency he hid the diagnosis from the public, issuing false medical bulletins and effectively making his cancer a state secret. Nevertheless, he survived until January 1996, over 14 years with metastatic prostate cancer, almost all spent as the French president. Following his death, his former personal physician, Dr Claude Gubler, wrote *Le Grand Secret,* a book disclosing Mitterrand's cancer. Gubler was stuck off the medical register for breach of confidentiality for revealing the truth but not for countersigning the 40 false medical bulletins describing the President's health as sound.

Epidemiology

Prostate cancer is the most common cancer in men in the Western world. In 2011, 41,736 men were diagnosed with prostate cancer and 10,793 died of the disease in the United Kingdom (Table 14.1).

Prostate cancer death rates have trebled in the last 30 years and the incidence figures have increased so strikingly that the number of men affected by this cancer has overtaken lung cancer as the most common of all male cancers in the United Kingdom and the United States. How do we explain this increase in prostate cancer incidence? Much of the increase has been attributed to the incidental discovery of prostate cancer because of rising numbers of transurethral resection of the prostate (TURP) operations and PSA testing. Prostate cancer risk increases with age and over the last 60 years the average age of death of men has increased from 65 to 79 years. However, after correcting for the ageing population, the rise in incidence of prostate cancer remains. Currently if you are a man your lifetime risk of getting prostate cancer is one in eight.

Pathogenesis

It is unlikely that there is a significant genetic basis to this recent change in incidence. No single gene has been found to cause prostate cancer although there are associations between risk and around 40 different genes. What is likely is that there are environmental risk factors. The impact of environmental factors in disease pathogenesis can be evaluated in migrating populations and their offspring. There were huge waves of migration from South East Asia to North America and Hawaii at the turn of the 19th century. Prostate cancer has a very low incidence in Asia (Figure 1.15). The incidence of prostate cancer in the generations that followed these waves of migration

---

Oncology: Lecture Notes, Third Edition. Mark Bower and Jonathan Waxman.
Companion Website: www.lecturenoteseries.com/oncology

Table 14.1 UK registrations for prostate cancer 2010

	Percentage of all cancer registrations	Rank of registration	Lifetime risk of cancer	Change in ASR (2000–2010)	5-year overall survival
	Male	Male	Male	Male	Male
Prostate cancer	25	1st	1 in 8	+22%	81%

increased, so that in two generations the incidence of prostate cancer was almost equivalent to that occurring in the Caucasian neighbours of these migrant families.

A second line of evidence for the significance of environmental factors comes from prospective and retrospective dietary studies, where it has been clearly shown that the incidence of prostate cancer in vegetarians is 50–75% that of the incidence in omnivores. There are inconsistent correlates between prostate cancer and diets containing smoked foods and dairy produce and protective benefits from diets that are rich in soy beans. For once neither smoking nor alcohol consumption appears to influence the risk of prostate cancer.

Heredity plays a minor role in prostate cancer accounting for less than one in twenty cases. The overall risk of developing prostate cancer is increased by just 1.3-fold for those men who have an affected father with the condition and by 2.5-fold for those with a brother affected. Germline mutations of the breast cancer susceptibility gene BRCA-2 increase the risk of prostate cancer. No consistent somatic genetic defect has been described within the tumour cells of prostate cancer; most have a multiplicity of mutations. These include a loss of heterozygosity around a number of chromosomes, the most common of which is a loss of genetic material on chromosome 10p. Known tumour suppressor genes are infrequently mutated in prostate cancer – for example, the retinoblastoma (RB) gene is mutated in just 5% of tumours.

Prostate cancer is strikingly hormone dependent. This is because the growth of prostatic tumours is regulated by the androgen receptor, which is a member of the steroid superfamily of transcription factors, and the majority of treatments for prostate cancer have their effect through this receptor. Steroids contain four linked cycloalkane rings and the 27-carbon precursor, cholesterol, is formed in humans from acetyl-CoA via the mevalonate or HMG-CoA reductase pathway that statins act on. Cholesterol is subsequently transformed into 21-carbon pregnanes (e.g. progesterone), 19-carbon androstanes (e.g. testosterone) and 18-carbon estranes (e.g. estradiol) (Figure 5.4).

Presentation

Patients with prostate cancer commonly present with urinary frequency, a poor urine flow or difficulty with starting and stopping urination. Other associated symptoms on presentation include bone pain and general debility. Weight loss is rare. Although patients with these symptoms are generally referred by GPs to a urologist, there is no real need for the urologist to be involved as diagnosis and treatment follows a medical pathway that rarely involves any surgery.

Patients with a potential diagnosis of prostate cancer usually have a blood test for prostate-specific antigen (PSA) performed by their GP. PSA levels are not necessarily diagnostic of prostate cancer. Where levels are raised above the normal range of 4 µg/L to between 4 and 10 µg/L, the chance of the patient having prostate cancer is approximately 25%. At levels over 10 µg/L, the chance of diagnosing prostate cancer increases to 40%. Levels of this antigen may be elevated in benign prostatic hypertrophy. Strangely, few people know much about PSA, and what is published in the Daily Mail and other newspapers about PSA is invariably wrong. PSA is a serine protease and acts like drain cleaner for the prostate, dissolving the prostatic coagulum.

In outpatients, a careful history should be taken, a full examination made and routine blood tests including PSA performed. In addition, plain X-rays of the chest and pelvis should be performed and a transrectal ultrasound and bone scan booked (Figures 3.4, 14.1 and 14.2).

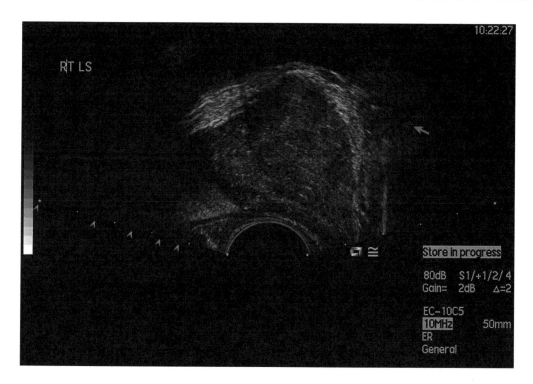

Figure 14.1 Transrectal ultrasound of the prostate gland showing extension of the primary tumour through the prostatic capsule (T3 disease).

Staging and grading

From the clinical findings an assessment can be made of the degree of prostate enlargement. If the prostate is malignant, it is staged as in Table 14.2. The tumour grade can be described as well, moderately or poorly differentiated. This is further elaborated in the Gleason scoring system. The Gleason system scores prostatic tumours on a 1–5 scale, where 5 is the most poorly differentiated. The combined Gleason grade describes the appearances of the two most common areas of prostatic malignancy. High-grade prostatic intraepithelial neoplasia (PIN), an acronym that coasts off the tongue with greater ease than prostatic intraepithelial neoplasia, has been suggested as a pre-malignant condition leading to invasive cancer, just as cervical intraepithelial neoplasia (CIN) leads to invasive cervical cancer. However, the evidence for this progression to malignancy is poor and surgeons should be discouraged from operative procedures in patients with PIN alone.

Transrectal ultrasonography (TRUS) should be combined with needle biopsy. As a standard, six cores are taken in general. Since diagnostic certainty is increased by carrying out more biopsies, 8 or even 12 needle cores are taken in many centres. Where the diagnosis is difficult and PSA levels are high, saturation biopsies are carried out but this procedure, which may involve 20 or more biopsies, may lead to yet further difficulties in defining treatment if a focus of low-grade cancer is found. If cancer is confirmed histologically, pelvic magnetic resonance imaging (MRI) is used to define extracapsular spread, involvement of the seminal vesicles or lymph nodes if radical therapy is contemplated. Radioisotope bone scanning is a sensitive method of detecting bone metastases but the high false positive rate lowers its specificity.

Treatment

Treatment of early-stage prostate cancer

The treatment of prostate cancer depends upon clinical stage and is surrounded by controversy. The approach to localized low-grade prostate cancer may be

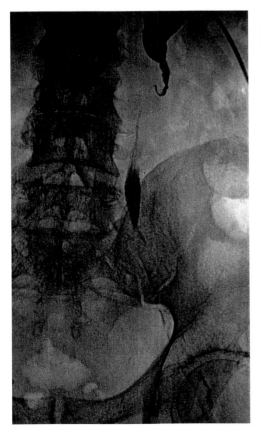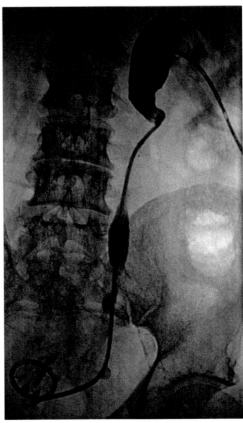

Figure 14.2 Antegrade nephrostogram showing irregular tapering and lack of contrast due to ureteric obstruction and hydronephrosis before and after the passage of a JJ stent to relive obstruction that was due to external compression by prostate cancer.

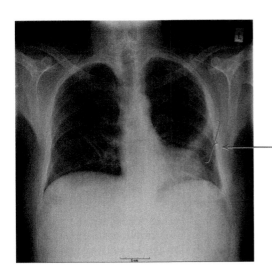

Sclerotic expanded left third rib due to metastatic prostate cancer

Figure 14.3 A the chest X-ray showing sclerosis and expansion of the anterolateral aspect of left third rib. This appearance was due to metastasis from prostate cancer, although the differential radiological diagnosis would include lymphoma, osteopetrosis and Paget's disease.

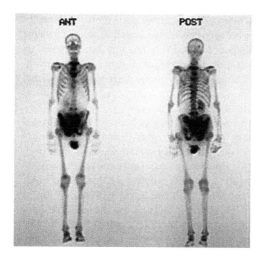

ANT   POST

Figure 14.4 Bone scan showing multiple hot spots in the axial skeleton due to bone metastases and a non-functioning left kidney due to long-standing obstruction. The patient had locally advanced and metastatic prostate cancer.

either surveillance or radical therapy. Radical treatment is advocated for high-grade localized prostate cancer in fit men, but here the debate surrounds the choice of therapy; radical prostatectomy, external beam radiotherapy (EBRT) or brachytherapy. The options for treatment depend upon the patient's overall state and preference. Observation involves regular follow-up without treatment, usually digital rectal examination and PSA measurement every 3–6 months. EBRT involves approximately 6 weeks of attendance at hospital for prostatic irradiation, which is given in an attempt to sterilize the tumour. Radiotherapy has morbidity. Acutely, it may be associated with symptoms of cystitis and proctitis; post-treatment it may produce impotence in up to 70% of patients. Newer techniques such as intensity-modulated radiotherapy (IMRT) enable higher doses of radiation to be delivered to the tumour whilst sparing the normal surrounding tissues. Radical prostatectomy involves major pelvic surgery, with removal of the prostate and associated lymph glands. The open surgical approach may be either perineal or retropubic. Modern anaesthetic techniques and surgical advances have meant that the morbidity is limited, but a degree of incontinence is reported in up to 25% of patients, and a degree of impotence, which is under-reported by surgeons, occurs in up to 90% of patients. It is agreed that morbidity has been reduced by the introduction of nerve-sparing techniques. There is an operative mortality of less than 1%. Surgeons delight in new toys and have been allowed to play with the Da Vinci robot; laparoscopic radical prostatectomy carried out by this procedure is said to lead to fewer problems with potency and certainly less blood loss than with standard open surgery. Nevertheless a recent study of men treated by radical surgery found that 80% were dissatisfied with their quality of life after robotic surgery.

The reason the patient can be offered the prospect of choice in determining what therapy he should have for early-stage disease is that observation, radiotherapy and radical surgery have all been shown to offer the patient with good or moderate histology tumours the same overall chance of long-term survival. The advantages of surveillance include a better quality of life and absence of treatment side effects but this may be offset by the anxiety of living with untreated cancer and the need for regular follow-up. For patients, with poor histology, surgery offers a marginally better survival chance than radiotherapy. The survival advantage is minimal. There has, however, been no randomized comparison of these three options involving significant patient numbers; and so this subject remains a matter for vociferous debate. A recent study of approximately 600 patients randomized to receive either watchful waiting or radiotherapy showed a better outlook for treated patients. The outlook for patients with low-grade Gleason 3 + 3 tumours is so good that in many ways this tumour group should be regarded as not being a malignant tumour. NICE, the most venerable body, advocate surveillance alone for patients with Gleason 3 + 3 tumours.

Table 14.2 TNM staging of prostate cancer

T (primary tumour)	N (nodal status)	M (metastatic status)
T0: No tumour palpable	N0: No nodes	M0: No metastases
T1: Tumour in one lobe of the prostate	N1: Homolateral nodes	M1: Metastases
T2: Tumour involving both prostate lobes	N2: Bilateral nodes	
T3: Tumour infiltrating out of the prostate to involve seminal vesicles	N3: Fixed regional nodes	
T4: Extensive tumour, fixed and infiltrating local structures	N4: Juxtaregional nodes	

In the early 1990s, investigations were initiated into the value of hormonal therapy given in addition to radiotherapy and surgery. No advantage to such "neoadjuvant" hormonal therapy has been found in those patients proceeding to radical surgery. In contrast, a number of randomized studies have shown an advantage to neoadjuvant hormonal therapy in patients receiving radiotherapy. The majority of studies have found a decreased risk of local relapse with hormonal therapy, and two major trials reported improved survival. There is controversy as to the suitable duration of treatment with adjuvant hormonal therapy.

Brachytherapy is a radiotherapy technique where the local intensity of radiation is increased by the implantation of radioactive seeds or wires (see Figure 3.11). This technique has been applied to localized prostate cancer. Up to 100 iodine-125 or palladium-103 radioactive seeds are permanently implanted directly into the prostate via transperineal needles under general or spinal anaesthetic. Excellent results have been claimed, but not proven in any randomized trial. Recent publications have shown that the incidence of major side effects of brachytherapy is the same as for conventional radiation, and the efficacy of brachytherapy is no doubt similar to conventional radiation treatment. Brachytherapy has additional side effects to radiotherapy and these include a 12% instance of urethral stricture requiring surgical intervention.

Treatment of locally advanced or metastatic prostate cancer

When patients have locally advanced, that is T3 or T4, prostate cancer or metastatic disease (Figures 14.3 and 14.4), the first-line treatment involves the use of hormonal therapy (see Figure 3.27). Urological surgeons have been heard to advocate radical surgery for T3 tumours, but 5-year "cure" rates are around 50% and so the authors of this book recommend systemic hormonal therapy or radiotherapy for this patient group. Again, this area is one of considerable debate and controversy.

Hormonal therapy for prostate cancer condition was first described in the 1940s, when the disease was found to be dependent upon testosterone. For this reason, the first treatments offered in the 1940s were orchiectomy, that is, removal of the testes or oestrogen therapy.

The results of treatment were first analysed in the 1960s by the Veterans Administration Cooperative Urological Research Group (VACURG). In their studies, the VACURG randomized patients to treatment with oestrogens or placebo, or with orchiectomy or placebo, respectively. The overall survival of patients treated or untreated was the same, but there was an excess mortality rate from cardiovascular deaths in the oestrogen-treated group. The reason for this is that oestrogens cause an increased coagulability of blood and increased blood volumes.

Because orchiectomy is barbaric and oestrogen therapy is associated with morbidity and mortality, medical treatments for this condition have been sought which are not so invasive and have no side effects. The most effective of these treatments, which has the least morbidity associated with its use, is a group of compounds called the gonadotropin-releasing hormone (GnRH) agonists. These include leuprorelin acetate, goserelin acetate and buserelin. These are currently given subcutaneously by monthly or 3-monthly injection. When treatment with GnRH agonists is started, there is a transient surge in luteinizing hormone (LH) before the levels fall, and this can lead to an initial rise in testosterone and flare of disease. Anti-androgens, such as flutamide and bicalutamide, can cover this flare by directly inhibiting the androgen receptor. Some doctors advocate continuing treatment with this combination or maximal androgen blockade of GnRH agonist plus anti-androgen. The evidence is overwhelming for the use of these agents in combination; survival is improved, osteoporosis is prevented and a chance is provided for an anti-androgen withdrawal response.

Prostate cancer is very responsive to endocrine treatment and 80% of patients improve subjectively. After an average period of approximately 1 year, however, most patients with metastatic cancer on presentation have PSA evidence of relapse. When biopsies from patients with recurrent tumour are examined and compared with biopsies on presentation, it is striking that up to 50% will show androgen receptor mutations. This is in contradiction to the situation in breast cancer, where hormone receptor amplification is the most commonly observed change. Over 700 mutations of the androgen receptor have been described, and these changes are a clue to the probable reason for the response to second-line hormonal therapy. This response is transient and is thought to occur because the mutation has led the tumour to depend upon the anti-androgen as a growth factor. The usual first approach to this is the addition of an anti-androgen to the GnRH agonist if initial treatment was GnRH monotherapy. Conversely if the first-line treatment was maximal androgen blockade, second-line treatment is the withdrawal of anti-androgen therapy, where cessation of anti-androgen treatment will lead to a response in up to 40% of patients.

Subsequent biochemical or clinical disease progression is usually described as hormone-refractory disease or castrate-resistant disease. An increasing number of approaches are available for hormone-refractory prostate cancer including interfering with the androgen pathway with oral abiraterone or enzalutamide, and intravenous taxane chemotherapy (docetaxel and cabazitaxel). Abiraterone inhibits androgen synthesis in both the testes and adrenal glands by inhibiting the CYP17 enzymes, 17,20-lyase and 17-α-hydroxylase. Corticosteroid replacement therapy is necessary for patients treated with abiraterone. Enzalutamide inhibits androgen receptor signalling. Chemotherapy is increasingly popular in patients with prostate cancer. Taxanes are the only chemotherapy agents that have been shown to significantly prolong overall survival in men with castrate-resistant prostate cancer. Unfortunately, because there are so many more urologists than oncologists in the United Kingdom, only limited numbers of men with prostate cancer are offered chemotherapy. A recent study has shown that only one man in seven who might be suitable for treatment with chemotherapy receives it. This is attributed to the reluctance of urologists to refer patients to oncologists. One can only speculate and wonder as to the psychological causes of this difficulty.

Until recently, men with prostate cancer represented a rather passive but extremely brave group of individuals who accepted their fate. The last two decades have seen significant changes in the way that men deal with their cancers and prostate cancer has now become, quite rightly, politicized with the cause championed to good effect.

The large number of men with advanced prostate cancer and the relatively prolonged natural history of the illness mean that palliative care plays an essential role. Moreover, the high frequency of metastases to bones reinforces the importance of palliative radiotherapy for pain control, bisphosphonates to reduce skeletal events and orthopaedic surgery for the management of pathological fractures (see Figure 3.6). Metastatic spinal cord compression is a relatively common occurrence in late-stage disease (Figure 14.5).

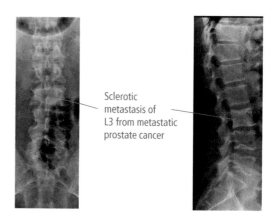

Sclerotic metastasis of L3 from metastatic prostate cancer

Figure 14.5 Sclerotic metastases of spine from prostate cancer.

all lead to an equivalent survival of 80% at 10 years for patients with small volume, well or moderately differentiated tumours. Patients with poorly differentiated, high Gleason grade tumours have a worse outlook with observation and radiotherapy than with surgery. Unfortunately only 15% of patients survive 15 years.

Prognosis for metastatic and large bulk localized disease

It has been shown in clinical trials that the addition of an anti-androgen to gonadotropin-releasing hormone agonist therapy leads to an improvement in survival rate. In the original studies, the median survival for patients with metastatic tumours treated with combination anti-androgen therapy was 3 years, as opposed to 2.5 years for patients treated with single-agent gonadotropin-releasing hormone agonist or by orchiectomy. Thanks to advances in drug development, the survival of patients with metastatic prostate cancer has been extended to around 6 years. The prospects for survival for a patient with bulky locally advanced disease without metastases are much better. The median survival of this group is 8 years. It is not known whether there is an advantage to combination gonadotropin-releasing hormone agonist and anti-androgen therapy in this patient group.

Prognosis

Prognosis for small bulk localized disease

The outlook for small bulk localized disease depends upon grade. Observation, radiotherapy and surgery

Screening

There is controversy also regarding the value of screening. It is important to recall that most men of

80 will have cancer cells in their prostate glands but only 1 in 25 will actually die of the prostate cancer. Furthermore, 25–40% of men with a raised PSA do not have prostate cancer. It is the substantial risk of over-diagnosis and treatment complications that detract from prostate cancer screening (see Box 3.5). There is no convincing evidence that earlier detection and treatment of prostate cancer (following detection by screening rather than symptoms) leads to improvements in mortality. Two large randomized screening trials have been recently published but have done little to clarify the issue. The European Randomized Study of Screening for Prostate Cancer (ERSPC) recruited 182,000 men aged 50–74 and allocated half to PSA screening. They reported a modest reduction in death from prostate cancer in the screened men, estimating that 1055 men needed to be screened to prevent one death from prostate cancer. The US prostate, lung, colorectal and ovarian screening programme (PLCO) study randomized 76,000 men aged 55–74 to annual PSA and DRE screening and reported increased number of prostate cancer diagnoses in the screened men but no fall in prostate cancer deaths. Unfortunately, overviews show that early detection of prostate cancer has not been found to save lives. A recent meta-analysis of screening in 350,000 normal men has concluded that screening increased the number of men diagnosed with prostate cancer but

did not reduce deaths from prostate cancer. Wouldn't it be nice if screening could be applied to normal population? Unfortunately meta-analyses such as this provide the reason why there is no national prostate cancer screening programme in the United Kingdom.

ONLINE RESOURCE

Case Study: The Rasta with a backache.

KEY POINTS

- Prostate cancer is the most common cancer in men and its incidence is rising even after adjustment for the ageing population
- Prostate cancer screening of well men by prostate-specific antigen measurement increased the number of men diagnosed but does not reduce deaths from prostate cancer
- Patients with prostate cancer commonly present with urinary flow symptoms or with bone pain from metastases
- The clinical management of prostate cancer is controversial at almost every stage and grade of disease with surgeons, radiotherapists and oncologists often interpreting the data differently

15

Testis cancer

Learning objectives

✓ Explain the epidemiology and pathogenesis of testis cancer
✓ Recognize the common presentation and clinical features of testis cancer
✓ Describe the treatment strategies and outcomes of testis cancer

Testicular cancer is one of the few solid cancers in adults that may be successfully cured even in the presence of metastases. This has only been achievable in the last 40 years, since the introduction of cisplatin chemotherapy. Cisplatin was discovered serendipitously by Barnett Rosenberg, a physicist at Michigan State University, in 1965. He studied the effects of electric currents on *Escherichia coli* using platinum electrodes in a water bath and found that they stopped dividing but not growing, leading to bacteria up to 300 times longer than normal. This was found to be due to cisplatin, a product from the platinum electrodes, which was interfering with DNA replication. Following this, Professor Sir Alexander Haddow, the then head of the Chester Beatty Institute in London, showed that cisplatin was active against melanoma in mice, and clinical trials with human patients began in 1972.

Epidemiology

The treatment of testis cancer represents one of the major and wonderful triumphs of oncology. The application of modern treatments has led to a fall in death rates by 70% over the last 10–15 years, and in 2011 only 68 men died of this condition in the United Kingdom compared to over 2207 patients that were diagnosed (Table 15.1).

Pathogenesis

A number of factors have been shown to increase the risk of developing testicular cancer:

- Cryptorchidism, or testicular maldescent (risk is less if orchidopexy is performed before puberty)
- Previous testicular cancer (risk in contralateral testis is 12-fold increased)
- Family history (father increases risk fourfold, brother ninefold)
- Caucasian (higher risk than other races)
- HIV (men living with HIV have a 35% higher risk)

There have been significant advances in the understanding of the molecular biology of adult male germ cell tumours. It is over 15 years since the original identification of the characteristic cytogenetic marker of adult male germ cell tumours: isochromosome 12p. An extra copy of chromosome 12p is present in 85% of all tumours, and in the remaining percentage there are tandem duplications embedded at other chromosomal locations. The cyclin D2 gene, which is concerned with the regulation of the cell cycle, is mapped to this area. This suggests that the aberrant expression of cyclin D2 leads to the dysregulation of the normal cell cycle and tumour development. This abnormality is present in both seminoma and teratoma. Testicular

Oncology: Lecture Notes, Third Edition. Mark Bower and Jonathan Waxman.
© 2015 by John Wiley & Sons, Ltd. Published 2015 by John Wiley & Sons, Ltd.
Companion Website: www.lecturenoteseries.com/oncology

Table 15.1 UK registrations for testicular cancer 2010

	Percentage of all cancer registrations	Rank of registration	Lifetime risk of cancer	Change in ASR (2000–2010)	5-year overall survival
	Male	Male	Male	Male	Male
Testis cancer	1	16th	1 in 190	+4%	97%

tumours also express c-KIT, stem cell factor receptor and platelet-derived growth factor (PDGF) α-receptor gene. Mutations in the KIT gene occur in 8% of all testicular germ cell tumours but are seen in 93% of patients with bilateral disease. These changes in the KIT gene appear to be specific to seminoma. These molecular findings suggest possible therapeutic options.

Presentation

Media campaigns have led to public awareness of testicular cancer as a curable condition and of the importance of early diagnosis. Generally, patients noticing testicular masses present to their GPs and are referred immediately to urology outpatients. There remain, however, a number of alarming instances where GPs have treated patients with testicular tumours for epididymitis rather than referring them on. Patients with teratoma present during the second and third decades of their lives, generally with swelling of the testes and less frequently with pain. Men with seminoma may present in their third to fifth decades. Men with testicular cancer may have gynaecomastia. This is due to the production of steroid hormones by the malignancy and clearly not to α-fetoprotein (AFP) or human chorionic gonadotropin (HCG) synthesis. Around 30% of patients with testicular cancer are oligozoospermic on presentation and another 30% have poorly motile sperm that render their manufacturers functionally sterile. An increasingly common presentation of testis cancer is therefore via the infertility services.

In urology outpatients, after examination, the patient should proceed to initial staging by routine haematology, biochemistry and measurement of AFP and HCG. A chest X-ray should be requested and an ultrasound examination of the testes ordered. The ultrasound will show features suggestive of testicular cancer, such as increased vascularity accompanying a mass. There may be additional features of microlithiasis, suggesting that the tumour has developed from carcinoma *in situ*. Carcinoma *in situ* is a bilateral condition with a 3% subsequent chance of development of a second testicular tumour. Rarely, patients with seminomas have very long histories of a testicular mass; the longest that the authors of this textbook have come across is 5 years and the patient with this history had stage 1 testis cancer.

Following these investigations, arrangements should be made for the patient to proceed to orchiectomy. This is performed through a groin rather than a scrotal incision, which would lead to an increased risk of the scrotal spread of testicular cancer, particularly in cases where there are embryonal elements to the tumour. The testis is removed by the surgeon, cut in half, examined and sent for pathological examination. Following the histological confirmation of malignancy, CT imaging of the chest abdomen and pelvis should be organized (Figure 15.1) and serial tumour marker levels measured post-operatively (Figure 15.2). Tumour markers fall to normal levels in localized testis cancer, but will not do so in disseminated disease. The half-life of HCG is around 48 hours and of AFP is 5 days.

Staging and grading

There are four main types of testicular tumour: seminoma, teratoma, lymphoma and small cell (Figure 15.2). Teratoma constitutes approximately 75% of all testicular malignancies and appears cystic when examined by the naked eye. Pure seminoma constitutes 20% of tumours and is uniform in appearance. Approximately 5% of all testicular tumours are lymphoma, the appearance of which is generally uniform but with some areas of necrosis. Less than 1% of tumours are of small cell origin. These tumours have no specific macroscopic features.

Microscopically, teratomas constitute a variety of different elements which may include cartilage, muscle, bone and virtually any other tissue. Subtypes of teratoma are described, and they are called undifferentiated, differentiated or choriocarcinoma (Figure 15.2). Seminoma consists of uniform and large cells with darkly standing nuclei.

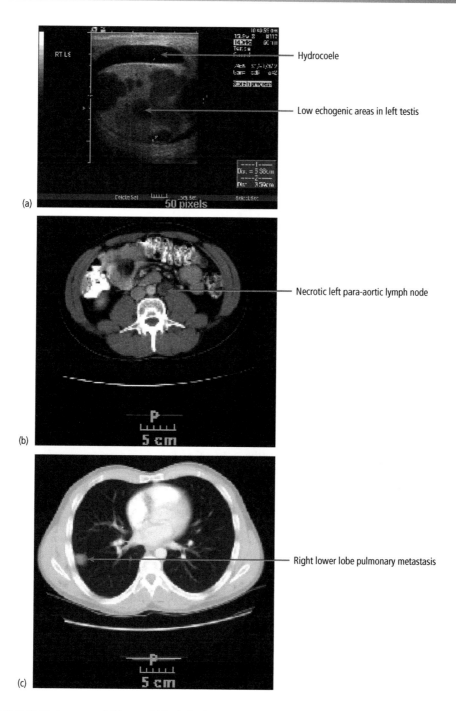

Figure 15.1 Testicular cancer. A 24-year-old Australian barman presented with a swollen testicle. (a) His ultrasound examination showed an enlarged left testicle with multiple low echogenicity areas and a small hydrocoele. (b) His body CT scan showed an enlarged and necrotic left para-aortic lymph node and (c) a right lower lobe peripheral lung nodule. His tumour markers were raised (serum AFP = 670 ng/mL; serum HCG = 56 IU/mL). Despite having metastatic disease at presentation, his chances of cure are over 90%.

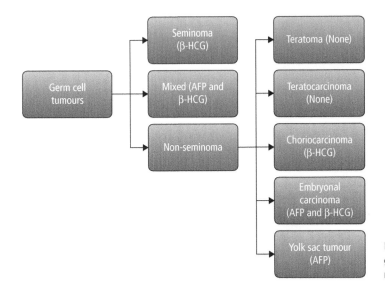

Figure 15.2 A classification of germ cell tumours and their tumour marker production.

Having made a histological diagnosis, treatment is initiated and depends upon the stage to which the tumour has advanced. The following stages are described and determined by CT imaging of the chest, abdomen and pelvis:

- Stage I: tumour confined to testes
- Stage II: tumour spread to abdominal lymph nodes
- Stage III: tumour spread to lymph nodes above the diaphragm
- Stage IV: tumour invading organs other than lymph nodes such as liver or lung

The disease is further sub-staged according to the size of the metastatic deposits and the number of pulmonary metastases. In the United States, retroperitoneal lymph node dissection is undertaken to stage testicular cancer, although this practice is disappearing. In our view, node dissection is not indicated as a routine staging procedure because of the major morbidity of the operation and also because of the side effects, which include retrograde ejaculation. Node dissection for staging purposes is not part of medical practice in the United Kingdom, which relies on imaging. Retrograde ejaculation is the ejaculation of sperm backwards into the bladder rather than forwards into the urethra. This phenomenon does not necessarily mean that the patient is functionally sterile, because sperm can be collected and artificial insemination techniques employed to successfully fertilize the patient's partner. In modern times, such *in vitro* fertilization (IVF) programmes require aspiration of sperm from the testes or testicular biopsy with sperm retrieval if collection of urine post-ejaculation with sperm retrieval is unsuccessful.

Treatment

Treatment of stage I testicular cancer

The tumour stage of testicular cancer defines its treatment. If the tumour is localized to the testis, two actions are available to the clinician. The first option for both seminoma and teratoma is observation without further therapy. If this policy is followed in the absence of poor prognosis pathology features, then the likelihood of any further treatment being required is 13% for testicular teratoma and 17% for seminoma. It should be noted that almost all patients who develop progressive disease during the period of observation without treatment are salvageable by chemotherapy. Active surveillance for stage I seminoma and stage I teratoma without lymphovascular invasion or embryonal elements is safe but requires regular follow-up with clinical examination, blood tests and radiology.

In the United Kingdom, many urologists refer patients with stage I seminoma for radiotherapy, following which the prognosis is excellent, with virtually no chance of relapse. The option of single-agent carboplatin is a vastly better alternative. A randomized trial has shown that chemotherapy with carboplatin is as effective as radiation therapy and without the morbidity, two infusions being given at

4-weekly intervals in contrast to 3 weeks of daily radiation therapy. Patients with stage I teratoma with high risk features are generally referred for adjuvant chemotherapy using bleomycin, etoposide and cisplatin (BEP) chemotherapy. Treatment in certain circumstances might be modified, dropping bleomycin from the treatment programme to reduce the risk of lung damage.

Treatment of stage II testicular cancer

For stage IIa seminoma, that is, with a nodal mass of less than 2 cm in diameter as defined by CT scanning, many clinicians in the United Kingdom advise treatment with radiotherapy. A consensus of opinion is now emerging, which follows the view that two courses of cytotoxic chemotherapy are equally as effective as radiation treatment in the control of this stage of disease. For stage IIb seminoma, that is, for patients with a disease mass of less than 5 cm, some clinicians, particularly radiotherapists, still treat with radiotherapy, but this is not generally advised in view of the side effects of large field radiotherapy. Chemotherapy should be given using cisplatin based combination chemotherapy.

For all patients with greater than stage IIb disease, whether it is seminoma or teratoma, cytotoxic chemotherapy is given. Before the advent of cytotoxic chemotherapy for teratoma, the disease was invariably fatal. The development of effective chemotherapy programmes has bought about a revolution in the management of patients with malignancy, and now virtually all patients are cured by treatment.

Treatment of advanced testicular cancer

Treatment with cytotoxic agents was originally introduced into medical practice by Li in the early 1960s. As a result, approximately 8% of patients with advanced disease were cured, using a combination of agents that included actinomycin and chlorambucil. In the early 1970s, Samuels treated patients with vinblastine and bleomycin and produced remissions in approximately 50% of men treated. This treatment was of considerable toxicity because of the large dosages of vinblastine and bleomycin used and the relative lack of support programmes for patients with neutropenic sepsis and thrombocytopenia, which occur as a result of the use of these agents. In 1976, Einhorn introduced the bleomycin, vinblastine and cisplatinum (BVP) programme for the treatment of malignant testicular tumours. The introduction of BVP was not in the context of a controlled clinical trial but in a speculative fashion and was found to work. Because BVP turned out to be such an effective regimen, it became widely used even before the results were published. This regimen was enormously successful, and 70% of patients with advanced disease were cured. By substituting etoposide for vinblastine, less toxicity resulted with equivalent effect.

Over the last decade, there have been further refinements in the way that treatment has been given. Drug treatment that initially required six courses of 5-day treatments has now been reduced to four courses of 3-day treatments. The expectation is that 95% of patients with good-prognosis tumour are cured with this regimen and 48% of patients with poor-prognosis disease are cured. Extraordinarily, there has been further change in the collective view with regard to chemotherapy for testicular cancer, and recently many oncologists have reverted to the original 5-day BEP programme. This is based upon analyses of huge numbers of patients and the realization of the superiority of this standard programme.

Treatment of residual tumour masses

At the end of treatment, one problem may be that of a persistent mass. By this we mean a residual tumour at the site of the original metastatic disease. The approach to this problem is to proceed to surgery. Surgery may be very extensive and involve both thoracotomy and laparotomy. At surgery, the residual mass of tumour is excised as completely as possible, and this may require dacron grafting of major vessels or removal of a kidney in order to take away the tumour completely. This operative procedure is extremely intricate. Histological examination of the excised mass shows that in one-third of cases there is necrotic tumour, in one-third of cases there is differentiated teratoma and in one-third of cases there is undifferentiated cancer. If necrotic tumour is found, no further action is taken. If undifferentiated tumour is found, further chemotherapy is given and 30–40% of patients will be cured by a combination of chemotherapy and surgery. In those patients who have residual differentiated tumour, it is important to remove the residual mass of the disease because over a 5-year period approximately 50% of differentiated tumours undergo further malignant change, transforming to undifferentiated malignancy.

Unfortunately, a significant number of patients still have progressive or unresponsive tumours and for these patients there is still a possibility of cure, which is in the range of 20–40%. Treatment programmes such as vinblastine, ifosfamide and cisplatin (VIP), paclitaxel, ifosfamide, cisplatin (TIP) or high-dose therapy with stem cell rescue are used to treat such patients.

Monitoring treatment

The effects of treatment are very closely monitored by measuring changes in the serum levels of the tumour markers AFP and HCG. These are hormones secreted by teratoma and seminoma. If the tumour is being treated effectively, then the levels of these hormones in the blood will decay over a known period: a half-life of 3–5 days for AFP and approximately 12–36 hours for HCG.

Side effects of treatment

There are specific toxicities that relate to treatment. Cisplatin will cause renal damage, deafness and peripheral neuropathy, which may manifest as numbness in the fingers or toes or complete loss of motor and sensory function in the limbs. Bleomycin unfortunately causes pulmonary toxicity, that is, an irreversible and progressive loss of lung function, which is fatal in approximately 2% of patients treated (see Figure 3.13). Bleomycin was omitted from Lance Armstrong's treatment for metastatic testicular cancer so that he would not lose lung function and of course he went on to win seven consecutive Tour de France titles, albeit with the assistance of doping. Testicular cancer and the drug regimen that is used generally causes sterility; by this we mean loss of functional spermatogenesis. In 80% of patients, however, there is recovery of spermatogenesis, which generally occurs at 18 months from the completion of treatment.

Prognosis

The treatment of teratoma and seminoma is highly complex and requires patient management in centres of excellence, where the delivery of chemotherapy and the maintenance of patients during neutropenic and thrombocytopenic episodes can be successfully achieved. In the best centres, 95% of patients with good-prognosis tumours are cured, which is without doubt a significant advance in medical science, as young men with this malignant tumour can be returned to an active life within the community after treatment.

Prognostic indices have been described in detail by many authors; one of the more commonly used is described by the International Germ Cell Cancer Collaborative Group. Patients with non-seminoma are classified as having good-prognosis disease with a 5-year survival of 92–95%, intermediate-prognosis tumours with a 72–80% 5-year survival and poor-prognosis tumours with a 48% 5-year survival. Patients with pure seminoma are described as having either good- or intermediate-prognosis disease. The classification into these categories is based on the presence or absence of non-nodal visceral metastases and serum levels of tumour markers. The influence of delay in diagnosis on prognosis is variably reported. Some authors link delay in excess of 1 year to a good prognosis, although this is described as being associated with a poor prognosis by other authors.

 ONLINE RESOURCE

Case Study: A tired suit.

 KEY POINTS

- Testis cancer is uncommon (1% of all cancers in men) but highly curable even when the disease has metastasized widely
- Cryptorchidism or testicular maldescent increases the risk of testis cancer but this risk is reduced if orchidopexy is performed before puberty
- Serum tumour markers (HCG and AFP) play an important role in the management of testis cancer, including diagnosis, prognosis and monitoring treatment

16

Gestational trophoblastic disease

Learning objectives

✓ Explain the epidemiology and pathogenesis of gestational trophoblastic disease (GTD)

✓ Recognize the common presentation and clinical features of GTD

✓ Describe the treatment strategies and outcomes of GTD

Gestational trophoblastic tumours originate from placental tissues and are among the few human cancers that can be cured, even in the presence of widespread metastasis. To a large extent the tumours are the father's fault as in most cases they contain chiefly paternal DNA. The term gestational trophoblastic disease (GTD) covers hydatidiform molar pregnancies, invasive moles, choriocarcinomas and placental site trophoblastic tumours. Half of the women with choriocarcinoma develop GTD after a molar pregnancy; the remainder have previously had non-molar gestations. Since GTD is relatively rare but can be treated with very high cure rates, all patients should be referred to specialist national units.

Epidemiology

The incidence of GTD varies geographically, with the highest rates reported from Asia and the risk rises with maternal age and a history of prior molar pregnancy. In the United Kingdom, hydatidiform moles account for one in 1000 pregnancies and about 10% of these will progress to persistent trophoblastic disease requiring chemotherapy.

Pathogenesis

Cytogenetic and molecular analysis of hydatidiform moles has provided a clue as to their origin (Figure 16.1). The majority of complete moles have a 46XX karyotype, with both X-chromosomes of paternal origin (androgenetic). They are believed to originate from fertilization of an empty ovum by a haploid sperm that then underwent duplication. In contrast, partial moles contain both maternal and paternal DNA and are typically triploid 69XXY, presumably as a result of fertilization of a single ovum by two sperm. It is thought that the developmental abnormality affecting uniparental diploid cells in complete moles (in this case androgenetic, 46XX) is due to genomic imprinting. The expression of some genes is determined by their parental origin – whether the allele was inherited from the mother or father – and this persists through multiple rounds of DNA amplification. This parent-of-origin effect is known as genomic imprinting and only affects a minority of genes. Genomic imprinting is an epigenetic phenomenon that does not rely on changes to the DNA base sequence but rather on methylation of individual bases. One

Oncology: Lecture Notes, Third Edition. Mark Bower and Jonathan Waxman.
© 2015 by John Wiley & Sons, Ltd. Published 2015 by John Wiley & Sons, Ltd.
Companion Website: www.lecturenoteseries.com/oncology

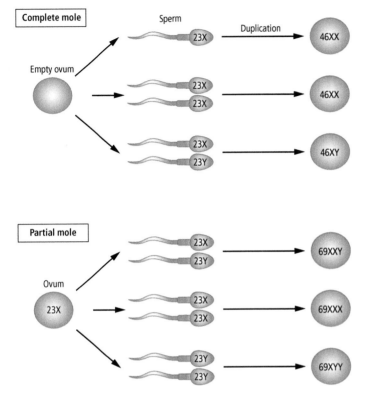

Figure 16.1 Possible chromosomal origin of complete and partial hydatidiform moles.

example of imprinting in humans is the insulin-like growth factor 2 (IGF2) gene. Only the paternal copy of IGF2 is expressed in foetal life; the silenced maternal gene is said to be "imprinted". The relaxation of this maternal imprinting results in congenital Beckwith–Wiedemann syndrome: gigantism, macroglossia, exophthalmos, neonatal hypoglycaemia and predisposition to childhood cancers, including Wilms' tumour, rhabdomyosarcoma and adrenal tumours. Imprinting is also responsible for paired congenital syndromes on chromosome 15q11. This region is differently imprinted in maternal and paternal chromosomes, and both imprintings are needed for normal development. In a normal individual, the maternal allele is methylated, while the paternal allele is unmethylated. Some individuals fail to inherit a properly imprinted 15q11 from one parent, either due to deletion of the 15q11 region from that parent's chromosome 15 or rarely due to uniparental disomy (in which both copies have been inherited from the one parent). If neither copy of 15q11 has paternal imprinting, the result is Prader–Willi syndrome (characterized by hypotonia, obesity and hypogonadism). If neither copy has maternal imprinting, the result is the Angelman syndrome (characterized by epilepsy, tremors and a perpetually smiling facial expression).

Presentation

Women with trophoblastic disease usually present with antepartum haemorrhage, passing grape-like particles during early pregnancy, anaemia and hyperemesis. Hyperthyroidism may occur because human chorionic gonadotrophin (HCG) acts as a weak thyroid-stimulating hormone (TSH) receptor agonist, due to homology between β-subunits of HCG and TSH, which has been called molecular mimicry. Metastases are typically haemorrhagic. The most frequent sites are the lungs and brain, where they mimic pulmonary thromboembolic disease and subarachnoid haemorrhage. It is therefore always worthwhile performing a pregnancy test in women with these presentations, since normal serum or urine HCG levels exclude this diagnosis. Choriocarcinoma, although rare, is an important diagnosis, as the tumour is exquisitely sensitive to chemotherapy and over 95% of women with this diagnosis can be cured. The definitive diagnostic investigations are a quantitative serum HCG assay and pelvic ultrasonography with colour Doppler flow measurement. Most cases of choriocarcinoma follow a hydatidiform molar pregnancy, although it may also occur after either spontaneous abortion or normal-term pregnancy. If choriocarcinoma follows a molar pregnancy, molecular analysis reveals that the tumour DNA is entirely androgenetic, being derived from the father, with the loss of all maternal alleles. In contrast, post-term choriocarcinoma has a biparental genotype, with DNA from both parents. Nonetheless, all cases of choriocarcinoma include paternal DNA sequences that are absent from the patient's genome and this may be used to confirm the diagnosis genetically if necessary.

Treatment

GTD was the first cancer to be cured by chemotherapy alone in the early 1960s. A scoring scheme has been devised that determines the risk of developing drug resistance to methotrexate and women at low risk can be successfully treated with single-agent methotrexate, with very high success rates and very few long-term sequelae. Women at higher risk of resistance require combination chemotherapy schedules, which, although still highly successful, run a small risk of causing a second malignancy. Serum HCG acts as the ideal tumour marker in this disease. HCG can be used:

- to screen women following a molar pregnancy
- to identify persistent trophoblastic disease that requires chemotherapy
- as a diagnostic investigation and in some circumstances obviates the need for a tissue diagnosis

- as part of the prognostic scoring index
- to determine the effectiveness of treatment
- to detect remission or chemoresistance
- in follow-up to identify relapse

Prognosis

The prognosis of gestational trophoblastic tumours is excellent, with the rare exceptions of placental site histological subtype. The cure rates exceed 95%, and much of the current focus of clinical research is aimed at minimizing the long-term side effects of any treatment rather than attempts to increase the cure rates.

 ONLINE RESOURCE

Case Study: The good casualty officer.

 KEY POINTS

- Gestational trophoblastic tumours originate from placental tissues
- The term gestational trophoblastic disease (GTD) covers hydatidiform molar pregnancies, invasive moles, choriocarcinomas and placental site trophoblastic tumours, and these tumours contain mostly paternal DNA
- The cure rate is very high even in the presence of widespread metastasis

17

Cervical cancer

Learning objectives

✓ Explain the epidemiology and pathogenesis of cervical cancer

✓ Recognize the common presentation and clinical features of cervical cancer

✓ Describe the treatment strategies and outcomes of cervical cancer

---

We are at a point where we may be able to consider the elimination of cervical cancer from our population. This is because of the development of effective vaccines against the cause of the vast majority of cervical cancers. The only major obstacles against the implementation of vaccination programmes are religious prejudice and the financial backing to support vaccination programmes in non-industrialized countries.

Cervical cancer cells are one of the most important of the tools in the laboratory armamentarium. The history of the development of cervical cancer cell lines tells a story that encapsulates research developments and contemporary attitudes to research. In 1951, George Otto Gey developed HeLa, the first human cancer continuous cell line. These cells proliferate in tissue culture and have been the basis of a great deal of research into cancer biology and drug development. The sample originated from the cervical cancer of a young black woman, Henrietta Lacks of Baltimore. Many thousands of tons of HeLa cells are now found in the incubators and freezers of laboratories around the world. Unfortunately the patient died less than a year after the cell line was established, and her family are said to be shocked by the development and proliferation of the cell line, which was obtained presumably without consent at the time.

Epidemiology

Cancer of the cervix is thought to affect over one-third of a million women worldwide and represents 10% of all female cancers (see Figure 1.15). Eighty per cent of all cases of cervical cancer occur in the developing world. The incidence in the United Kingdom, as in many developed countries, is decreasing. In 2011, 3064 women were diagnosed and 972 women died of cervical cancer in the United Kingdom (Table 17.1).

Pathogenesis

Invasive cervical cancer is believed to be the final stage in a continuum that starts with infection of the cervix by high-risk genotypes of human papillomavirus (HPV) and progresses via cervical intraepithelial neoplasia (CIN) to invasive cancer (see Box 1.2). CIN is a cytological diagnosis and is divided into three grades (CIN1–3). The histological equivalent of CIN is the squamous intraepithelial lesion (SIL), which is divided into low-grade SIL (LGSIL) that is similar to CIN1 and high-grade SIL (HGSIL)

Oncology: Lecture Notes, Third Edition. Mark Bower and Jonathan Waxman.
© 2015 by John Wiley & Sons, Ltd. Published 2015 by John Wiley & Sons, Ltd.
Companion Website: www.lecturenoteseries.com/oncology

Table 17.1 UK registrations for cervical cancer 2010

	Percentage of all cancer registrations	Rank of registration	Lifetime risk of cancer	Change in ASR (2000–2010)	5-year overall survival
Cervical cancer	2	12th	1 in 139	+10%	67%

analogous to CIN2 and CIN3. There are over 100 genotypes of HPV and some are associated with a higher risk of cancer than others (see Chapter 2). Three-quarters of cervical cancers contain either HPV 16 or HPV 18 the two most common high risk HPV genotypes and a further 10% harbour HPV 31 or HPV 45. It is thought that cervical cancer only occurs in the presence of HPV and that HPV is the first identified example of a "necessary cause" of a human cancer. The risk of acquiring HPV infection rises with the number of sexual partners, whilst the risk of CIN3 increases with age at first sexual intercourse and with smoking. Smoking is not a risk factor for HPV infection but appears to co-operate with HPV infection in the pathogenesis of CIN and cervical cancer. HPV infection is also associated with cancers of the vulva, vagina, penis, anus and oropharynx. HPV infection has been estimated to cause 4.8% of the world's cancers.

Screening

In 1928, a Greek cytopathologist Georgios Papanicolau invented a cervical cytology smear test to detect cancer cells that has saved thousands of lives. Despite living until 1962, Papanicolau never received a call from the Nobel committee in Stockholm, although he did appear on the 10,000 drachma banknote before Greece adopted the Euro. Cervical smear screening was introduced in the United Kingdom in 1964 and the current programme is for women aged 25–49 to have screening every 3 years and women aged 50–65 to have smears every 5 years. Around 80% of women attend for their screens and 4.5 million women are screened every year. Screening has reduced the incidence of cervical cancer by over 50%. Of the women who have an abnormal smear test, 0.1% have cancer, 7% CIN3, 11% CIN2 and 25% CIN1. Screening by smear cytology is a subjective process, which, although well regulated, may be subject to human error. The introduction of liquid cytology has improved the diagnostic accuracy and this may be further improved when testing for HPV infection is added to the screening. It has been estimated that cervical cancer screening saved over 8000 lives in the United Kingdom in the decade 1988–1997.

Prevention (vaccination)

The central role of HPV infection in the pathogenesis of cervical cancer led to vaccination strategies. Recombinant HPV viral coat proteins self-assemble into hollow virus-like particles that lack DNA so are unable to replicate but are immunogenic. A quadrivalent vaccine made up of VLP of HPV 6, 11, 16 and 18 protects against 98% of CIN and cancer caused by HPV 16 and 18. In the United Kingdom, girls aged 12–13 years have been offered this vaccine since 2008. The quadrivalent vaccine also confers immunity against HPV 6 and 11, the main causes of genital warts.

Presentation

Women with cervical cancer usually present to their doctors with inter-menstrual bleeding, post-coital bleeding or painful intercourse. There may be a vaginal discharge that can be bloody or offensive or symptoms suggestive of a urinary infection such as urinary frequency or urgency. When the cancer has spread, common symptoms include back pain due to enlarged abdominal lymph nodes or referred pain in the legs due to involvement of the nerve plexuses of the pelvis. These symptoms may be accompanied by loss of weight. The examination should include an assessment of the patient's general state of health together with palpation of the abdomen and a vaginal assessment. This may confirm the presence of a discharge and reveal a cervical mass (Figure 17.1).

Outpatient diagnosis

The GP should refer the patient to a gynaecologist who will repeat the examination, take smears from the cervix for cytological examination and then organize admission for examination under anaesthesia and cervical biopsy. Colposcopy should be performed as an outpatient procedure prior to admission. This technique allows direct visualization of the cervix with

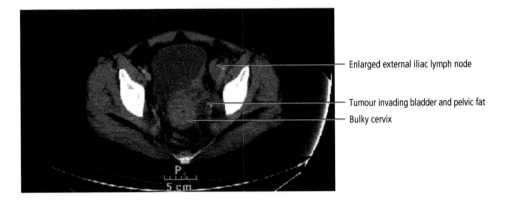

Enlarged external iliac lymph node

Tumour invading bladder and pelvic fat

Bulky cervix

5 cm

Figure 17.1 Cervical cancer with extensive, locally infiltrating tumour. This CT scan of a 65-year-old woman who had never had a cervical smear shows a bulky cervix with loss of the normal fat plane that separates it from the bladder. There is extension of the invasive cervical cancer into the posterolateral bladder wall anteriorly and into the pelvic fat laterally. There is also an enlarged left external iliac lymph node. The staging was therefore T4N1M0 (Stage 4A).

properly directed biopsies. After these assessments have been performed and a histological diagnosis has been obtained, staging investigations should be organized. These should include a full blood count, profile, chest X-ray and a CT or magnetic resonance scan of the abdomen and pelvis.

Staging and grading

Carcinoma of the cervix is staged as a result of these findings as follows:

- Stage 0: carcinoma *in situ*. Intraepithelial carcinoma (CIN) grades 1–3

- Stage 1A: microscopic disease confined to the cervix
- Stage 1B: clinically visible disease confined to the cervix
- Stage 2A: carcinoma extending beyond the cervix without parametrial involvement
- Stage 2B: parametrial involvement
- Stage 3A: extension to the pelvic side wall
- Stage 3B: extension to the pelvic wall with hydronephrosis or a non-functioning kidney
- Stage 4A: extension beyond the true pelvis to adjacent organs
- Stage 4B: spread to distant organs (Figure 17.2)

Sixty-six per cent of cervical cancers are squamous cell tumours. These are graded as G1, G2 or G3

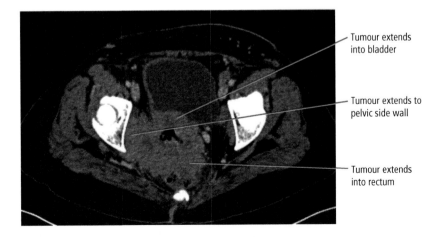

Tumour extends into bladder

Tumour extends to pelvic side wall

Tumour extends into rectum

Figure 17.2 Stage 4B cervical cancer. Tumour invasion into the bladder and rectum denotes T4 disease but in addition there was spread to regional lymph nodes (N1) and to retroperitoneal lymph nodes (M1). Hence the FIGO stage is 4B.

tumours, according to their microscopic appearance: G1 tumours are well differentiated, G2 tumours moderately and G3 tumours poorly differentiated. Fifteen per cent are adenocarcinomas, and these are also graded G1–3. Other rarer tumours include small cell cancers and lymphomas. Carcinomas *in situ* are graded I–III and abbreviated to CIN or cervical glandular intraepithelial neoplasia (CGIN), depending on whether squamous or adenocarcinoma cells are present.

Treatment

The treatment of cervical cancer depends upon the stage of disease. Stage 0 carcinoma of the cervix should be treated by cone biopsy or by surgical excision. Stage 1A disease is usually treated by hysterectomy, although more limited approaches with cone biopsy, local excision or radical trachelectomy have their advocates. Stage 1B and 2A cervical cancer is usually treated by either radical hysterectomy with pelvic lymphadenectomy or by pelvic irradiation. Both methods are equally effective in the long-term control of the disease. Stage 2B and 3 carcinoma of the cervix should be treated by pelvic radiotherapy and stage 4 carcinoma with chemotherapy.

Patients treated with pelvic radiotherapy with curative intent are frequently prescribed additional concurrent adjuvant chemotherapy. Typically, patients will be treated with weekly courses of single-agent cisplatin. Chemoradiation has been subjected to a number of randomized trials, and it has been concluded that concomitant chemoradiation appears to improve overall survival and progression-free survival in locally advanced cervical cancer. Consideration is also given to treatment with neo-adjuvant chemotherapy in some centres, but its role is not defined in cervical cancer.

The side effects of radiotherapy include an early menopause and radiotherapy-related bowel and bladder toxicity. Ovarian conservation is offered to younger patients treated by hysterectomy. Progressive or metastatic cervical carcinoma is treated with combination chemotherapy usually using a regimen that includes cisplatin.

Cervical intraepithelial neoplasia

As a result of treatment, virtually 100% of patients with CIN disease are cured. Approximately 0.05–0.3% of treated women subsequently develop invasive carcinoma. If CIN is left untreated, then over a 30-year follow-up period, 10–40% of patients will develop invasive cancer. The evidence for this is based on data from a single study carried out in New Zealand of untreated patients with CIN, by a clinician who apparently was convinced that CIN did not progress. The standard management for CIN is colposcopy with local ablation by cone biopsy, cryotherapy, laser therapy or loop electrosurgical excision procedure (LEEP).

Prognosis

Approximately 5% of patients treated for stage 1A carcinoma of the cervix will progress to develop advanced disease. Sixty-five to eighty-five per cent of all patients with stage 1B and 2A carcinoma of the cervix survive 5 years after treatment by a radical hysterectomy or radiation. The chance for a cure is smaller in stage 2B disease, and the expectation is that approximately 50–65% survive with radiotherapy alone. About 40–60% of patients with stage 3A disease and 25–45% of patients with stage 3B disease survive 5 years and are treated with radiotherapy and frequently with chemotherapy.

These statistics are relevant to patients with squamous cancers or adenocarcinomas. Variant histologies, such as small cell carcinomas, are associated with a poor prognosis, with the expectation that, even at an early stage, survival is less than 5% at 5 years.

Patients with stage 4 cervical cancer do very poorly. In this situation, it is very unlikely that a cure will be achieved. Chemotherapy is the treatment of first choice. A number of agents have activity in the order of 15% and their combination is accompanied by some synergy of effect. Cisplatin is the single agent with the greatest activity, but it is commonly used in combination with paclitaxel or topotecan. About 30–40% of patients will respond to treatment, but durable responses are rare. Chemotherapy is associated with toxicity, and this includes nausea and vomiting, hair loss, infections and kidney failure. Because of the toxicities of treatment, an alternative approach is to palliate symptoms with pain killers alone.

Terminal care

In the terminal phases of illness, patients with cervical cancer may have a number of problems that prove difficult to manage. These include fistulae from the vagina to bladder and from the rectum to vagina or bladder, as a result of local progression of the tumour.

Obstruction of kidney function may occur as a result of blockage of the ureters, either by enlarged lymph nodes or by tumour from the cervix growing within the pelvis, blocking the ureters. These situations can be treated surgically, in which case a colostomy or ileostomy may be formed, relieving bowel or ureteric obstruction or radiologically by the passage of a stent to reverse obstructive damage to the kidneys. A good life quality can be obtained by limited interventions.

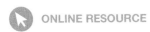

ONLINE RESOURCE

Case Study: The dignified Rwandan.

 KEY POINTS

- Cervical cancer is caused by human papillomavirus (HPV) infection and as such is preventable by vaccination
- Cervical smear screening cytology identifies pre-invasive cervical intraepithelial neoplasia (CIN) that can be treated before it progresses to invasive cancer
- Cervical cancer usually presents with inter-menstrual bleeding, post-coital bleeding or painful intercourse

18

Endometrial cancer

Learning objectives

✓ Explain the epidemiology and pathogenesis of endometrial cancer
✓ Recognize the common presentation and clinical features of endometrial cancer
✓ Describe the treatment strategies and outcomes of endometrial cancer

---

Uterine cancer has lagged behind other cancers in the search for new approaches to treatment. Thinking about this as we do, it is likely that the reason for this is that the patients who suffer from this disease do not have a voice. Patients with uterine cancer are generally elderly women and unlike their younger and perhaps more strident sisters with breast cancer are not empowered to stimulate the changes needed to effect outcome. Endometrial cancer is associated with a hormonal predisposition, age and obesity. Increases in obesity and life expectancy have led to significant increases in the incidence of this cancer. Menarche for modern women is usually around the age of 12 years and menopause 52 years; during these 40 years the average parity is 2 and the average length of breast feeding per birth only 3 months. Thus women have approximately 456 ovulatory cycles. By comparison, women in the nomadic hunter-gatherer societies of 15,000 years ago had later menarche, more pregnancies, longer breast feeding and earlier menopause. It is estimated that these women only had 150 ovulatory cycles with the associated pulses of oestrogen and progesterone and as a consequence may have been less susceptible to breast and endometrial cancers.

Epidemiology

In 2011, 8475 women were diagnosed with cancer of the endometrium in the United Kingdom and 1930 died of this disease, making it the fourth commonest cancer in women (Table 18.1).

Pathogenesis

The key to endometrial function lies in the effects of oestrogen and progesterone on the endometrium, enabling it to progress through the normal menstrual cycle and to prepare for embryo implantation. Oestrogen stimulates proliferation in the glands and stroma. Progesterone inhibits mitotic activity and stimulates secretion in the glands and decidualization of the stroma, where the cells acquire more cytoplasm. It is therefore perhaps not surprising that unopposed oestrogens will promote continuous mitotic activity, leading to cancers, whilst progestogens provide some protective effect. Thus high oestrogen levels, whether endogenous or exogenous, and low progestogen levels are risk factors for endometrial cancer. High endogenous oestrogen levels can occur because of increased aromatization of androgens to oestrogens. Thus, endometrial cancer is 10 times more common in obese women because the peripheral conversion of androstenedione to oestrone happens in the adipose tissue. Exogenous oestrogens also increase the risk of endometrial cancer. The use of unopposed oestrogens carries a fourfold to eightfold relative risk, especially in hormone replacement therapy (HRT), which is abrogated almost completely by combining

---

Oncology: Lecture Notes, Third Edition. Mark Bower and Jonathan Waxman.
© 2015 by John Wiley & Sons, Ltd. Published 2015 by John Wiley & Sons, Ltd.
Companion Website: www.lecturenoteseries.com/oncology

Table 18.1 UK registrations for endometrial cancer 2010

	Percentage of all cancer registrations	Rank of registration	Lifetime risk of cancer	Change in ASR (2000–2010)	5-year overall survival
Endometrial cancer	5	4th	1 in 43	+22%	77%

progesterone with oestrogen. A great deal of attention has been paid to the induction of endometrial cancer by tamoxifen and has led to the development of new selective oestrogen receptor modulators, including raloxifene. Although the benefit of tamoxifen therapy for breast cancer outweighs the potential increase in endometrial cancer, the relative risk is sixfold to sevenfold. Screening for endometrial cancer in women with breast cancer, taking tamoxifen, has no proven benefit, but abnormal bleeding should prompt rapid investigation. Low progestogen levels are also a risk factor for the development of endometrial cancer and occur with the polycystic ovarian syndrome (Stein–Leventhal syndrome) as well as early menarche, late menopause and nulliparity.

In addition to the hormonal factors that increase the risk of cancer of the endometrium, inherited genetic factors play a role in about 5% of cases. Germline mutations of the DNA mismatch repair genes (see Chapter 2) are responsible for the Lynch syndrome (hereditary non-polyposis coli cancer) and lead to microsatellite instability. Microsatellites are short repetitive base sequences of DNA, and although they vary between individuals, they are the same length in every cell of the body. They are the basis for DNA fingerprint analysis, and the most frequent microsatellite is the CA dinucleotide sequence that occurs tens of thousands of times in the genome. Inherited mutations of mismatch repair genes cause errors in replication of microsatellites, especially changes to their length, to go uncorrected and this is called microsatellite instability. Endometrial cancer is a feature of hereditary Lynch syndrome and the lifetime risk in women is 50%.

Presentation

Endometrial cancer rarely develops before the menopause, and, since it causes abnormal vaginal bleeding, it can usually be diagnosed at an early stage. Postmenopausal bleeding is always abnormal and requires prompt investigation. Hysteroscopy, which allows visual inspection of the uterine lining, is often used for diagnosis and can detect abnormalities in 95–100% of cases. The probability of endometrial cancer among women with postmenopausal bleeding who do not use HRT is 10%. If the transvaginal ultrasound scan is normal, this probability falls to 1%, so ultrasound allows the majority of women to be quickly reassured. Outpatient endometrial biopsy methods are now as accurate as dilatation and curettage (D&C), which requires a general anaesthetic.

Treatment and prognosis

The optimum treatment for endometrial cancer depends on the stage and grade of the disease and on the risk of tumour in lymph nodes. When the cancer is confined to the inner half of the myometrium (stage IA and IB), the lymph nodes are likely to be clear and total hysterectomy is usually sufficient as treatment. This applies to about 70% of women with endometrial cancer, and their 5-year survival exceeds 85%. Surgical colleagues are inclined to eagerness to wield their scalpels, but they should be dissuaded from proceeding to lymphadenectomy. A recent Cochrane analysis has shown an increase in morbidity with no survival benefit. In women with tumour that extends beyond the inner half of the myometrium or with regional lymph node involvement, adjuvant pelvic radiotherapy is widely used. This has been shown to reduce the rate of local recurrence but may have long-term sequelae, including lymphoedema. Radiotherapy is also valuable in the management of pelvic recurrence and in palliating bone metastases. Extrapelvic disease and distant metastases may be treated with platin-based combination chemotherapy or endocrine treatment.

Two subtypes of endometrial cancers are recognized, with contrasting outlook (Table 18.2). Type 1 endometrial tumours strongly express the receptors for oestrogen, progesterone and gonadotrophin-releasing hormone. They occur in perimenopausal women with oestrogen excess and generally have an excellent prognosis. Type 2 tumours often occur in elderly women with endometrial atrophy, who have

Table 18.2 Comparison of type 1 and type 2 endometrial cancer

	Type 1	Type 2
Age	Perimenopausal (50s–60s)	Postmenopausal (70s)
Endometrium	Hyperplastic	Atrophic
Parity	Nulliparous	Parous
Tumour growth	Slow-growing	Rapid progression
Tumour histology	Endometrioid	Papillary serous, clear cell
Tumour grade	Low	High
Tumour stage	Usually early	Often disseminated
Unopposed oestrogen	Present	Absent
Receptor expression by tumour	Oestrogen receptor, progesterone receptor	None
Tumour genetics	Diploid	Aneuploid
Tumour molecular biology	PTEN, KRAS mutation, microsatellite instability	TP53, HER-2 mutation
Prognosis	Good	Poor
Recurrence	Loco-regional	Extrapelvic

atypical high-grade histology, who are poorly responsive to hormonal therapy and who have a poor outlook. Endometrial cancer expression of hormone receptors leads to opportunities for palliative endocrine treatment most commonly with progestogens. Conversely, in type 2 tumours, palliation can be achieved with combination chemotherapy.

 KEY POINTS

- Endometrial cancer is common and is associated with high oestrogen and low progestogen levels
- Endometrial cancer presents with postmenopausal bleeding which is always abnormal and requires prompt investigation

 ONLINE RESOURCE

Case Study: The headmistress' family.

19

Ovarian cancer

Learning objectives

✓ Explain the epidemiology and pathogenesis of ovarian cancer
✓ Recognize the common presentation and clinical features of ovarian cancer
✓ Describe the treatment strategies and outcomes of ovarian cancer

---

In 1962, three men (Francis Crick, James Watson and Maurice Wilkins) were awarded the Nobel Prize for work on DNA including the discovery of the double helix structure. However, the X-ray crystallography images crucial to the model were made by the biophysicist Rosalind Franklin in 1953. In 1956, she developed ovarian cancer and died in 1958 at the age of just 37 years. The contribution of occupational radiation exposure and her Ashkenazi Jewish hereditary are uncertain, although other women in her family suffered with both breast and ovarian cancers. Although many have accused the Nobel committee of misogeny, no more than three people can be awarded a single prize and it is never awarded posthumously. Four hundred years earlier in 1558, our first Queen regent, Mary I also succumbed to (presumed) ovarian cancer after having been repeatedly misdiagnosed as pregnant on account of a combination of pelvic mass and amenorrhoea.

Epidemiology

Carcinoma of the ovary is a common tumour affecting 7116 women in the United Kingdom in 2011 and leading to the death of 4272 women (Table 19.1). The average age at which the disease occurs is 63 years.

Pathogenesis

There are three main types of ovarian cancer: epithelial (representing 90% of patients), germ cell (5%) and sex cord–gonadal stromal tumours (5%) (Figure 19.1). By far the most common pathological subtype of ovarian cancer is epithelial, and this chapter concentrates virtually exclusively upon ovarian epithelial malignancy.

The relatively uncommon ovarian germ cell tumours originate from embryonic germ cells and resemble testicular germ cell tumours in their histology, tumour marker production, treatment and good prognosis. The four most common histological types are:

- dysgerminoma (resembling seminoma in men)
- immature teratoma
- yolk sac tumours (also named endodermal sinus tumours)
- mixed tumours

Sex cord–stromal tumours arise from stromal elements in ovaries and generally are indolent tumours with favourable prognoses. Most are granulosa cell tumours that secrete inhibin, which can be used as a tumour marker, and oestradiol that is responsible for postmenopausal bleeding which is the most common

---

Oncology: Lecture Notes, Third Edition. Mark Bower and Jonathan Waxman.
© 2015 by John Wiley & Sons, Ltd. Published 2015 by John Wiley & Sons, Ltd.
Companion Website: www.lecturenoteseries.com/oncology

Table 19.1 UK registrations for ovarian cancer 2010

	Percentage of all cancer registrations	Rank of registration	Lifetime risk of cancer	Change in ASR (2000–2010)	5-year overall survival
Ovarian cancer	4	5th	1 in 51	−11%	43%

presentation. Less common sex cord–stromal tumours are thecomas and fibromas which originate from gonadal stromal cells. Most thecomas secrete oestrogens, but some produce androgens causing hirsutism and virilization.

The pathogenesis of epithelial ovarian cancer includes hereditary predisposition and environmental factors particularly relating to the total lifetime number of ovulatory cycles. There is a familial association between breast and ovarian cancers. This relates to germline mutations in the BRCA1 and BRCA2 genes, which are associated with a risk approaching 60-80% of developing ovarian cancer. The prevalence of BRCA mutations is about 1 in 500; however; in some populations such as in the Ashkenazi Jews, it is 1 in 40. The Ashkenazis represent

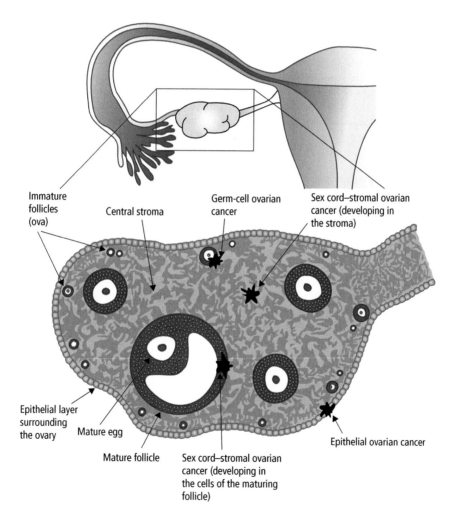

Immature follicles (ova)

Central stroma

Germ-cell ovarian cancer

Sex cord–stromal ovarian cancer (developing in the stroma)

Epithelial layer surrounding the ovary

Mature egg

Mature follicle

Sex cord–stromal ovarian cancer (developing in the cells of the maturing follicle)

Epithelial ovarian cancer

Figure 19.1 The origins of the histological subtypes of ovarian cancer.

about 75% of Jews, total around 11 million worldwide and included Sigmund Freud, Albert Einstein, Gustav Mahler and Franz Kafka. The lifetime risk of ovarian cancer in a woman carrying a BRCA1 mutation is 40% and a BRCA2 mutation is 10–20%. Ovarian cancer is also a feature of Lynch syndrome (hereditary non-polyposis colon cancer (HNPCC)) and Peutz–Jeghers syndrome (see Table 2.3).

Early menarche, late menopause and nulliparity are all associated with a higher risk of ovarian cancer. Similarly the oral contraceptive pill reduces the risk of ovarian cancer. There is controversy as to other associated risk factors for the development of ovarian cancer, especially postmenopausal hormone replacement therapy (HRT). For example, long-term oestrogen replacement therapy may be associated with the development of these tumours, and in one prospective study of over 31,000 postmenopausal women, the increased risk for the development of ovarian cancer was 1.7-fold. This effect may be diminished with combined oestrogen–progesterone HRT. The UK Million Women Study suggests that risk was only increased in current HRT users and that this risk only became significant after 7 or more years of HRT.

Screening

Because ovarian cancer patients generally present with late-stage tumours, attempts have been made to reduce this mortality by population screening. The results of multimodality screening of transvaginal ultrasound (TVUS) and serum CA-125 tumour marker measurement have been inconsistent. The large US PLCO screening trial (prostate, lung, colon and ovary) included 68,000 postmenopausal women who were randomized to annual multimodality screening or usual care. During follow-up there was no difference in the incidence, tumour stage at diagnosis or mortality of ovarian cancer between the screened and unscreened women. Furthermore 5 times as many women had surgery for false-positive screening results as for cancer. In contrast, ongoing two studies, one from the United Kingdom, are reporting that the ovarian cancers diagnosed in the screened women are in earlier stage at diagnosis and this may translate into improved survival. At present no routine screening for ovarian cancer is advocated outside of a clinical trial. A recent meta-analysis of 10 screening trials has shown no survival benefit for screening normal populations. There may be hope that new screening technologies using molecular markers for ovarian cancer might be proved more successful than conventional screening with ultrasonography and measurement of serum CA-125 levels.

Presentation

Patients with ovarian cancer usually present to their GPs with non-specific abdominal symptoms such as abdominal discomfort and swelling. There may be associated urinary frequency, alteration of bowel habit, tenesmus, colicky abdominal pain or postmenopausal bleeding. Patients with disseminated disease may have loss of appetite and weight. Early repletion is another common finding in the history. A patient with these symptoms should be examined by her GP, and if there is abdominal swelling or a pelvic mass, the patient should be referred on to a specialist gynaecologist for his or her views as to the patient's management. It is unfortunately the nature of ovarian cancer to present late, and almost 70% of patients have advanced disease at diagnosis. Patients with early-stage, localized tumours are often diagnosed as a result of the investigation of another medical condition.

The specialist should see the patient in an outpatient clinic and take a full clinical history and examine the patient. The examination should include a pelvic assessment. If the patient is thought clinically to have ovarian cancer, the investigations organized should include a full blood count, routine biochemistry, chest X-ray, a pelvic ultrasound and an abdominal and pelvic CT scan, together with measurement of serum levels of CA-125 (Figures 19.2, 19.3 and 19.4).

Ovarian cancer secretes CA-125, which is a glycoprotein. Approximately 80% of patients with advanced ovarian cancer have elevated CA-125 levels in the blood. Raised CA-125 levels may also occur in patients with almost any gynaecological, pancreatic, breast, colon, lung or hepatocellular tumour. CA-125 levels also are elevated in a number of benign conditions including endometriosis, pancreatitis, pelvic inflammatory disease and peritonitis. So, a raised CA-125 level is not sufficient for a diagnosis of ovarian cancer, but changing levels may be used to monitor treatment and in follow-up after treatment.

If the tumour is operable, the patient should then be booked for a laparotomy. Surgery should be undertaken in specialist centres by a surgical gynaecological oncologist. At operation, the abdominal contents are examined and, where possible, tumour debulking should be undertaken. This should include removal of the omentum, ovaries, fallopian tubes and uterus, with excision of all visible peritoneal deposits (total abdominal hysterectomy with bilateral

Omental cake of metastatic ovarian cancer

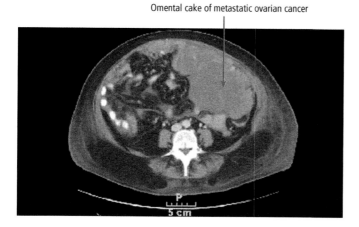

Figure 19.2 CT scan showing an omental cake of metastatic ovarian cancer deposits anteriorly with a large lobulated mass that extends from the midline to the left flank. The term omental cake refers to infiltration of omental fat by tumour.

salpingo-oophorectomy and omentectomy). The aim of surgery is to remove as much tumour as possible, optimally reducing the maximum diameter of any tumour deposit to 1 cm or less. Effective cytoreductive surgery is the most significant correlate for survival.

Staging and grading

Ninety per cent of ovarian cancers are epithelial tumours. The classification of tumours is given in Table 19.2.

An attempt should be made to stage the patient's tumour. The staging used is the FIGO classification, which is as follows:

- Stage 1: growth limited to the ovaries
    - Stage 1A: one ovary, no malignant ascites
    - Stage 1B: both ovaries, no malignant ascites
    - Stage 1C: tumour on ovarian surface or capsular rupture or ascites positive for malignant cell (Figure 19.5)
- Stage 2: growth involving one or both ovaries with pelvic extension

Lobulated heterogeneous ovarian cancer mass extending from the pelvis

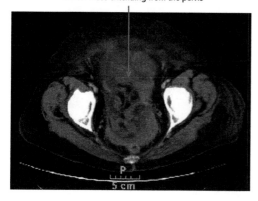

Figure 19.3 The CT scan shows a huge, lobulated, heterogeneous pelvic mass that extends anteriorly. This mass was due to epithelial ovarian cancer.

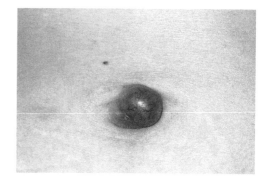

Figure 19.4 Umbilical nodule metastasis known as Sister Mary Joseph nodule, which usually denotes transcoelomic spread from an ovarian or gastric primary. The eponym appears to have been given for Sister Mary Joseph Dempsey (1856–1929) who was a surgical assistant to Dr William Mayo. This eponym is one of the very few given for a nurse.

Table 19.2 Pathological classification of ovarian tumours	
A. Epithelial	Serous
	Mucinous
	Endometrioid
	Clear cell
	Brenner
	Mixed
	Undifferentiated
	Unclassified
B. Sex cord/stromal	Granulosa
	Androblastoma
	Gynandroblastoma
	Unclassified
C. Lipid cell	
D. Gonadoblastoma	
E. Soft tissue	
F. Germ cell	Dysgerminoma
	Endodermal sinus
	Embryonal
	Polyembryonal
	Teratoma
	Mixed
G. Unclassifiable	
H. Metastatic	

- Stage 3: growth involving one or both ovaries with peritoneal implants or superficial liver metastases or abdominopelvic lymph node involvement (Figure 19.6)
- Stage 4: tumour metastazing to liver parenchyma, pleura or other visceral metastatic sites

Treatment

Treatment is defined by the FIGO staging system. If the tumour is confined to one ovary, the gynaecological oncologist may choose to observe the patient after definitive surgery. For stage 1A and 1B ovarian cancer, patients derive no benefit from adjuvant chemotherapy, and studies suggest that all patients with more advanced stages can be offered chemotherapy with benefit. Most specialists would agree that stage 1A or 1B well-differentiated tumours can be observed, but adjuvant chemotherapy is increasingly offered to most patients with grade 2 and upwards disease irrespective of stage, and stage 1C and upwards irrespective of grade because it offers a survival benefit. Ovarian cancer is chemosensitive, and there is

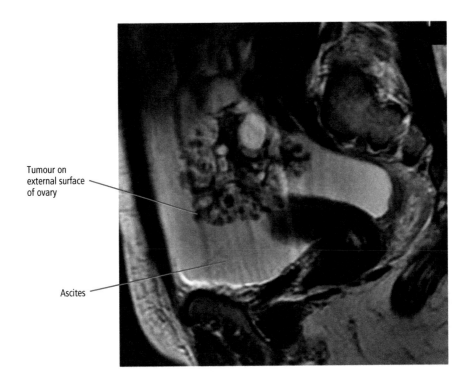

Tumour on external surface of ovary

Ascites

Figure 19.5 MRI scan showing tumour on the external surface of the ovary (stage 1C). Ascites is also present.

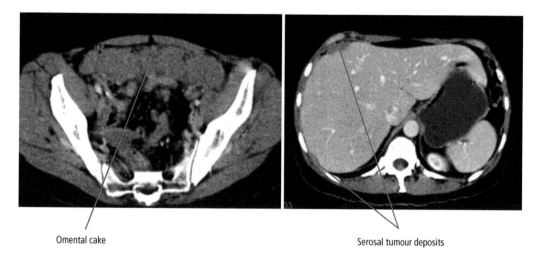

Omental cake

Serosal tumour deposits

Figure 19.6 CT scan showing both peritoneal disease (omental cake) and deposits on liver serosa. Both features denote FIGO stage 3C ovarian cancer.

a long history of the use of chemical agents in the treatment of this condition. The discovery of responsiveness to single-agent treatments led to the use of combination chemotherapy programmes. Intensive treatment using multiple drug regimens was advocated throughout the 1970s and early 1980s.

For patients with advanced ovarian cancer it was thought during the early 1990s that single-agent therapy carboplatin was just as effective as combination treatments in terms of overall survival, although it was thought that there might be a minor advantage in terms of initial response rates and response duration to combination programmes. In the late 1990s, fashions changed again and treatment involved the use of combination therapy. There was evidence from randomized studies that combination therapy with cisplatin and paclitaxel had the highest response rates and in two high-profile studies showed superiority over another platinum-based regimen in terms of disease-free result and overall survival. In this century, treatment recommendations have come full circle, and in the ICON 3 study, a large trial conducted in the United Kingdom and Italy, single-agent carboplatin was not shown to be inferior to carboplatin and paclitaxel together. Ovarian cancer is, however, a highly heterogeneous condition of many entities, and current advice from the National Institute for Health and Clinical Excellence (NICE) is that the patient and oncologist should discuss whether better benefit might be obtained from single-agent carboplatin or carboplatin and paclitaxel on a case-by-case basis.

At relapse patients are divided into those with platinum-sensitive disease and those with platinum refractory disease on the basis of a platinum-free interval of greater or less than 6 months. Those with platinum-sensitive relapses are usually retreated with a platinum-based chemotherapy regimen. The management of those with refractory disease requires the introduction of new lines of chemotherapy. Agents such as pegylated liposomal doxorubicin, gemcitabine, topotecan, pemetrexed, trabectedin, oxaliplatin and ixabepilone have been shown to be effective. Chemotherapy resistance is one of the major features of patients with end-stage ovarian cancer, and this may be due to clonal evolution with gains of chromosomal material on the chromosomes 1 and 17 and losses at chromosome 3.

Patients with relapsed ovarian cancer are commonly troubled by recurrent pelvic and abdominal disease that obstructs bowel and kidneys and causes ascites (Figure 19.7). The treatment of recurrence involves a combined approach between oncologists, surgeons and interventional radiologists in order to provide the patient with good quality of life. Interventions may include further attempts at cytoreductive surgery, the formation of stomas, renal stenting and the use of agents such as octreotide to relieve intestinal obstruction. In what seems to be a rehearsal of treatments investigated in the 1980's peritoneal chemotherapy appears to be undergoing a resurgence.

However, the explosion of targeted biotherapies informed by the results of the Human Genome Project is

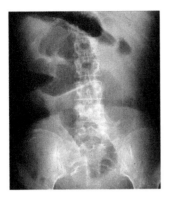
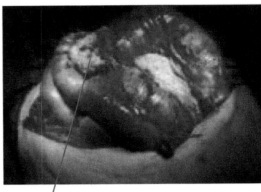

Peritoneal metastases on
large bowel omentum

Figure 19.7 Large bowel obstruction due to peritoneal metastases of ovarian cancer.

beginning to find its way into ovarian cancer clinical trials. The main target under consideration currently is vascular endothelial growth factor (VEGF) and its receptor and poly-ADP ribose phosphorylase (PARP) an enzyme involved in repairing single strand breaks in DNA. These molecules are targeted in ovarian cancer by small molecular weight inhibitors (nibs) and monoclonal antibodies (mabs). In the case of VEGF, both the monoclonal antibody bevacizumab that binds VEGF and the kinase inhibitor cediranib that inhibits VEGF receptors 1, 2 and 3 have shown promise in ovarian cancer. For patients with BRCA mutation associated cancers including ovarian cancer, olaparib, a PARP inhibitor, has been shown to be effective. It would seem that if there is to be a bright future for these modern novel agents then it is most likely to be in combination with conventional chemotherapy.

Non-epithelial ovarian cancer (germ cell tumours and sex cord–stromal tumours) is treated initially, where possible, by surgery. The procedures may range from oophorectomy to extensive tumour debulking. In relapse, or where a patient has presented with gross metastatic disease, treatment for non-epithelial ovarian cancers may involve similar chemotherapy programmes to those used for testicular cancer. Occasional responses are seen to hormonal therapy, using luteinizing hormone-releasing hormone (LHRH) agonists for those patients with ovarian malignancies secreting sex steroids.

cancer have an excellent outlook, with a 95% chance of survival. The survival of patients with stage 1C disease with ovarian cyst rupture is variably reported and depends on tumour grade. In one series, just 63% of patients survived 5 years. Approximately 60–80% of patients with advanced ovarian cancer respond to suitable chemotherapy. The median survival for this group of patients is 2.5 years, with less than 30% of patients surviving for 5 years.

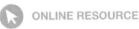 ONLINE RESOURCE

Case Study: The sister's cyst.

KEY POINTS

- Ovarian cancer is the fifth most common cancer in women and frequently is advanced stage at the time of diagnosis
- The symptoms of ovarian cancer are relatively non-specific abdominal complaints such as swelling and discomfort
- Screening for ovarian cancer with ultrasound and serum CA-125 measurement does not reduce mortality
- The management of ovarian cancer depends on the stage of disease but for advanced disease usually involves a combination of debulking surgery and chemotherapy

Prognosis

Localized ovarian cancer constitutes 24% of all presenting patients. Patients with stage 1A and 1B ovarian

20

Head and neck cancers

Learning objectives

✓ Explain the epidemiology and pathogenesis of head and neck cancers

✓ Recognize the common presentation and clinical features of head and neck cancers

✓ Describe the treatment strategies and outcomes of head and neck cancers

There have been advances in our understanding of the causes of head and neck cancers and changes in the standard of care that have come from developments in molecular biology that have been applied to this diverse tumour group. Students who are worried about biodiversity or just simply fans of the Looney Tunes cartoon character Taz may be concerned to learn that the carnivorous marsupial, the Tasmanian devil, has become an endangered species because of a head and neck tumour that threatens the survival of the whole species. Devil facial tumour disease is a parasitic tumour allograft transmitted between individual devils. The tumours are all derived from the same original cancerous cells and spread from animal to animal. Transmissible cancer is extremely rare. The only other well-described example is canine transmissible venereal tumour in dogs, where again it is the actual cancer cells themselves that are spread from dog to dog rather than transmission of an infection that causes the cancer. Occasional similar cancer transmission has been described in humans. For example, organ transplant recipients very rarely develop cancers that are shown genetically to derive from the donor. Transplacental transmission of malignancy has also been described with the spread of melanoma from mother to child.

It was announced in 2010 that the actor Michael Douglas had been diagnosed with throat cancer (which subsequently turned out to be base of tongue cancer). In an interview with the Guardian newspaper in 2013, the actor attributed the cancer to human papillomavirus (HPV) infection acquired by cunnilingus. Around 40% of cases of head and neck cancer are associated with high-risk genotypes of HPV, and it has been shown that people with a higher number of sexual partners, particularly oral sex partners, are at an increased risk for oropharyngeal, tonsil and base of tongue cancers. Of course drinking and smoking also contribute. It is intriguing that the actor who portrayed Gordon Gekko in Wall Street turns out to be a political activist advocating nuclear disarmament and gun control and is a UN messenger of peace. Sigmund Freud succumbed to cancer of the head and neck in 1939, but in his case it was attributed to smoking rather than sex.

To the oncologist, the head and neck means anything between the brain and the clavicles, excluding the thyroid gland and the skin. It comprises seven regions (Figures 20.1, 20.2, 20.3 and 20.4):

1. The nasopharynx (the area behind the nose and pharynx)
2. The oral cavity (including the lips, floor of the mouth, tongue, cheeks, gums and hard palate)
3. The oropharynx (the base of the tongue, the tonsillar region, the soft palate and pharyngeal walls)
4. The hypopharynx (the lower throat)
5. The larynx (including the vocal cords and both supraglottis and subglottis)
6. The paranasal sinuses cavity (the maxillary, ethmoid, sphenoid and frontal sinuses)
7. The salivary glands (the parotid, submandibular and minor salivary glands)

Oncology: Lecture Notes, Third Edition. Mark Bower and Jonathan Waxman.
© 2015 by John Wiley & Sons, Ltd. Published 2015 by John Wiley & Sons, Ltd.
Companion Website: www.lecturenoteseries.com/oncology

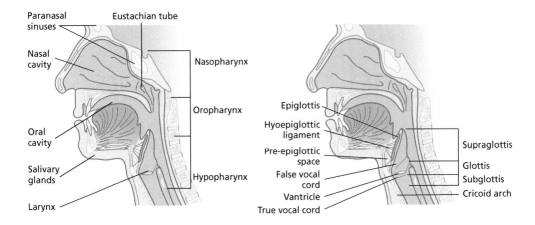

Figure 20.1 The anatomy of head and neck cancers.

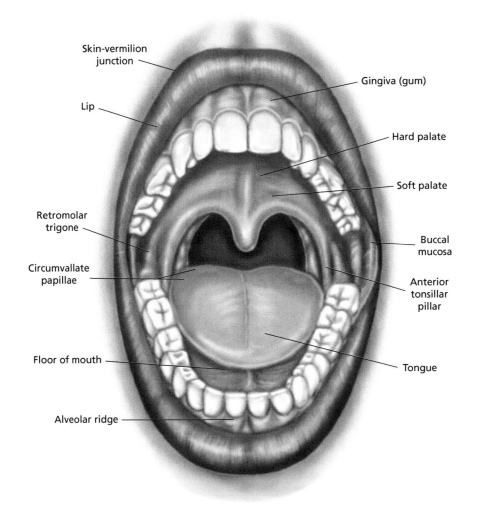

Figure 20.2 The anatomy of the oral cavity.

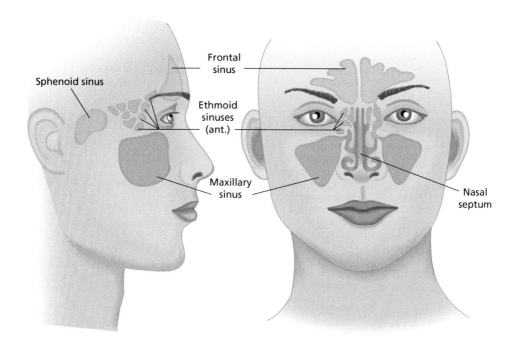

Figure 20.3 The anatomy of the paranasal sinuses.

The International Statistical Classification of Diseases and Related Health Problems (ICD) is the full list of diseases recognized by the WHO and is currently in its 10th revision (ICD-10). Cancers of the head and neck include more than 30 different ICD-10 codes. Although lymphomas, sarcomas, melanomas and other tumours may affect these regions, the term "head and neck cancers" generally refer to squamous tumours, which make up 90% of cancers at these sites. Cancers of the nasopharynx include not only squamous cancers but also non-keratinizing transitional cell cancers and undifferentiated lymphoepitheliomas. The latter are the most common tumours in the nasopharynx, and, unlike most other head and neck cancers, they

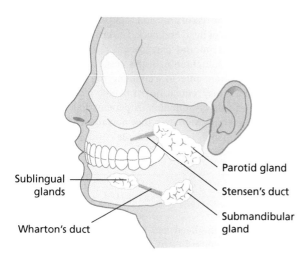

Figure 20.4 The anatomy of the major salivary glands.

Table 20.1 Frequency and survival in head and neck cancer by primary tumour site

	Sites	Proportion of head and neck cancers	5-year survival
Nasopharynx	Nasal cavity	2%	50%
Oral cavity	Buccal mucosa	40%	50%
	Retromolar triangle		
	Alveolus		
	Hard palate		
	Anterior $^2/_3$ tongue		
	Floor of mouth		
	Mucosal surface of lips		
Oropharynx	Base of tongue	25%	45%
	Tonsil		
	Soft palate		
Hypopharynx	Postcricoid area		20%
	Pyriform sinus		
	Posterior pharyngeal wall		
Larynx	Supraglottis	30%	95%
	Glottis		
	Subglottis		
Paranasal sinuses	Maxillary sinus	1%	50%
	Ethmoidal sinus		
Salivary glands	Parotid glands	5%	80%
	Submandibular glands		
	Sublingual glands		
	Minor salivary glands		

frequently spread to distant sites. Tumours of the salivary glands are the most heterogeneous group of tumours of any tissue in the body, with almost 40 histological subtypes of salivary gland tumours. Salivary gland tumours are more often benign than malignant.

Epidemiology

Head and neck cancers comprise 5% of all cancers in the United Kingdom and account for 2.5% of cancer deaths (Table 20.1). They are twice as common in men as in women and generally occur in those over 50 years of age. Over 90% are squamous carcinomas.

Pathogenesis

The incidence of head and neck cancers varies geographically, as does the most common anatomical site of these cancers. Smoking, high alcohol intake and poor oral hygiene are well-established risk factors for the development of head and neck tumours. In addition, the Epstein–Barr virus is implicated in the aetiology of nasopharyngeal carcinoma in southern China, betel nut chewing in oral cancer in Asia and wood dust inhalation by furniture makers, who may contract nasal cavity adenocarcinomas. In the United Kingdom, the incidence and mortality are greater in deprived populations, most notably for carcinoma of the tongue.

Primary prevention by smoking cessation and alcohol abstention are the most effective methods of reducing the risk of head and neck cancers. Increasing awareness of head and neck cancers may encourage earlier referral and diagnosis at a stage when the cancer is still curable. In this respect, dentists play an important role in examining the oral mucosa. Retinoids may reduce the risk of both recurrence and second primary tumours in patients following primary therapy. Moreover, they may reduce malignant transformation in precancerous conditions such as leukoplakia.

Clinical presentation

Cancer of the head and neck is often preventable, and, if diagnosed early, is usually curable. Patients, however, frequently have advanced disease at the time of diagnosis. This is incurable or requires aggressive treatment, which leaves them functionally disabled. The optimum management of these tumours requires a multidisciplinary approach, including oncologists, otorhinolaryngologists, oromaxillofacial surgeons and plastic surgeons, along with clinical nurse specialists, speech and language therapists, dieticians and prosthetics technicians.

Most head and neck tumours present as malignant ulcers with raised indurated edges on a surface mucosa. Oral tumours present as non-healing ulcers with ipsilateral otalgia (earache). Oropharyngeal tumours present with dysphagia (difficulty swallowing), pain and otalgia. Hypopharyngeal tumours present with dysphagia, odynophagia (painful swallowing), referred otalgia and neck nodes. Laryngeal cancers present with persistent hoarseness, pain, otalgia, dyspnoea and stridor. Nasopharyngeal cancers present with a bloody nasal discharge, nasal obstruction, conductive deafness, atypical facial pain, diplopia, hoarseness and Horner's syndrome. Nasal and sinus tumours present with a bloody discharge or obstruction. Salivary gland tumours present as painless swellings or facial nerve palsies. Cervical lymph node enlargement as the presenting feature is not uncommon, particularly when the primary tumour lies in certain hidden sites, such as the base of the tongue, supraglottis and nasopharynx. Systemic metastases are uncommon at presentation (10%). Synchronous or metachronous tumours of the upper aerodigestive tract occur in 10–15% of patients.

A number of criteria for urgent referral have been established (Table 20.2). Diagnostic surgical resection of cervical nodes, without first determining

Table 20.2 Indications for urgent referral for suspected head and neck cancer

Hoarseness persisting for >6 weeks

Ulceration of oral mucosa persisting for >3 weeks

Oral swellings persisting for >3 weeks

All red or red-and-white patches on the oral mucosa

Dysphagia persisting for >3 weeks

Unilateral nasal obstruction, particularly when associated with purulent discharge

Unexplained tooth mobility, not associated with periodontal disease

Unresolved neck masses for >3 weeks

Cranial neuropathies

Orbital masses

the site of the primary tumour, may compromise subsequent therapy, increases the morbidity and worsens the outcome. Before biopsying an upper cervical lymph node, nasendoscopy and laryngoscopy and clinical examination should be performed to identify a primary tumour site. For lower cervical and supraclavicular lymph nodes, panendoscopy (laryngoscopy, bronchoscopy, oesophagoscopy) may be required.

Treatment

The approach to managing these tumours varies according to their site, but in general the primary site and potential for cervical lymph node metastases should be considered. Small early-stage tumours, where there are no regional lymph node metastases, should be treated with surgery or radiotherapy, with 60–69% cure rates. The decision between surgery and radiotherapy is often determined by the anatomical site and the long-term morbidity. Function is generally better after radiotherapy but requires daily attendance for 4–6 weeks, whilst surgical treatment is quicker, but patients need to be fit for anaesthesia (see Figure 3.9).

Conventional radiotherapy is delivered by photons or occasionally electron beams (β-radiation) for superficial tumours. However, particle beam radiotherapy uses hadrons (colour charge neutral collections of quarks bound by the strong nuclear force) usually protons, neutrons or positive ions. Proton beam therapy is the most commonly used of these techniques but is only available in one institution in the United Kingdom currently. The theoretical advantage of proton beam radiotherapy is that the higher mass of protons results in less scatter and a more concentrated delivery of energy to the tumour and greater sparing of normal adjacent tissues. Proton beam therapy offers promise in the management of head and neck cancers as well as other tumours located in anatomically challenging sites such as intraocular melanoma and retinoblastoma. In recent times it has been suggested that antiprotons (a fermion formed of two anti-up quarks and one anti-down quark) and pi-mesons (formed of an up and an anti-down quark) could be used as particle beam radiotherapy (Box 3.2).

More advanced tumours are usually managed surgically, provided that the tumour is resectable. This is followed by adjuvant radiotherapy if the margins are insufficient, or if there is extranodal spread, multiple lymph node involvement or poorly differentiated histology. The resection of large tumours may leave sizeable defects, requiring myocutaneous flaps. Inoperable or recurrent disease may be treated with combinations of chemotherapy and radiotherapy, but outcomes generally remain poor, and in many cases of advanced disease symptomatic palliation is a more valued approach.

If cervical lymph node metastases are present, surgical resection is recommended, and, recently, more limited and selective neck dissection has been advocated. This preserves function, especially in relation to the accessory nerve, which, if sacrificed, usually gives rise to a stiff and painful shoulder. A scoring index can be used to predict the likelihood of metastasis to cervical lymph nodes. If the expected incidence of lymph node involvement exceeds 20%, neck dissection is usually recommended.

The addition of chemotherapy to radiotherapy, the use of hyperfractionated radiotherapy as well as intensity-modulated radiotherapy have all improved the delivery of radiotherapy for patients with advanced head and neck tumours, resulting in modest improvements in survival and declines in morbidity. The addition of the monoclonal antibody cetuximab, which targets epidermal growth factor receptor (EGFR), to radiotherapy has been shown to double survival in advanced head and neck cancers, especially tumours of the oropharynx. However, this widely quoted landmark phase III trial did not use cisplatin chemoradiotherapy, the gold standard therapy, as the control arm. Recurrent or metastatic tumour may be palliated with further surgery or radiotherapy to aid local control, and systemic chemotherapy has a response rate of around 30%. The addition of cetuximab to platinum-containing regimens is superior to platinum-containing chemotherapy alone in patients with recurrent disease. Other treatments targeting receptors that have shown promise in these tumours include afatinib, an irreversible ErB blocker, and gefitinib, the EGFR inhibitor.

Second malignancies are frequent in patients who have been successfully treated for head and neck tumours, with an annual rate of 3%, and all patients should be encouraged to give up smoking and drinking to lower this risk. In addition, a number of studies have addressed the role of retinoids and β-carotene as secondary prophylaxis, but none have proved to have any significant effect.

Quality of life issues are especially important in head and neck cancers, given the anatomical site of the disease and the consequences of treatment, which can affect facial appearance, speech, swallowing and breathing. These cancers have enormous sociopsychological impact and may result in physical disability. These concerns must be addressed sympathetically with patients. Rehabilitation following treatment for head and neck cancers needs input from many professionals, particularly speech and language therapists, dieticians and prosthetics technicians. Rehabilitation, furthermore, requires enormous patience and effort on behalf of the patient. For example, 40% of patients will achieve communication by oesophageal speech following total laryngectomy.

Prognosis

Five-year survival rates for patients with head and neck tumours are listed in Table 20.1.

Salivary gland tumours

Salivary gland tumours represent around 5% of all head and neck cancers and affect both genders equally. They are most common in the sixth and seventh decades of life. Over half of the tumours are benign, and 80% originate in the parotid gland. Approximately 25% of parotid tumours, 40% of submandibular tumours and over 90% of sublingual gland tumours are malignant. Histologically, the most common benign tumour is the pleomorphic adenoma, and the most common malignant tumour is the mucoepidermoid carcinoma. Most patients present with painless swelling of the parotid, submandibular or sublingual glands. Facial numbness or weakness due to cranial nerve involvement usually indicates malignancy and is an ominous sign. Pleomorphic adenomas, although not malignant, often recur if not completely excised, and a small proportion may become malignant if left untreated. Early-stage, low-grade malignant salivary gland tumours are usually curable by surgical resection alone. The prognosis is best for parotid tumours, then submandibular tumours; the least favourable sites are the sublingual and minor salivary glands. Larger or high-grade tumours require postoperative radiotherapy. Complications of surgical treatment for parotid neoplasms include facial nerve palsy and Frey's syndrome. Frey's syndrome is gustatory flushing and sweating of the ipsilateral forehead because the sympathetic nerve fibres to the sweat glands of the scalp and parasympathetic fibres to the parotid gland have reconnected wrongly after the auriculotemporal branch of the trigeminal nerve was severed in surgery; instead of salivating the patient sweats.

ONLINE RESOURCE

Case Study: The priest with bad breath.

 KEY POINTS

- Cancers of the head and neck include all tumours arising between the brain and the clavicles except skin and thyroid cancers.

- Ninety per cent are squamous cancers and most are associated with smoking, high alcohol intake and poor oral hygiene.

- Most head and neck tumours present as malignant ulcers with raised indurated edges on a surface mucosa.

- The management of head and neck cancers requires a large multidisciplinary team.

21

Thyroid cancer

Learning objectives

✓ Explain the epidemiology and pathogenesis of thyroid cancer

✓ Recognize the common presentation and clinical features of thyroid cancer

✓ Describe the treatment strategies and outcomes of thyroid cancer

---

Epidemiology

Thyroid cancers are relatively uncommon malignancies. In 2011, there were 2727 patients registered in the United Kingdom with this condition and 343 deaths reported in the last national statistics publication (Table 21.1). There is a 3:1 ratio of women to men affected with thyroid malignancies.

Pathogenesis

Radiation exposure is the most common predisposing factor to the development of thyroid cancer. This included the treatment of childhood tinea capitis and tonsilar and thymus enlargement in the past. It also includes populations exposed to nuclear fallout such as the survivors of the atomic bombs dropped on Hiroshima and Nagasaki, the Marshall Islanders who were exposed during nuclear bomb tests and those exposed by nuclear power plant accidents at Chernobyl, Three Mile Island and Fukushima (see Box 2.3). Children exposed to nuclear fallout are most at risk and develop papillary thyroid cancers with a particular molecular signature; these radiation-induced tumours are characterized by RET gene translocations but absence of point mutations of the BRAF gene. Potassium iodide prevents the uptake of radioactive iodine by the thyroid and lowers the risk of

radiation-induced thyroid cancer in exposed people; so it would be helpful to have a supply of potassium iodide close at hand.

Thyroid cancer includes a number of clinical entities, ranging from the classical papillary, follicular and anaplastic tumours to the atypical Hurthle and medullary cell carcinomas, as well as thyroid lymphoma. The different histological subtypes are associated with different molecular abnormalities. Papillary thyroid cancer is the most common type accounting for around 75% of tumours. These cancers frequently carry gene mutations and rearrangements that activate the mitogen-activated protein kinase (MAPK) pathway. Amongst these changes are rearrangements of the genes of the tyrosine kinase receptors RET and NTRK1 and activating mutations of signal transduction proteins BRAF and RAS. An individual papillary thyroid cancer usually only carries one of these MAPK-activating genetic alterations. Follicular thyroid cancer accounts for 10–15% thyroid cancers and is associated with a chromosomal translocation t(2:3)(q13:p25). The consequence of this translocation is the fusion of the DNA-binding domain of the thyroid transcription factor PAX8 gene and the peroxisome proliferator-activated receptor (PPAR) gene. The hybrid fusion protein is thought to block differentiation and stimulate cell division in thyroid follicular cells. The third most common and most aggressive cancers are anaplastic thyroid cancers. The anaplastic thyroid cancers carry mutations of p53 tumour suppressor that are not found in papillary or follicular thyroid cancers. They also commonly have

---

Oncology: Lecture Notes, Third Edition. Mark Bower and Jonathan Waxman.
© 2015 by John Wiley & Sons, Ltd. Published 2015 by John Wiley & Sons, Ltd.
Companion Website: www.lecturenoteseries.com/oncology

Table 21.1 UK registrations for thyroid cancer 2010

	Percentage of all cancer registrations		Rank of registration		Change in ASR (2000–2010)		5-year overall survival	
	Female	Male	Female	Male	Female	Male	Female	Male
Thyroid cancer	1	<1	18th	>20th	+67%	+53%	79%	74%

mutations of the beta-catenin gene (CTNNNB1). Beta-catenin protein plays a role in cell adhesion and signalling through the Wnt pathway. Finally, medullary thyroid carcinoma is associated with multiple endocrine neoplasia (MEN) types 2A and 2B (see Table 25.1). The RET gene encodes a transmembrane tyrosine kinase receptor. This gene is mutated in almost 100% of all MEN 2A patients and in 85% of patients with familial medullary thyroid carcinoma.

Presentation

The most common presentation of thyroid malignancy is with a thyroid nodule or with cervical lymphadenopathy. Much less frequently, patients will present with features suggestive of advanced disease, such as vocal cord paralysis or with symptoms due to metastases.

Investigations

The diagnosis of a thyroid malignancy is made following routine investigations, which should include thyroid function, thyroid isotope scanning and thyroid ultrasound. Under ultrasound control, fine-needle aspiration biopsy is used to obtain a cytological diagnosis and thereby defines treatment. Other staging investigations should include CT scanning of the neck and thorax. Serum calcitonin levels are measured in patients with medullary thyroid carcinomas, while serum thyroglobulin can be used to monitor relapse in well-differentiated carcinomas after thyroid ablation.

Treatment

After initial staging, patients with thyroid malignancies proceed to surgery. In the majority of patients with thyroid cancers, the surgical options are either subtotal thyroid resection, removing the lobe bearing the tumour together with the thyroid isthmus or total thyroidectomy. Care must be taken to avoid damaging the parathyroid glands and the recurrent laryngeal nerves. Generally, partial thryoidectomy is only considered in those patients with low-risk tumours, for example those with a single focus of papillary carcinoma measuring less than 1 cm in diameter. There is no evidence that routine lymph node dissection has any added survival advantage. Subsequent to surgery, patients are treated with thyroid replacement, aiming to suppress thyroid-stimulating hormone (TSH) completely, which may be a driver for the development of recurrence.

When patients with thyroid tumours develop recurrent disease, further options for management may include surgery or radiation therapy. Surgery is the treatment of choice for patients with recurrent medullary carcinoma of the thyroid, which is relatively resistant to radiation therapy and chemotherapy. Radiation treatment is given both by using external beam radiotherapy and by treating with radioiodine (^{131}I), which localizes to thyroid tissue. Differentiated thyroid cancer (papillary or follicular) that no longer responds to radioiodine and TSH suppression may respond to anti-angiogenic tyrosine kinase inhibitors. Sorafenib is an inhibitor of multiple receptor tyrosine kinases including RET; VEGFR1, 2 and 3; Flt3; cKIT; and wild-type and mutated BRAF. An overview of seven trials of patients with papillary, follicular and poorly differentiated thyroid cancer,

Table 21.2 Five-year survival rates for thyroid cancers

Tumour	Relative frequency	5-year survival
Papillary thyroid cancer	70–80%	80%
Follicular thyroid cancer	10–20%	60%
Anaplastic thyroid cancer	5%	10%
Medullary thyroid cancer	<5%	50%

medullary thyroid cancer and anaplastic cancer has concluded that the partial response rate to sorafenib is 21% and that a further 60% of treated patients have stable disease. Cabozantinib, another small-molecule tyrosine kinase inhibitor, targets hepatocyte growth factor receptor, VEGFR2 and RET, and has clinical activity in medullary carcinoma of the thyroid. In studies, the duration of response to cabozantinib is reported as "progression free survival" and is around 10 months.

Prognosis

Table 21.2 shows the 5-year survival rates for thyroid tumours according to histological subtype.

 ONLINE RESOURCE

Case Study: An old lady with a lump in her neck.

 KEY POINTS

- Thyroid cancer is relatively uncommon and radiation exposure and genetic predisposition are acknowledged risk factors
- Thyroid cancer usually presents with a thyroid nodule, cervical lymphadenopathy or less frequently features of advanced disease, such as vocal cord paralysis or metastases

22

Adrenal cancers

Learning objectives

✓ Explain the epidemiology and pathogenesis of adrenal cancer
✓ Recognize the common presentation and clinical features of adrenal cancer
✓ Describe the treatment strategies and outcomes of adrenal cancer

Epidemiology of adrenal cortical cancers

Adrenal cortical cancers occur with an incidence of approximately one per million of population per annum. Adrenal cortical cancers are derived from the adrenal cortex and may be secretory. The major adrenal hormone products of these tumours include androgens, aldosterone and cortisol. Serum levels of these hormones may be elevated, and 24-hour urinary cortisol secretion may be increased.

Presentation of adrenal cortical cancers

Patients with adrenal cortical cancers generally present with non-specific symptoms, such as weight loss and general fatigue, or specific symptoms relating to their anatomical position, which include abdominal or loin pain. Adrenal cortical cancers may also produce symptoms related to the hormones that they secrete. Women may be virilized by the excessive production of androgenic hormones. Occasionally, adrenal cortical cancers are picked up as a result of an abdominal ultrasound or CT scan carried out for another reason.

Investigations of adrenal cortical cancers

The patient with a suspected diagnosis of adrenal cortical cancer will generally be investigated in an endocrinological or surgical outpatient setting where routine blood testing together with specific endocrinological investigations will be arranged. These will include measurement of the adrenal androgens, adrenocorticotrophic hormone (ACTH) levels, 24-hour urinary cortisol levels, plain X-rays and CT scans of the abdomen, pelvis and chest (Figure 22.1).

Initial treatment of adrenal cortical cancers

Once staging investigations have been completed, the patient with a suspected diagnosis of an adrenal cortical cancer should be referred on to a specialist endocrine surgeon. The patient will proceed to

Right adrenal phaeochromocytoma

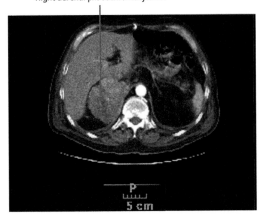

Figure 22.1 Adrenal tumour. This CT scan was performed on a 28-year-old man with hypertension and shows a lobulated heterogeneous right adrenal mass which was due to phaeochromocytoma.

laparotomy, and an attempt is made to resect the tumour. Surgery is complex, and there may be a major morbidity and mortality associated with the procedure. There is no clinical advantage to any adjuvant treatment.

Treatment of metastatic or locally advanced adrenal cortical cancer

The secretory symptoms of adrenal cortical tumours are unpleasant. Secretory symptoms are most unpleasant in women because of virilization caused by androgenic steroid production. These symptoms may include acne, hirsutism, change in habitus and increased libido. Attempts are made to block the production of hormones by an adrenal cortical cancer, using blocking agents such as metyrapone and ketoconazole, which inhibit steroidogenesis. Treatment may be given using o,p′-dichlorodiphenyl-dichloroethane (o,p′DDD), which is also called "mitotane". Mitotane is a selective adrenal poison that is structurally related to the chlorinated insecticide dichlorodiphenyltrichloroethane (DDT). DDT is a cheap insecticide developed in the 1940s that has cumulative toxicity in mammals. It is estimated that DDT saved 500 million people globally from malaria. In 1962, however, Rachel Carson published The Silent

Spring, in which she attributed the declining songbird population to widespread DDT use, and there have since been calls to ban DDT globally. The alternative insecticides are far more expensive, however, as they remain subject to patents owned by the pharmaceutical industry. Patients with adrenal cortical cancers are also prescribed chemotherapy. Approximately 40% of patients will respond and the most effective agents include doxorubicin, etoposide and cisplatin. The secretory symptoms of adrenal carcinoma can be controlled with octreotide. This agent has no effect on survival and does not lead to reductions in tumour bulk. The wingless-related integration (Wnt) and insulin-like growth factor (IGF) signalling pathways may be dysregulated in adrenal cortical cancers. Cixutumumab, an antibody directed against IGF1-receptor, may have activity in this tumour group, but trials petered out due to poor patient accrual in this rare tumour. The FIRM-ACT trial results suggest that treatment with mitotane, etoposide and cisplatin is the standard of care for patients with metastatic adrenal cortical cancer.

Prognosis of adrenal cortical cancers

The outlook for the majority of patients with adrenal cortical cancers is very poor, except in the patients with localized, small bulk disease. For this group of patients, the expectation is for a 70% chance of complete cure following surgery. For patients with bulky tumours, the expectation is for a median survival of 1 year. Patients with metastatic tumours survive a median period of 4 months.

Adrenal medullary tumours

These uncommon tumours occurring in association with multiple endocrine neoplasia are a rare cause of hypertension. Phaeochromocytomas of the adrenal medulla produce their effects by the secretion of catecholamines, resulting in intermittent, episodic or sustained hypertension, anxiety, tremor, palpitations, sweating, flushing, headaches, gastrointestinal disturbances and polyuria. Twenty-four-hour urinary collection for urinary free catecholamines (epinephrine, norepinephrine and dopamine) is now the most

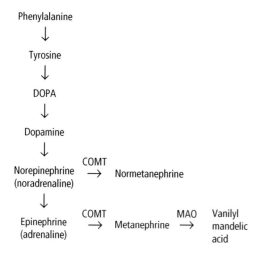

Phenylalanine
↓
Tyrosine
↓
DOPA
↓
Dopamine
↓

Norepinephrine $\xrightarrow{\text{COMT}}$ Normetanephrine
(noradrenaline)
↓

Epinephrine $\xrightarrow{\text{COMT}}$ Metanephrine $\xrightarrow{\text{MAO}}$ Vanilyl mandelic acid
(adrenaline)

Figure 22.2 Synthesis and breakdown of catecholamines. COMT, catechol o'methyl transferase; MAO, monoamine oxidase.

widely employed diagnostic test, although some centres also measure catecholamine metabolites such as metanephrines and vanillylmandelic acid (VMA). In 15% of patients with phaeochromocytomas, there may be changes in the RET, VHL and succinic dehydrogenase subunit B and D genes. Not a lot of people know about this, and the authors of this textbook are numbered amongst the ignorant. The treatment is surgical, and the results of treatment are generally excellent. Metastatic phaeochromocytoma may be treated with ^{131}I-MIBG (meta-iodobenzyl guanidine), a catecholamine precursor, which may also be used to image the tumour (see also Chapter 45). Treatment is generally only successful in those patients with small volume disease owing to the limited penetration of the ionizing radiation.

 ONLINE RESOURCE

Case Study: The Lebanese man with a sweet tooth.

 KEY POINTS

- Adrenal cortical cancers are rare and present with local symptoms or occasionally because they secrete androgens, aldosterone or cortisol
- Adrenal medullary cancers are occasionally familial and include phaeochromocytomas that secrete catecholamines, resulting in intermittent, episodic or sustained hypertension, anxiety, tremor, palpitations, sweating, flushing, headaches, gastrointestinal disturbances and polyuria
- The diagnostic investigation for phaeochromocytoma is now 24-hour urinary collection for urinary free catecholamines (epinephrine, norepinephrine and dopamine)

23

Carcinoid tumours

Learning objectives

✓ Explain the epidemiology and pathogenesis of carcinoid tumours

✓ Recognize the common presentation and clinical features of carcinoid tumours

✓ Describe the treatment strategies and outcomes of carcinoid tumours

---

Carcinoid syndrome appears frequently amongst Dr House's differential diagnoses but only turns out to be the final correct diagnosis in one episode ("Here Kitty"). This episode also includes the nursing home cat that only seems to visit people shortly before they die. House concludes that the cat is attracted to the warmth of the heated blankets on the beds of dying patients, but what does House know about medicine? The term carcinoid was coined by a German pathologist Siegfried Oberndorfer in 1907, meaning carcinoma-like, because of the relatively benign behaviour of these tumours despite their malignant appearance down a light microscope.

Carcinoid tumours are neuroendocrine tumours that may arise in numerous anatomical sites, particularly the gastrointestinal tract and lungs (Table 23.1). These are usually well-differentiated tumours, although carcinoids also include the rarer high-grade neuroendocrine tumours. Much of their medical notoriety derives from their secretion of vasoactive compounds that give rise to the carcinoid syndrome. This usually follows the development of liver metastases, when first-pass metabolism of these products is bypassed. Carcinoid tumours are much more common than previously recognized but the true incidence is not clearly known. It is estimated that around 1200 people are diagnosed with carcinoid tumours each year in the United Kingdom.

Presentation

Patients with carcinoid tumours may be asymptomatic or may present with symptoms due to the secretory products of their tumour. These metabolic products cause diarrhoea, flushing and occasionally bronchospasm (Figure 23.1). These symptoms are so specific that there is little difficulty in making a diagnosis, which is often achieved in general practice (see Chapter 45). The carcinoid syndrome of symptoms usually occurs with small bowel carcinoid tumours after the development of liver metastases but may occur without metastatic spread from bronchial carcinoid tumours. Carcinoid heart disease develops in up to half patients with 5HT-producing neuroendocrine tumours. It is due to the formation of fibrous plaques within the heart, causing valvular dysfunction. Classically, the valves affected are right-sided. Right-sided heart failure due to valve disease is treated surgically by valve replacement. In view of the underlining excellent prognosis for carcinoid tumours, this condition is actively treated. Carcinoid tumours also lead, because of their secreted products, to fibrosis at other sites, such as in the retroperitoneum, where it may lead to small bowel obstruction.

Oncology: Lecture Notes, Third Edition. Mark Bower and Jonathan Waxman.
© 2015 by John Wiley & Sons, Ltd. Published 2015 by John Wiley & Sons, Ltd.
Companion Website: www.lecturenoteseries.com/oncology

Table 23.1 Comparison of carcinoid tumours by site of origin

	Foregut	Midgut	Hindgut
Site	Respiratory tract, pancreas, stomach, proximal duodenum	Jejunum, ileum, appendix, Meckel's diverticulum, ascending colon	Transverse and descending colon, rectum
Tumour products	Low 5HTP, multihormones*	High 5HTP, multihormones*	Rarely 5HTP, multihormones*
Blood	5HTP, histamine, multihormones,* occasionally ACTH	5HT, multihormones,* rarely ACTH	Rarely 5HT or ACTH
Urine	5HTP, 5HT, 5HIAA, histamine	5HT, 5HIAA	Negative
Carcinoid syndrome	Occurs but is atypical	Occurs frequently with metastases	Rarely occurs
Metastasizes to bone	Common	Rare	Common

ACTH, adrenocorticotrophic hormone; 5HIAA, 5-hydroxyindole-acetic acid; 5HT, 5-hydroxytryptamine (serotonin); 5HTP, 5-hydroxytryptophan.
*Multihormones include tachykinins (substance P, substance K, neuropeptide K), neurotensin, PYY, enkephalin, insulin, glucagon, glicentin, VIP, somatostatin, pancreatic polypeptide, ACTH and α-subunit of human chorionic gonadotropin.

Investigations

The presence of symptoms is likely to indicate that the patient with a carcinoid tumour has metastatic disease. The examination of such a patient should be confined to establishing the extent of disease and obtaining a histological diagnosis. The investigations that are required include a blood count, liver function test, chest X-ray and a CT scan of the chest and abdomen (Figure 23.2). Twenty-four-hour urinary 5-hydroxyindole acetic acid (5HIAA) levels should be measured. This is because 5HIAA is the excretory product of the metabolites produced by carcinoids and results from the breakdown of

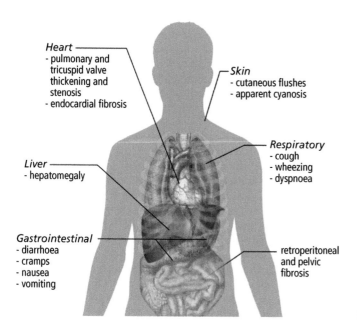

Figure 23.1 Carcinoid syndrome.

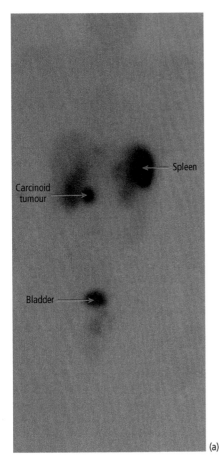

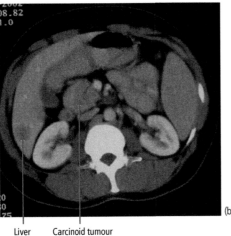

Figure 23.2 (a) Indium-113-labelled somatostatin scan demonstrating a focus of carcinoid tumour in the pancreas as well as normal tracer uptake in the spleen and bladder. (b) Matched CT scan showing a tumour in the head of the pancreas and liver metastases.

5-hydroxytryptamine (5HT) or serotonin. There has been interest in the use of both chromagranin A and B as serum markers for carcinoid. This is a neurosecretory product that is of value because we can monitor carcinoid using this as a blood test, rather than having to carry out 24-hour urinary collections to measure 5HIAA. Tumours may be localized by specialized isotope scanning with either an octreoscan or DOTATATE scan. Octreoscan uses a radiolabelled somatostatin analogue, [111]indium pentetreotide and scintigraphy, whilst the newer and more sensitive DOTATATE scan uses [68]gallium-DOTA-Octreotate and CT/PET imaging.

Treatment

Surgical resection of non-metastatic carcinoid tumours is usually curative, whilst the management of metastatic disease is focussed on a combination of pharmacological control of the carcinoid syndrome. The latter includes agents that block the synthesis, release and peripheral blockade of circulating tumour products. The list of drugs used in the treatment of carcinoid symptoms include inhibitors of 5HT synthesis such as parachlorophenylalanine, peripheral 5HT antagonists such as cyproheptadine, antihistamines and inhibitors of 5HT release such as somatostatin and its long-acting analogues. The most frequently used somatostatin analogue is octreotide, and this leads to a relief of symptoms in 80% of patients for a median duration of 10 months. Interferon has been used to treat patients with metastatic carcinoid tumours that have become refractory to somatostatin analogues. Symptom relief will occur in 50–70% patients, but fewer than 5% of patients achieve any significant tumour regression. Treatment with interferon is associated with significant side effects, which may include flu-like symptoms; for this reason, it is not generally given.

When metastatic disease in the liver is extensive, hepatic artery embolization, chemoembolization or radioembolization may be considered. This involves selective cannulation of the artery with injection of embolic material. Amongst the substances injected are radiolabelled analogues of somatostatin such as [90]yttrium DOTA-octreotide and [90]yttrium-embedded microspheres (see Figure 3.12). This will lead to sustained symptom relief in the majority of patients. There may be significant side effects from embolization, and so this procedure is not entered into without due consideration of the benefits. In some clinical series, mortality rates are 3–5%.

A "landmark" trial comparing treatment with octreotide with everolimus and octreotide was published in 2011. Everolimus is an orally active inhibitor of the mammalian target of rapamycin, an "mTOR inhibitor". The progression-free survival of the patients treated with combination therapy was 16 months and for those treated with single-agent octreotide was 11 months. As a result of this excellent study of 429 patients, the combination of octretoide and everolimus is now the "standard of care" for patients with metastatic carcinoid syndrome.

Prognosis

The prognosis for patients with metastatic carcinoid tumour is relatively good in comparison to that for most metastatic tumours. Patients with metastatic carcinoid tumour commonly survive a considerable time and the expectation, even in the presence of liver disease, is that approximately 36% of patients will survive 5 years and 20% for 10 years. In the absence of metastases and following resection of the primary, the outlook is excellent. Carcinoid tumours of different primary sites are thought to have different outlooks, but this is very much debated.

 ONLINE RESOURCE

Case Study: The blushing bride.

 KEY POINTS

- Carcinoid tumours are neuroendocrine tumours arising in various anatomical sites, most frequently the gastrointestinal tract and lungs
- Carcinoid syndrome (diarrhoea, flushing and occasionally bronchospasm) usually follows the development of liver metastases and is due to secretion of vasoactive compounds
- Carcinoid syndrome is diagnosed by measuring 24-hour urinary 5HIAA levels because 5HIAA is the breakdown product of 5HT

24

Pituitary tumours

Learning objectives

✓ Explain the epidemiology and pathogenesis of pituitary tumours

✓ Recognize the common presentation and clinical features of pituitary tumours

✓ Describe the treatment strategies and outcomes of pituitary tumours

---

Epidemiology and pathology

Pituitary tumours are common, and the most common are prolactinomas with an incidence of up to 1 in 3000 of the population per annum. Pituitary tumours arise from the anterior lobe and produce their effects by uncontrolled production of specific hormones, by destruction of normal pituitary tissues, leading to hypopituitarism or by compressing adjacent structures such as the optic chiasm, hypothalamus and bony structures (Table 24.1). Secretory tumours produce syndromes that cause gross clinical signs and symptoms. The local symptoms include headaches and visual field loss. The systemic symptoms produced depend upon the secreted product and range from acromegaly to pituitary Cushing's disease.

There are no classical oncogene mutations in pituitary tumours. However, there are clues to the development of this group of malignancies that come from dysregulation of the inhibitory components of the β-catenin pathway, and the relationship of this pathway to the cadherins. Both the Akt and MAPK pathways appear to be overexpressed in many pituitary tumours, and this blocks the inhibitors of the cell cycle. This is equivalent to snapping the brake cable as you are bicycling down a steep hill. The role of epigenetic modulation of gene expression in the aetiology of pituitary tumours is a cause for considerable excitement in endocrinologists, but oncologists have remained calm because in their view there is a lack of specificity to the changes described.

Treatment

Treatment options for pituitary tumours include blocking agents, such as bromocriptine and other dopamine agonists, neurosurgery and radiotherapy. The mainstay of therapy, however, is surgery, which is important in establishing the histological diagnosis, in decompressing the optic chiasm and in relieving obstructive hydrocephalus, as well as providing the possibility for completely excising the tumour. A transfrontal approach is required for large tumours with extrasellar extension, while for smaller tumours a trans-sphenoidal approach with dissecting microscope to the fore is safer and tolerated better. Radiotherapy may be used as the primary treatment for intrasellar tumours and as an adjunct to surgery for larger tumours. Surgery is more likely to control pituitary tumours than radiotherapy. The outlook is generally excellent with 5-year overall survival rates in excess of 85%.

Oncology: Lecture Notes, Third Edition. Mark Bower and Jonathan Waxman.
© 2015 by John Wiley & Sons, Ltd. Published 2015 by John Wiley & Sons, Ltd.
Companion Website: www.lecturenoteseries.com/oncology

Table 24.1 Comparison of clinical features of pituitary tumours

Tumour	Percentage of tumours	Morphology	Endocrine features	Neurological features
Prolactin-secreting adenoma	40	Macroadenoma	Amenorrhoea, galactorrhoea, hypopituitarism in men	Headache, visual field defects
Non-secretory adenoma	20	Macroadenoma	Hypopituitarism	Headache, visual field defects
Growth hormone-secreting adenoma	20	Macroadenoma	Gigantism in children, acromegaly in adults	Headache, visual field defects
Corticotrophin-secreting adenoma	15	Microadenoma	Cushing's disease	Usually none
Gonadotrophin-secreting adenoma	5	Macroadenoma	Panhypopituitarism	Headache, visual field defects
Thyrotropin-secreting adenoma	<1	Microadenoma	Hyperthyroidism	Usually none

In the treatment of pituitary Cushing's disease, where first-line therapies have failed and disease progression on first-line agents such as bromocriptine has occurred, the role of alternative agents blocking metabolic pathways becomes important; metyrapone, ketoconazole, mitotane and etomidate all inhibit enzymes involved in steroid synthesis and are used. Additionally drugs that affect ACTH production including the dopamine receptor D2 agonist cabergoline and the somatostatin analogue pasireotide are occasionally used with some benefit.

 ONLINE RESOURCE

Case Study: The infertile banker with a headache.

 KEY POINTS

- Pituitary tumours are common, 40% secrete prolactin, 20% growth hormone, 15% corticotrophin and 20% are non-secretory
- Pituitary tumours present with features related to hormone secretion or local destruction, leading to hypopituitarism or visual field defects
- Neurosurgical tumour resection is the primary treatment, although blocking agents, such as bromocriptine and other dopamine agonists, and radiotherapy may be required
- Five-year survival exceeds 85%

25

Parathyroid cancers

Learning objectives

✓ Explain the epidemiology and pathogenesis of parathyroid cancers

✓ Recognize the common presentation and clinical features of parathyroid cancers

✓ Describe the treatment strategies and outcomes of parathyroid cancers

---

Epidemiology and pathology

Parathyroid carcinomas are extremely rare, with an annual incidence of 0.5–1 per million of the population and account for only 1–2% of all cases of primary hyperparathyroidism. A rare familial syndrome of ossifying fibromas of the jaw, cystic and neoplastic renal tumours, uterine cancers and parathyroid cancers has been described. This familial hyperparathyroidism-jaw tumour syndrome is caused by a germline mutation in the HRPT2 tumour suppressor gene. It turns out that the majority of sporadic parathyroid cancers have somatic mutations of this same gene that encodes a protein parafibromin of uncertain function. A trawl through PubMed shows that research into the causes of parathyroid cancer reflects waxing and waning fashions in scientific research, but there is little that is likely to yield a true insight into this rare cancer. Non-coding RNAs, histone ubiquination and germline mutations in CDC73 are picked up in the net but inspection of the catch, to extend the clumsy metaphor, reveals tiddlers rather than trout.

Multiple endocrine neoplasia

Parathyroid cancers occur in the context of multiple endocrine neoplasia (MEN), which comprises a group of tumours whose clinical manifestations seem to delight old-fashioned physicians. In particular, the products they secrete give rise to many unusual syndromes. The majority of endocrine tumours are rare, with an incidence of 0.5 per million of the population per annum. But others are more common, such as carcinoid tumours, which have a reported incidence of 1.5 per 10^5 of people per annum. These tumours, including parathyroid cancers, are frequently listed as occurring in the context of MEN. MENs are due to gene mutations. The MEN 1 gene is encoded at chromosome 11q13. The gene product is called, imaginatively, menin and encodes a nuclear protein that partners with JunD, NF-κB and many other proteins. The function of menin is, however, not known, but is lost in MEN 1. Mutations in MEN 2 lead to changes in the RET proto-oncogene. The RET gene encodes a receptor tyrosine kinase and mutations at different

---

Oncology: Lecture Notes, Third Edition. Mark Bower and Jonathan Waxman.
© 2015 by John Wiley & Sons, Ltd. Published 2015 by John Wiley & Sons, Ltd.
Companion Website: www.lecturenoteseries.com/oncology

Table 25.1 Features of multiple endocrine neoplasia syndromes

	MEN 1 (Werner's syndrome)	MEN 2A (Sipple's syndrome)	MEN 2B (also known as MEN 3)
Components	Parathyroid hyperplasia or adenoma (90%)	Medullary thyroid cancer (100%)	Mucosal neuromas (100%)
	Pancreatic islets adenoma, carcinoma or more rarely diffuse hyperplasia (80%)	Phaeochromocytoma (50%)	Medullary thyroid cancer (90%)
	Pituitary anterior adenomas (65%)	Parathryoid hyperplasia or adenoma (40%)	Marfanoid habitus (65%)
	Adrenal cortex hyperplasia or adenoma (40%)		Phaeochromocytoma (45%)
Genetic locus	Chromosome 11q13	Chromosome 10q11	Chromosome 10q11
	Menin gene	RET gene	RET gene

sites within the RET gene are associated with MEN type 2A and type 2B, Hirschsprung's disease (congenital aganglionic megacolon) and medullary thyroid carcinoma. This one-gene source of multiple diseases is of course a blow to traditional paradigms of genetic disease but should perhaps be seen in the context of the shrinking genome. The number of genes postulated for the human genome has steadily fallen from the early days of the Human Genome Project, when it was speculated that 50,000–75,000 genes were present in the human genome, to the present "post-genomic" era, when estimates have decreased to 20,000 genes only. By comparison it requires 5000 components to make a Mercedes class C car.

The MEN syndromes are described in Table 25.1.

Presentation and treatment

Parathyroid cancers secrete parathormone (PTH), and for this reason the majority of patients present with hypercalcaemia. The hypercalcaemia is usually gross and, rather oddly, patients may be asymptomatic, with a calcium level that would normally be associated with death in the acute situation. The reason for this is that this condition generally has a long natural history and may have been present for many years prior to diagnosis. Calcium levels in excess of 4 mmol/L are frequently reported and the patient's cellular processes will have adapted to this level of hypercalcaemia.

The primary treatment for this condition is surgical. The prognosis for patients with parathyroid cancer depends on a number of pathological features of the surgical specimen. These include vascular invasion, and spread to lymph nodes and adjacent organs. There is no role for adjuvant therapy with either radiation or chemotherapy. Modern imaging techniques used to stage the disease include radioactive technetium-labelled Sestamibi scanning. Sestamibi is a compound made up of six (sesta in Italian) methoxyisobutylisonitrile (MIBI) ligands. The outlook for patients with metastatic disease is awful and the hypercalcaemia is often highly refractory to treatment. Death is usually due to the complications of hypercalcaemia on the kidney or heart.

 ONLINE RESOURCE

Case Study: An achy Iranian woman in a chador.

 KEY POINTS

- Parathyroid cancer is very rare and occurs as part of MEN 1 and MEN 2a
- Parathyroid cancers secrete PTH and present with profound hypocalcaemia
- The mainstay of treatment for parathyroid cancer is surgery
- The prognosis for metastatic parathyroid cancer is particularly poor

26

Lung cancer

Learning objectives

✓ Explain the epidemiology and pathogenesis of lung cancer

✓ Recognize the common presentation and clinical features of lung cancer

✓ Describe the treatment strategies and outcomes of lung cancer

---

In a celebrated television documentary *Death in the West*, produced in 1976 by Thames Television, the vice president of the tobacco company Philip Morris attempted to dismiss established links between tobacco and cancer. During the interview he said: "Too much of anything can kill you. Too much apple sauce can kill you". And: "If there were something harmful in tobacco smoke, we could remove it". Despite numerous court cases, the tobacco industry continues to target the young and encourage smoking. It took until 1999 for the Royal Family to withdraw its royal warrant from the tobacco multinational Gallaher, which entitled them to display "By Appointment" on packs of Benson & Hedges cigarettes. This was despite the death of the last three kings from tobacco-related disease, including King George VI, who died of lung cancer.

Epidemiology

Lung cancer is the second most common tumour of both men and women in the United Kingdom (Figure 26.1). The overall prospects for survival are poor: fewer than 10% of patients survive 5 years from diagnosis (Table 26.1). In the United Kingdom, there were 43,463 new diagnoses and 35,184 deaths from lung cancer in 2011.

Smoking and prevention

The most important cause of lung cancer is smoking, and the incidence of lung cancer is directly related to the number of cigarettes smoked (see Box 2.5). It is estimated that smoking is responsible for 86% of lung cancers and that smoking causes a total of 102,000 deaths a year in the United Kingdom. Smoking contributes to the risk of many different cancers including:

- lung cancer
- upper aerodigestive system cancers (oral cavity, nasal cavity, sinuses, pharynx, larynx and oesophagus)
- stomach cancer
- pancreas cancer
- liver cancer
- kidney cancer
- cervical cancer
- colorectal cancer
- mucinous ovarian cancer
- myeloid leukaemias

At present there are 10 million smokers in the United Kingdom having declined from a peak in the mid 1970s. In 1974, there were 10 cigarettes smoked each day per adult male and 5 cigarettes smoked per

---

Oncology: Lecture Notes, Third Edition. Mark Bower and Jonathan Waxman.
© 2015 by John Wiley & Sons, Ltd. Published 2015 by John Wiley & Sons, Ltd.
Companion Website: www.lecturenoteseries.com/oncology

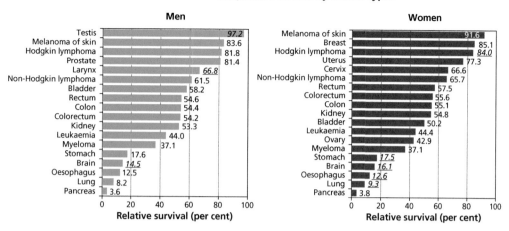

Comparative survival by tumour types

Men

	Relative survival (per cent)
Testis	97.2
Melanoma of skin	83.6
Hodgkin lymphoma	81.8
Prostate	81.4
Larynx	66.8
Non-Hodgkin lymphoma	61.5
Bladder	58.2
Rectum	54.6
Colon	54.4
Colorectum	54.2
Kidney	53.3
Leukaemia	44.0
Myeloma	37.1
Stomach	17.6
Brain	14.5
Oesophagus	12.5
Lung	8.2
Pancreas	3.6

Women

	Relative survival (per cent)
Melanoma of skin	91.6
Breast	85.1
Hodgkin lymphoma	84.0
Uterus	77.3
Cervix	66.6
Non-Hodgkin lymphoma	65.7
Rectum	57.5
Colorectum	55.6
Colon	55.1
Kidney	54.8
Bladder	50.2
Leukaemia	44.4
Ovary	42.9
Myeloma	37.1
Stomach	17.5
Brain	16.1
Oesophagus	12.6
Lung	9.3
Pancreas	3.8

Figure 26.1 Lung cancer – the second most common cancer and the second worst survival.

day per adult woman in the United Kingdom (Figure 26.2). One in two regular smokers will eventually be killed by the habit and half of them will die before the age of 70. The link between smoking and lung cancer was established 50 years ago and since then 6.5 million people have died in the United Kingdom because of tobacco-related disease (Figure 26.3).

The Department of Health has adopted six strategies to try and reduce the deaths from smoking:

1. Reducing exposure to environmental tobacco smoke
2. Educating people on risks of smoking
3. Increasing taxation on tobacco products
4. Limiting tobacco advertising and promotion
5. Regulating tobacco products
6. Providing assistance for individuals to quit smoking

Examples of these strategies include the introduction of smoke-free legislation in 2007 and public education through graphic television anti-smoking advertisements. Raising duty on cigarette sales also

reduces consumption; a 10% price rise reduces consumption by 4%. However, this is undermined by increasing levels of tobacco smuggling, which is estimated to account for 16% of the current UK cigarette market. Tobacco advertising promotion and sponsorship is banned in the United Kingdom and plain packaging of cigarettes should be introduced in 2015, unless the government makes another U-turn on this policy.

Public policy on smoking has been led by a complex cost–revenue balance. It is said that if all smoking ceased, the loss of revenue from tobacco taxation coupled to increases in pension payments because of reduced mortality would bankrupt UK Plc. Others argue that the revenue generated by smoking pays for the cost of care to the NHS of smoking-related illness. These are not great arguments.

In 1999, an NHS stop smoking service was established. In addition to encouragement advice and avoidance strategies, most clients are provided with pharmacological support: usually nicotine replacement therapy, bupropion or varenicline. Nicotine replacement therapy is meant to be used for a short

Table 26.1 UK registrations for lung cancer 2010

	Percentage of all cancer registrations		Rank of registration		Lifetime risk of cancer		Change in ASR (2000–2010)		5-year overall survival	
	Female	Male	Female	Male	Female	Male	Female	Male	Female	Male
Lung cancer	12	14	2nd	2nd	1 in 18	1 in 14	−13%	−14%	9.3%	7.8%

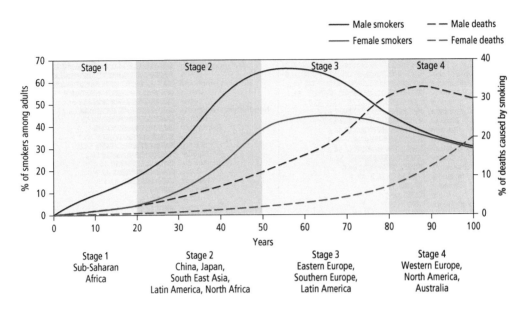

Figure 26.2 The evolving global epidemic of smoking. Source: Edwards R. The problem of tobacco smoking. BMJ, 2004;328(7433):217. Reproduced with permission of BMJ Publishing Group Ltd.

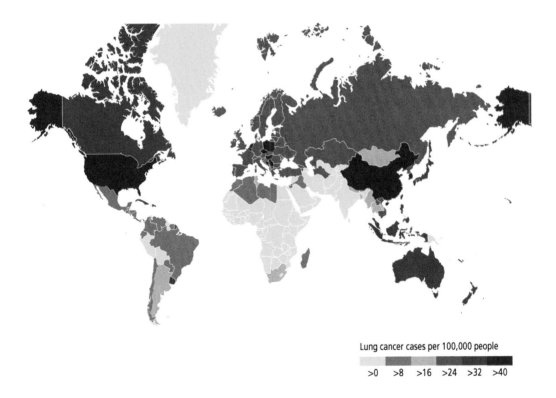

Figure 26.3 The evolving global epidemic of lung cancer.

length of time with gradual tapering off of the dose. It is available as transdermal patches, gum, lozenges, sprays and inhalers. Nicotine replacement therapy increases the chances of stopping smoking by 50% compared to placebo but the vast majority of over-the-counter users will relapse within 6 months.

The antidepressant bupropion (Zyban) reduces nicotine craving and is generally used for 12 weeks with advice to stop smoking 10 days into the course. The most important side effect is epileptic seizures and both headaches and insomnia are common. Bupropion is about as effective as nicotine replacement therapy but fewer people will return to smoking after completing the course. Varenicline (Champix) is a partial nicotinic acetylcholine receptor agonist that reduces both craving and enjoyment of tobacco. It causes nausea and less frequently neuropsychiatric disturbances. It is more likely to result in smoking cessation, with a 1-year complete abstention rate of 23%. Despite all these efforts and advances, the rate of decline in smoking in the United Kingdom is only 0.4% per year.

Pathogenesis

Smoking causes cancer because tobacco smoke contains at least 19 pyrolytic carcinogens. These include polycyclic aromatic hydrocarbons (PAH) such as benzopyrenes that are metabolized in the liver into potent epoxides that bind irreversibly to the bases of DNA resulting in mutations. Similarly, acrolein in cigarette smoke alkylates guanine bases but this does not require prior metabolism in the liver.

In addition to smoking, there are other risk factors for developing lung cancer. These include exposure to asbestos and heavy metals, such as nickel, and fibrotic disease of the lung. Air pollution is a significant factor in the development of lung cancers, and it is often said that living in London has the equivalent effect on lung cancer incidence to smoking five cigarettes a day. Similarly, proximity to industrial pollution has a significant impact upon mortality rates. Radiation, both therapeutic radiotherapy and background radon levels, increases the risk of lung cancer.

As with so many other tumour groups, there is significant interest in the molecular biology of lung cancer. Amongst the first observations of the molecular changes in lung cancer were mutations in the Ras family of oncogenes, which have guanosine triphosphatase (GTPase) activity and are important as second messengers linking events between the cell membrane and nucleus. The history of the molecular biology of lung cancer reads almost like a contemporaneous commentary on the development of our understanding of the molecular biology of cancer, and the next alterations to be discovered were mutations in the tumour suppressor genes Rb and p53 present in at least 80% of all small cell lung cancers. Loss of heterozygosity of a number of chromosomes has also been observed in small cell lung cancer. These include chromosomes 3, 9, 12, 13 and 17. The changes in chromosome 17 involve the c-erb-B2 oncogene and this has led to the development of new therapeutic approaches to the management of lung cancer.

More recently, observations of abnormal DNA methylation of the cyclin D2 gene has been described in approximately 60% of small cell lung cancer cell lines. The cyclin D2 gene has a primary function in cell cycle regulation and has recently been brought to the general public's attention because of the awards of the 2001 Nobel Prizes to the scientists involved in this discovery who included Sir Paul Nurse. Sir Paul Nurse according to *The Sun* is "the David Beckham of science". He later became the director of CRUK (Cancer Research UK) but that did not stop him saying that Margaret Thatcher did "a good job of ruining British science".

Screening

The survival for early stage lung cancer is much better than if the disease is diagnosed late, so early detection by screening has long been advocated. Neither plain chest X-rays nor sputum cytology has been found to be sufficiently sensitive, but there is hope that low-dose CT scans may be. The potential disadvantages of this approach include the cost, the high false positive rate and the radiation exposure. There are currently two large randomized controlled trials underway of low-dose CT screening.

Presentation

Patients with lung cancer generally present with a cough or haemoptysis. This may be associated with weight loss and symptoms of metastatic cancer (Box 2.2(e)), such as bone pain (Figure 26.4) or jaundice. Patients with symptoms suggestive of lung cancer should be referred promptly by their general practitioner to a specialist chest physician. One of the concerns of oncologists in the 1990s was the lack of referral on from specialist chest physicians to oncologists,

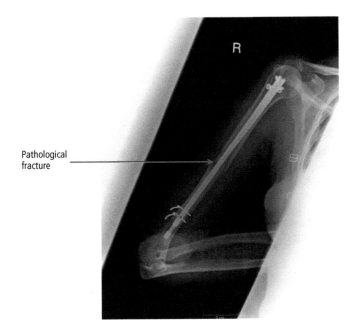

Pathological
fracture

with patients regarded somewhat as property. One of the major changes that we have seen in the third millennium has come about as a consequence of the central promotion of the philosophy of the multidisciplinary team. As a result, there is multispecialty input into the management of lung cancer patients and it is the view of these authors that the care of lung cancer patients has generally improved throughout the country.

The signs of lung cancer are many and of particular interest is the observation of clubbing of the fingers occurring in squamous cell lung cancer. The aetiology of finger clubbing, which is associated with hypertrophic osteoarthropathy and polyarthralgias, has been postulated as including the secretion of parathormone (PTH) by tumours and also, more recently, the ectopic secretion of platelet-derived growth factor (see Figures 39.6 and 39.7). Other clinical abnormalities may include Horner's syndrome (Figure 26.5) or hoarseness, which are pointers to inoperability as a result of nerve entrapment by the tumour of the sympathetic chain and recurrent laryngeal nerves, respectively. Dysphagia may occur as a result of mediastinal lymph node enlargement. Paraneoplastic syndromes are commonly associated with lung cancer, particularly the small cell carcinoma variant. These include cutaneous syndromes of dermatomyositis and acanthosis nigricans, the neurological complications of peripheral neuropathy,

cerebellar ataxia and the Eaton–Lambert syndrome (see Chapter 39). The endocrine features of ectopic PTH, adrenocorticotrophic hormone (ACTH) and antidiuretic hormone (ADH) secretion are all spectacular in their presentations.

Investigations should include a full blood count, liver function tests, chest X-ray (Figure 26.6) and sputum cytology. Bronchoscopy is organized and should proceed within a few days (Figure 26.7). Biopsies and washings are then obtained and examined microscopically. By these means, a histological diagnosis will be achieved. Diagnosis may not be achieved in the context of peripheral lesions and if this is the case, then needle biopsies under CT scanning or fluoroscopic imaging should be arranged (see also Figures 2.6, 40.1, 40.2, 40.3, 40.4, 40.5, 40.6b, 40.10 and 40.11).

Pathology

There are a number of different variants of lung cancer, and these histological classifications are important in that they define the patient's further treatment. The main histological variants are squamous cell carcinoma, small cell carcinoma, adenocarcinoma and large cell carcinoma (Figures 1.6, 1.7, 26.8, 26.9, 26.10 and 26.11). For treatment purposes, tumours are described as being either small or non-small cell lung

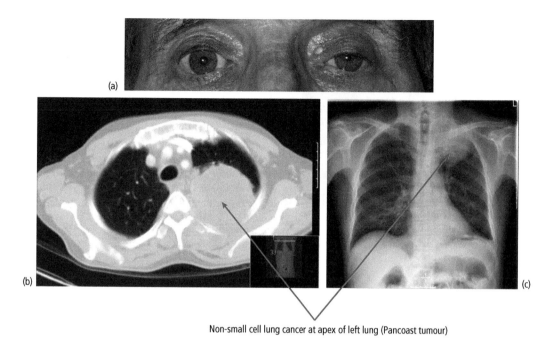

Non-small cell lung cancer at apex of left lung (Pancoast tumour)

Figure 26.5 (a) Left unilateral ptosis and miosis (constricted pupil). The other features of Horner's syndrome are enophthalmos (sunken eye) and anhidrosis (no sweating). It is due to loss of sympathetic innervation due in this case to a Pancoast tumour of the left lung apex affecting the T1 nerve root (b, c) (also associated with ipsilateral wasting of the small muscles of the hand). Horner (1831–1886) was a Swiss ophthalmologist; Pancoast (1875–1939) was an American radiologist.

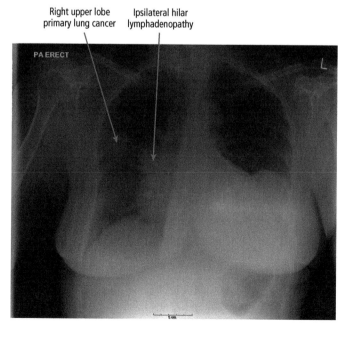

Right upper lobe primary lung cancer

Ipsilateral hilar lymphadenopathy

Figure 26.6 Chest X-ray of a 67-year-old woman with T2N2M0 small cell lung cancer showing a right upper lobe primary lesion with extensive ipsilateral and contralateral hilar lymphadenopathy.

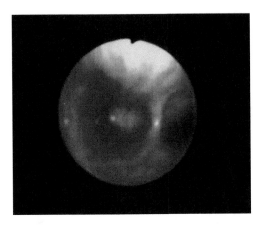

Figure 26.7 Appearance at bronchoscopy of a primary non-small cell lung tumour blocking the right main bronchus.

cancers. These constitute 95% of primary lung neoplasms. Squamous cell carcinoma accounts for approximately 20% of lung cancers, with adenocarcinoma accounting for 40% and small cell carcinoma for 15% of all lung tumours. Approximately 10% of lung cancers are of mixed histology. Rarer variants include carcinoid tumours, lymphomas and hamartomas.

Staging and grading

Lung cancer staging is determined usually by the TNM classification. Staging should include a CT scan of the chest and abdomen, a radioisotope bone scan, a liver ultrasound and ideally a positron emission tomography (PET) scan. Although not carried out routinely, examination of the bone marrow by aspiration and trephine in small cell lung cancer shows the presence of metastases in 95% of patients. Pulmonary function tests to assess vital capacity are essential, both to assess operability, and to ensure that the patient is not left with profound breathlessness following lung resection.

Treatment

Treatment of non-small cell lung cancer

Non-small cell lung cancer may be treated with either surgery or with radiation treatment. Surgery is only possible for patients with limited stage disease; that is, T1N0M0 and T2N0M0 disease, and a small number

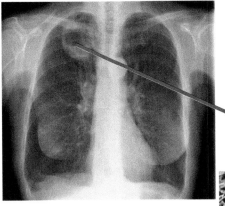

Right upper lobe cavitating mass caused by squamous cell lung cancer

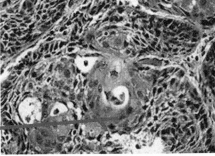

Well differentiated squamous cell lung cancer with characteristic keratin whorls

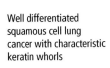

Figure 26.8 Squamous cell lung cancer.

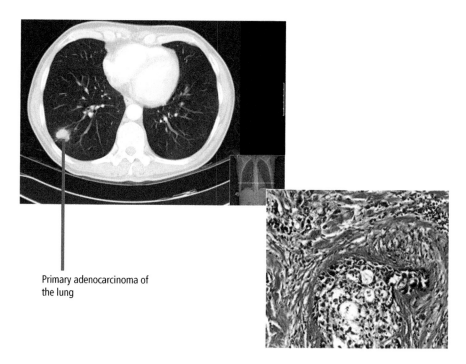

Primary adenocarcinoma of
the lung

Figure 26.9 Adenocarcinoma of lung.

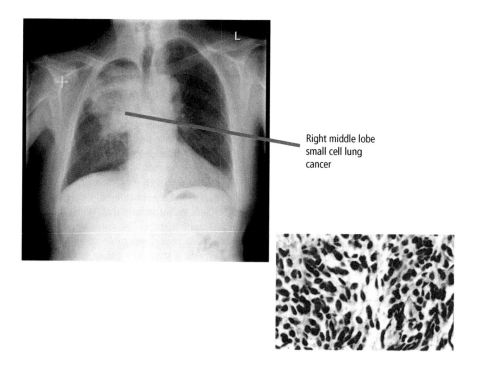

Right middle lobe
small cell lung
cancer

Figure 26.10 Small cell lung cancer.

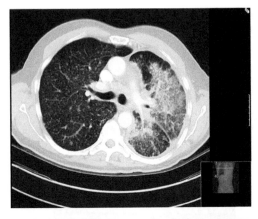

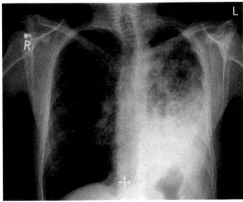

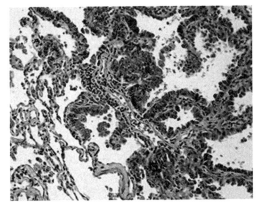

Figure 26.11 Bronchoalveolar cancer of the lung. Bronchoalveolar cancer is now often known as adenocarcinoma with lepidic growth. Lepidic means scaly and refers to the pattern of tumour growth in the terminal airways of the lungs.

with T2N1M0 tumours. There is increasing surgical enthusiasm for operating on more extensive tumours, and it is not uncommon to find patients with T3 disease proceeding to surgery. However, the results of this approach are usually poor. The increasing use of CT–PET scanning prior to surgery provides more accurate tumour staging and has reduced the number of patients undergoing "open and shut" thoracotomies for inoperable tumours.

The United Kingdom falls below the European average in terms of the number of people proceeding to surgery because of issues of resource availability in terms of scans and surgeons. Surgery has a significant morbidity and mortality, and operability depends upon lung function prior to resection, together with cardiac status and the presence of other major illnesses. It is estimated that approximately 30% of patients with non-small cell carcinoma of the lung have operable tumours. The 5-year survival for this group of patients is variably quoted at between 5% and 40%. A review of 2675 patients gave a five-year survival of

30%. There is a subgroup variation in survival, depending upon pathological staging and histology. For example, if those operable patients with adenocarcinoma are considered, the expectation for survival ranges between 38% and 79% and averages 65% at 5 years. If, on the other hand, operable patients under 40 years of age are considered, survival rises to 70%.

Radical radiotherapy, that is, radiotherapy given with curative intent, is considered for those patients who have inoperable disease by virtue of a poor medical state rather than spread of the cancer. Five-year survival figures of 6% were reported in a review of 1487 patients. Conventionally, patients receive 6000cGy over a 6-week period. More rapid treatment regimens are used, particularly in the north of England, and similar survival figures are found. For the majority of patients with more advanced cancer, radiotherapy is only used to palliative symptoms, which might include haemoptyses, breathlessness or chest pain. Radiotherapy is given according to various prescriptions; some radiotherapists advise a single dose of 1000–1500 cGy, others 3000 cGy in 10 fractions over 2 weeks. Radiotherapy, too, has side effects, and these include tiredness, oesophagitis and skin changes.

There is an increasing role for chemotherapy in the management of lung cancer, both as adjuvant therapy following surgery, neoadjuvant treatment prior to surgery, in combination with radiotherapy in stage III disease and as palliative therapy for advanced disease. The optimum treatment for advanced lung cancer depends upon the histological classification (non-squamous or squamous) and the presence of driver mutations of genes such as epidermal growth factor receptor (EGFR) and anaplastic lymphoma kinase (ALK) for which specific inhibitors are available. This approach has been rather grandly named "personalized genotype directed therapy". In general in the absence of a specific mutation, chemotherapy is given as a doublet of two drugs, one of which is permetrexed and cisplatin if the tumour is nonsquamous. For tumours harbouring activating mutations of EGFR, oral tyrosine kinase inhibitors such as erlotinib and gefitinib are indicated as first-line therapy. Side effects are reported, the most common of which is an erythematous skin reaction, and the occurrence of this rash seems to be associated with tumour responsiveness. Tumours with an ALK fusion oncogene may be treated with crizotinib, an oral tyrosine kinase inhibitor that targets ALK. What was once a Cinderella disease waiting for her prince has now emerged from the shadows with the availability of several new drugs of promise to be bestowed upon her, provided her dowry is bountiful, as the cost of these new drugs is considerable.

Treatment of small cell lung cancer

Small cell lung cancer is an entirely different disease from non-small cell lung cancer. It is very rare for patients to have localized small cell lung cancer, and approximately 95% of patients with small cell lung cancer have metastatic disease at presentation.

The most important modality of treatment for small cell lung cancer is chemotherapy. The current chemotherapy programme of first choice is etoposide and cisplatin. Approximately 80% of patients have an initial response to chemotherapy with this and similar programmes, and this generally includes a complete remission rate of up to 60% of patients. However, the great majority of small cell lung cancers will recur

after chemotherapy. Untreated, the median survival is 3 months. With treatment, 10–20% of patients will survive for 2 years and 5% for 5 years.

Treatment of paraneoplastic syndromes

Small cell lung cancer is associated with many paraneoplastic syndromes, due to secretion by the tumour of specific growth factors and hormones. One of the most common is hyponatraemia, due to inappropriate secretion of ADH. This is treated by water restriction, tetracyclines or the vasopressin receptor antagonist, tolvaptan. Steroids are prescribed in high dose for the treatment of polymyositis, Eaton–Lambert syndrome and the peripheral neuropathies associated with small cell lung cancer. Ectopic ACTH secretion may require high-dose therapy with adrenal enzyme-blocking drugs such as metyrapone and ketoconazole. Unfortunately, these two agents have toxicity in the dosages used and may make the patient feel awful. In this context, adrenalectomy may be rarely required.

 ONLINE RESOURCE

Case Study: A charlady with a rash.

 KEY POINTS

- Do not smoke
- Lung cancer is the second most common cancer in the United Kingdom and the second most common cause of cancer deaths
- Smoking accounts for most cases of lung cancer and the modest decline in lung cancer incidence reflects the decline in smoking since the 1970s
- Lung cancer usually presents with a cough, haemoptysis or the symptoms of metastatic cancer, such as bone pain or jaundice
- Treatment of lung cancer depends on the histopathological subtype and now increasingly on the molecular analysis of the tumour
- A minority of patients have surgically resectable disease at diagnosis but most patients have advanced disease and are treated with palliative systemic anticancer therapy or radiotherapy
- Overall fewer than 1 in 10 patients is alive 5 years after diagnosis

27

Mesothelioma

Learning objectives

✓ Explain the epidemiology and pathogenesis of mesothelioma
✓ Recognize the common presentation and clinical features of mesothelioma
✓ Describe the treatment strategies and outcomes of mesothelioma

---

Stephen Jay Gould was an evolutionary paleontologist at Harvard University and a prolific essayist. In 1982, he was diagnosed with peritoneal mesothelioma, which had a quoted median survival of 8 months. In response to this information he wrote an essay entitled "The median is not the message", which wisely and humanely explains the statistics of cancer survival. We urge students and patients to read it. Gould survived a further 20 years, dying in 2002 of a second primary lung cancer.

Epidemiology

In 2011, 2540 people were diagnosed and 2310 died of mesothelioma in the United Kingdom (Table 27.1). Three quarters of all mesotheliomas are pleural in origin and the remainder are peritoneal or pericardial. This tumour was originally described by occupational health doctors working in the asbestos factories in the East End of London around the time of the end of the First World War. It would appear, however, that this information was suppressed, and it was not until the 1960s that the association between mesothelioma and asbestos exposure was clearly publicized. The incidence of mesothelioma rose markedly in the last quarter of the 20th century and appears to mirror asbestos exposure rates 20–30 years previously. In the 1970s, after the risk of exposure was recognized, rigorous controls on the handling of asbestos were introduced in the United Kingdom. For this reason the rate

of rise of mesothelioma is expected to peak in 2015 and decline thereafter. But this is a global problem and touches countries all over the world from North Korea to South Africa.

Pathogenesis

The development of mesothelioma is generally related to asbestos exposure, but this may not always be the case. The risk of mesothelioma is not related to the amount of exposure. It may not only occur in the asbestos workers but also in family members exposed to the fibres of asbestos brought home in their spouse's, father's or mother's clothes. There are no specific chromosomal changes associated with the development of mesothelioma, but there are a host of abnormalities that may occur, which are entirely nonspecific. Different asbestos fibres have different properties and carcinogenicity. The most carcinogenic fibres tend to be the needle-shaped blue (crocidolite) and brown (amosite) asbestos rather than the commoner corkscrew-shaped white asbestos (chrysotile) (Table 27.2).

Presentation

Mesothelial tumours take their origins in the pleura or peritoneum. Patients with mesothelioma characteristically present with pleural effusions or ascites.

Oncology: Lecture Notes, Third Edition. Mark Bower and Jonathan Waxman.
© 2015 by John Wiley & Sons, Ltd. Published 2015 by John Wiley & Sons, Ltd.
Companion Website: www.lecturenoteseries.com/oncology

Table 27.1 UK registrations for mesothelioma cancer 2010

	Percentage of all cancer registrations		Rank of registration		Lifetime risk of cancer		Change in ASR (2000–2010)		5-year overall survival	
	Female	Male	Female	Male	Female	Male	Female	Male	Female	Male
Mesothelioma	<1	1	>20th	17th	1 in 773	1 in 150	+24%	+4%	<10%	<10%

Investigations

The diagnosis of mesothelioma may be suspected from a chest X-ray (Figure 27.1), where a patient may have pleural plaques and an effusion. CT scanning will show the extent of the pleural or peritoneal tumour. The next step in the investigatory process is to carry out a pleural or peritoneal biopsy. Multiple biopsies are frequently needed to make the diagnosis, and video-assisted thoracoscopy (VATS) may be required. A further complication of invasive diagnostic procedures for mesothelioma is the risk of seeding the tumour along the biopsy site resulting in chest wall recurrences. This risk can be reduced by prophylactic radiotherapy to the biopsy track or scar. Recurrent effusions are a dramatic problem for patients, and the intervention of a thoracic surgeon may be required to strip the pleura and provide an effective pleurodesis.

Possibly the most important aspect of the care of patients with mesothelioma is to ensure that the appropriate compensatory mechanisms are put in place. In the United Kingdom, industrial compensation is usually arranged for patients by their union officers and involves an examination of the tumour by a pathology panel. It is enormously important for the patient and his or her family that the clinician signposts this process. In the United Kingdom, two possible benefits are available: compensation from an employer linked to exposure to asbestos and industrial injuries disablement benefit from the Department of Works and Pensions.

Treatment

Unfortunately, the majority of patients with mesothelioma present with incurable disease. Treatment options are limited. Chemotherapy is generally ineffective, with response rates in the order of less than 10%, although newer combinations of cisplatinum and permetrexed (a dihydrofolate reductase inhibitor) offer promise. Radiation therapy may be helpful in controlling pain. Multiple pleurodeses are often required, with installation into the pleural cavities of materials such as talc, and VATS pleurodesis is the most effective at palliating pleural effusions. For operable patients, some clinicians advocate a trimodality approach incorporating radical surgery with extrapleural pneumonectomy (en bloc removal of both the parietal and visceral pleura, involved lung, mediastinal lymph nodes, diaphragm and pericardium with mesh reconstruction), coupled with neoadjuvant systemic chemotherapy and adjuvant hemithorax intensity modulated radiotherapy (IMRT). Nevertheless, disease progression rates are high and in one series the rate was 77% at 1 year. There is no randomized data to support this aggressive approach and most of the few patients who have been treated in this way experience severe side effects.

One potential approach is chemoprevention for people at risk of mesothelioma as a consequence of asbestos exposure. Currently there are no clinical studies of chemoprevention, although celecoxib, the COX2 selective non-steroidal anti-inflammatory drug (NSAID), has shown promise in laboratory models.

Table 27.2 Types of asbestos and cancer risk

Type	Colour	Morphology	Usage	Cancer risk	Location of mining
Crocidolite	Blue	Amphibole needles	10%	+++	South Africa, Australia
Amosite	Brown	Amphibole needles	5%	++	South Africa
Chrysotile	White	Serpentine corkscrew	85%	+	Canada

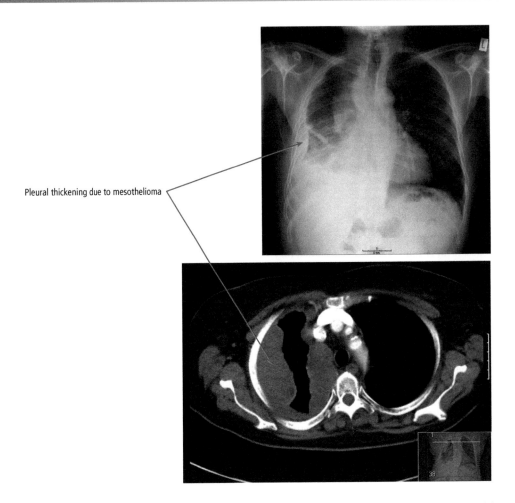

Pleural thickening due to mesothelioma

Figure 27.1 This chest X-ray and CT scan of a retired boiler-maker show diffuse circumferential pleural thickening of the right hemithorax, extending to the mediastinal pleura. In addition, there is substantial volume loss of the right hemithorax. The appearances are due to mesothelioma.

Prognosis

Unfortunately, the outlook for patients with mesothelioma is poor, with survival for patients with advanced disease ranging between 6 and 18 months. Three histological subtypes of mesothelioma exist: epithelial (55%), mixed (35%) and sarcomatoid (10%). The prognosis for these three subtypes is bad (epithelial), worse (mixed) and even worse (sarcomatoid).

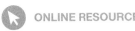 **ONLINE RESOURCE**

Case Study: The builder who could not climb his ladder.

KEY POINTS

- Mesothelioma is an uncommon cancer most commonly related to prior occupational asbestos exposure
- Most mesotheliomas are pleural in origin and present with dyspnoea, pleural effusion and thickening
- Even with aggressive approaches the outlook is poor, the survival with advanced disease is only 6–18 months

28

The leukaemias

Learning objectives

✓ Explain the epidemiology and pathogenesis of leukaemia

✓ Recognize the common presentation and clinical features of leukaemia

✓ Describe the treatment strategies and outcomes of leukaemia

---

Haematological malignancies are amongst the success stories in cancer treatment, with major advances in the second half of the 20th century. The first description of "white blood" was by Rudolf Virchov in 1845 when he was a 24-year-old junior doctor. He went on to become the father of modern pathology as well as a strong supporter of democracy during 1848, the year of European revolutions (see also Chapter 7). Cancer chemotherapy started with the treatment of haematological malignancies in the 1940s, following the demonstration by Alfred Gilman and Louis Goodman at Yale of lymphoma regression in mice with nitrogen mustard and their treatment of the first patient in 1944. Shortly afterwards, Sidney Farber at Harvard began to use folate antagonists in children with acute leukaemia, and in 1947 he reported temporary remissions with aminopterin. In the early 1960s, Emil Freireich and Emil Frei successfully used combination chemotherapy to cure childhood leukaemia and also started the trend of using acronyms for chemotherapy regimens. Theirs was VAMP (Vincristine, Amethopterin (methotrexate), Mercaptopurine and Prednisolone). Since that era, when childhood acute leukaemia was universally fatal, the long-term remission rate has risen to over 80%. Perhaps because of this success, medical oncologists and haematologists often fight over the management of haematological malignancies in the United Kingdom. Compared to some cancers, leukaemia is a clean, non-disfiguring disease and no fault can be attributed in any way to the patient. Perhaps that is why Jennifer (played by Ali MacGraw, one time wife of Steve McQueen), the heroine of Erich Segal's romantic drama film "Love story" dies of leukaemia. One witty critic defined "Ali MacGraw's disease as an illness in which the only symptom is that the patient grows more beautiful before finally dying".

Epidemiology

Leukaemias are relatively common with a preponderance of men affected (Table 28.1). In the United Kingdom, 8616 people were diagnosed with leukaemia and 4603 died of the disease in 2011.

The leukaemias are described generally as either acute or chronic. The main variants are lymphoid and myeloid leukaemia, which account for almost 95% of leukaemia. Myeloid neoplasms are derived from bone marrow progenitor cells that normally develop into erythrocytes, granulocytes (neutrophils, basophils and eosinophils), monocytes or megakaryocytes. The myeloid proliferations are divided into four groups:

- acute myeloid leukaemia (AML) defined as >20% myeloid blast cells in the blood or bone marrow, often associated with chromosomal rearrangements;
- myeloproliferative neoplasms are a group of clonal proliferations of one or more myeloid lineages, often associated with tyrosine kinase mutations;

Oncology: Lecture Notes, Third Edition. Mark Bower and Jonathan Waxman.
© 2015 by John Wiley & Sons, Ltd. Published 2015 by John Wiley & Sons, Ltd.
Companion Website: www.lecturenoteseries.com/oncology

Table 28.1 UK registrations for leukaemia cancer 2010

	Percentage of all cancer registrations		Rank of registration		Lifetime risk of cancer		Change in ASR (2000–2010)		5-year overall survival	
	Female	Male	Female	Male	Female	Male	Female	Male	Female	Male
Leukaemia	2	3	10th	9th	1 in 96	1 in 66	+0%	+0%	45%	44%

- myelodysplastic syndromes are disorders with ineffective production of blood cells and a variable risk of transformation to acute leukaemia;
- myelodysplastic/myeloproliferative neoplasms are disorders sharing dysplastic and proliferative features.

Examples of each group are shown in Figure 28.1.

Lymphoid neoplasms derive from cells that develop into B lymphocytes or T lymphocytes and are further divided into those originating from lymphoid precursors (such as acute lymphoblastic leukaemia (ALL)) and those deriving from mature lymphocytes

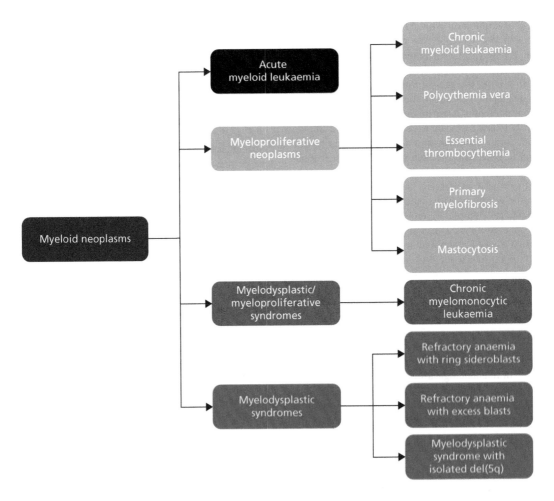

Figure 28.1 Classification scheme for myeloid malignancies.

and plasma cells. ALL is far more common in childhood than acute myeloid leukaemia (AML); whilst in adults approximately 80% of all the acute leukaemias are myeloid. In adults, chronic lymphocytic leukaemia (CLL) outnumbers chronic myeloid leukaemia (CML).

Pathogenesis

Radiation is the best recognized risk factor for the development of leukaemia and is estimated to account for 9% of cases in the United Kingdom including secondary leukaemias following radiotherapy. Smoking increases the risk of AML and may be responsible for a further 6% of all cases of leukaemia in the United Kingdom. Chemical carcinogens causing leukaemia include cytotoxic chemotherapy itself, and benzene and formaldehyde used in rubber production. Children with Down's syndrome are at increased risk of leukaemia, as are patients with certain other conditions with a chromosomal basis, such as Klinefelter's syndrome, Fanconi's syndrome and ataxia telangiectasia.

The biology of leukaemia has been studied intensively over the last 30 years. With this investigation, the idea of a single cell origin of leukaemia has developed as originally described in 1976 by Peter Nowell who also discovered the Philadelphia chromosome (the truncated chromosome 22 found in CML). The leukaemic clone is thought to have a survival advantage over normal haematological cells. One of the first leukaemias to be characterized at a molecular level was CML, where there is a fusion between chromosomes 9 and 22 that juxtaposes the BCR and ABL genes, which is observed cytogenetically as the "Philadelphia" chromosome. This molecular abnormality may be seen in other haematological cells, such as platelet and red cell precursors. The protein product of a fusion gene may have aberrant function. For example, the BCR–ABL protein is thought to activate cell cycle controlling proteins, thus speeding up cell division. BCR–ABL also inhibits DNA repair checks causing genomic instability, which may result in blast crisis in CML.

Hybrid fusion genes caused by reciprocal chromosomal translocations that join half a gene from one chromosome to half a gene from another chromosome occur relatively commonly in leukaemias. For example, acute promyelocytic leukaemias (APMLs) are characterized by a translocation between chromosomes 15 and 17. The resultant fusion gene is formed between part of the promyelocytic leukaemia (PML)

Table 28.2 Chromosomal abnormalities and their products

Abnormalities	Disease	Fusion gene
Altered transcription regulators		
t(12;21)	ALL	TEL/AML1
t(8;21)	AML	AML1/ETO
t(15;17)	APML	PML/RARA
Activated kinases		
t(9;22)	CML, ALL	BCR/ABL
t(5;12)	CMML	TEL/PDGFRB

gene on chromosome 15 and the retinoic acid alpha receptor gene (RARA) on chromosome 17. This hybrid gene interacts with histone deacetylase complexes that regulate gene transcription (see Chapter 3). Treatment with retinoic acid leads to dissociation of this complex and a transient remission of the leukaemia. Some examples of the fusion genes seen in leukaemia are described in Table 28.2.

Point mutations and gene deletions are also seen in leukaemias involving oncogenes such as p53 and RAS. P53 mutations are seen in ALL and blast crisis of CML, and N-RAS and c-KIT mutations are found in AML. Similarly, the myeloproliferative neoplasms are associated with mutations of tyrosine kinase genes. For example, polycythemia rubra vera, essential thrombocythemia and primary myelofibrosis are associated with mutations of JAK-2 (Janus kinase 2). It should be noted that the predominant molecular change in leukaemia is chromosomal translocation. This is in contrast with solid tumours, where the predominant changes are gene deletions and amplifications.

Although there is a greater understanding of the molecular biology of leukaemia, the reason for the genetic changes observed is not known. The exceptions are those rare leukaemias that occur in the context of exposure to radiation or as secondary events following chemotherapy. Such secondary leukaemias are commonly associated with chromosomes 5, 7 or 11 abnormalities (see Figure 3.25).

Presentation

The presentation of patients with acute leukaemia is remarkable in its dramatic onset. It is usual to obtain a history that dates back only a few days, with features of anaemia, thrombocytopenia and leucopenia, although some people date their symptoms back for much longer periods. Chronic leukaemia may

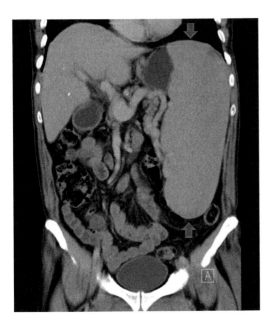

Figure 28.2 Massive splenomegaly due to CML (red arrows). The differential diagnosis of massive splenomegaly is myeloproliferative disease (including CML), malaria, myelofibrosis (including ET and PRV) and visceral leishmaniasis.

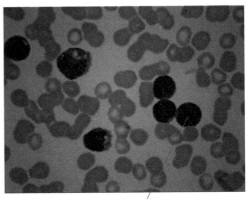

myeloblasts

Figure 28.4 Peripheral blood film of acute myeloid leukaemia demonstrating myeloblasts. Occasionally Auer rods, needle-like granules in the cytoplasm, are seen.

be diagnosed as an incidental finding, for example, when a blood count is performed as part of a routine screen for another medical problem. Patients with chronic leukaemia may have abdominal discomfort due to splenomegaly or present with anaemia or lymphadenopathy (Figure 28.2). Such presentations generally tend to be insidious; this is particularly the case for CLL. The situation is a little different for CML, which progresses from a chronic to an accelerated to a blast phase. The diagnosis can be made at any point in this clinical course.

Investigations and classification

The diagnosis of acute leukaemia is made by an examination of the peripheral blood and bone marrow (Figures 28.3, 28.4, 28.5, 28.6). In ALL, a lumbar puncture will be performed in order to investigate the possibility of CNS infiltration. Two common cytochemical stains are used to distinguish between AML and ALL. These are the Sudan black, which is usually

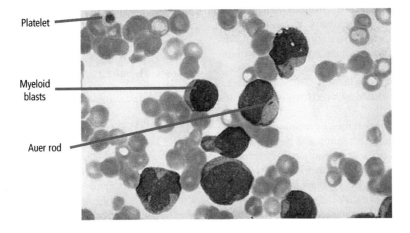

Platelet

Myeloid blasts

Auer rod

Figure 28.3 Acute leukaemia (AML-M4).

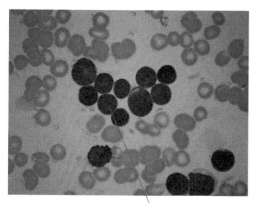

lymphoblasts

Figure 28.5 Peripheral blood film of acute lymphoid leukaemia demonstrating lymphoblasts with a very high nuclear to cytoplasmic ratio.

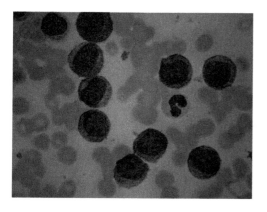

Figure 28.6 Bone marrow aspirate showing acute myeloid leukaemia with monocytic differentiation (AML-M5). This acute myelomonocytic subtype of AML is occasionally associated with gum infiltration and hypertrophy.

positive in AML and negative in ALL, and the periodic acid–Schiff (PAS) test, which is usually positive in ALL and negative in AML. These stains are outmoded and have been largely replaced by immunophenotyping.

The classification of acute leukaemias usually follows the French–American–British (FAB) classification, which essentially describes the degree of differentiation and maturation. AML are described as M1 to M7, and ALL as L1 to L3 (Table 28.3).

Immunophenotyping is also carried out in suspected ALL, where the presence of B- and T-cell markers is sought out. More than 70% of adult ALL are of B-cell origin. Following immunophenotyping, cytogenic and molecular analysis is carried out in order to define chromosomal and molecular abnormalities,

Table 28.3 The FAB classification of acute leukaemia

M0	Acute myeloid leukaemia with minimal evidence of differentiation
M1	Acute myeloid leukaemia without maturation
M2	Acute myeloid leukaemia with maturation
M3	Acute promyelocytic leukaemia
M4	Acute myelomonocytic leukaemia
M5	Acute monocytic leukaemia
M6	Acute erythroleukaemia
M7	Acute megakaryoblastic leukaemia
L1	Small monomorphic
L2	Large heterogeneous
L3	Large homogeneous (Burkitt)

which provide prognostic information (Figure 28.7). Cytogenetic analysis is useful in the diagnosis of CML and the prognosis of CLL.

The t(8;21) translocation in AML is associated with a good prognosis and occurs in about 8% of patients. The inversion or reciprocal translocation t(16;16) of chromosome 16 is associated with the M4 phenotype and again confers a favourable response. Translocations with an 11q23 breakpoint is a poor prognostic feature. The presence of the Philadelphia chromosome is found in about 5% of childhood and 25% of adult ALL, and is thought to perhaps indicate transformation from CML: this is an adverse prognostic feature.

CLL is a tumour of B-cell origin in 95% of patients (Table 28.4 and Figures 28.8, 28.9 and 28.10). Cytogenetic changes are described in up to 80% of patients with CLL. Although there is no particular pattern that emerges to characterize this leukaemia, five or six abnormalities are usually observed. Trisomy 12, for example, the most common cytogenetic abnormality, is found in just one-third of patients. Patients with CLL are classified using a number of different systems, most of which are helpful in describing survival related to lymphocytosis, lymph node involvement and the presence or absence of anaemia or thrombocytopenia.

Treatment

Acute leukaemia

The management of acute leukaemia is complex. It requires psychological support of the individual and of

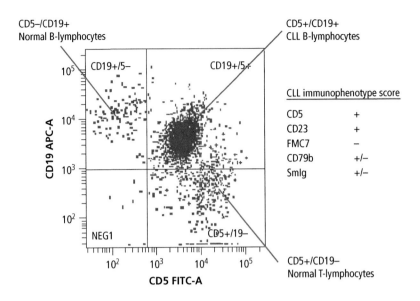

Figure 28.7 Immunophenotype by flow cytometry of peripheral blood in CLL. The majority of cells shown are CLL blasts that express both CD5 and CD19 (top right quadrant).

the family, and active and urgent treatment, particularly for the acute leukaemias. Initial treatment involves attempts to stabilize the patient by transfusion of red cells and platelets, combined with treatment of infection by antibiotics to limit the complications that may occur with the initiation of chemotherapy. These mainly revolve around the tumour lysis syndrome. Rehydration is required, and the patient is started on allopurinol and rasburicase to prevent the metabolic abnormalities that are described in detail in Chapter 40.

The chemotherapy that is given to patients with leukaemia has evolved as a result of many clinical trials over very many years, involving the Medical Research Council (MRC) in the United Kingdom, and the Cancer and Leukaemia Group B in the United States. The mainstay of induction chemotherapy in adult has been the use of daunorubicin and cytosine arabinoside given in a daily schedule, the dosage and duration of which is varied and repeated upon recovery of haematological parameters.

During treatment, patients require supportive therapies with blood products such as platelets and red cells. Platelet support is given to keep platelet counts above 10×10^9/L, which limits the risk of spontaneous haemorrhage (Figure 3.22). There is a risk of immunization against platelets, which may require human leucocyte antigen (HLA) matched transfusions rather

Table 28.4 Chronic lymphocytic leukaemias

B-cell	T-cell
B-cell chronic lymphocytic leukaemia/small lymphocytic lymphoma	T-cell chronic lymphocytic leukaemia (large granular lymphocytic leukaemia)
B-cell prolymphocytic leukaemia	T-cell prolymphocytic leukaemia
Hairy-cell leukaemia and variant	Adult T-cell leukaemia/lymphoma
Splenic marginal zone lymphoma, including splenic lymphoma with villous lymphocytes	Leukaemic phase of mycosis fungoides/Sézary syndrome
Leukaemic phase of mantle cell lymphoma	
Leukaemic phase of follicular lymphoma	
Leukaemic phase of lymphoplasmacytoid lymphoma	

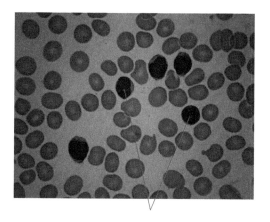

Figure 28.8 Peripheral blood film of chronic lymphocytic leukaemia showing multiple small B-cell lymphocytes with dense nuclei.

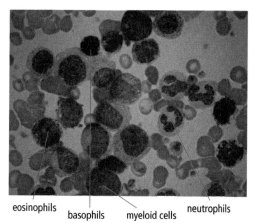

eosinophils   basophils   myeloid cells   neutrophils

Figure 28.10 Peripheral blood film showing chronic myeloid leukaemia with a spectrum of myeloid cells including eosinophils, basophils and segmented neutrophils as well as immature myeloid cells.

than random donor platelet transfusion. There is also a risk of graft versus host reactions in these heavily immunosuppressed patients who are also candidates for stem cell transplantation (Figure 28.19). This risk, from lymphocytes in blood donations, is reduced by irradiating blood prior to transfusion. Patients are of course at risk from neutropenic sepsis, which is treated with intravenous antibiotics. Prolonged neutropenia may be associated with fungal infection. In the context of persistent fever, particularly following transplantation, antifungal therapy is instituted. CT scanning may be appropriate in order to diagnose *Aspergillus* pneumonia. There is little evidence to

suggest that any prophylactic antifungal treatment is of value, but randomized studies have shown that prophylaxis with antibiotics such as co-trimoxazole reduces the risk of *Pneumocystis* infection.

With recovery of the marrow, a further bone marrow examination is carried out. The majority of patients will have entered complete remission just before the second course of chemotherapy. Generally, four to six cycles of treatment are given in all, and this may be followed by post-remission treatment using an allogenic stem cell transplant ideally from a closely matched relative. These approaches are used in younger patients who have entered their first remission. Approximately 50–55% of patients who receive a transplant will be cured, but there is no evidence of better survival after transplantation in the good-prognosis patients.

The management of patients in transplant programmes is, of course, highly specialized, and medical training is focussed on the recognition of the problems associated with profound and prolonged immunosuppression (see Box 28.1). The management of transplant patients has completely changed in recent years, because of the availability of recombinant growth factors. The use of granulocyte colony-stimulating factor (G-CSF) in transplant programmes has reduced the period of profound neutropenia such that the average duration of stay on a transplant ward has decreased from 28 to 17 days. One of the major complications of allogeneic transplantation is the development of graft versus host disease (GVHD), which is associated with a significant morbidity and

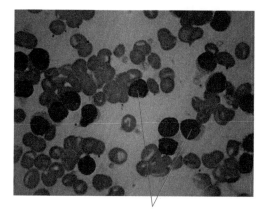

Figure 28.9 Bone marrow aspirate of an elderly asymptomatic man with a total white cell count of 28 × 10^9/L. There are many small lymphocytes present, which were CD19- and CD5-positive B-cells. The diagnosis is CLL.

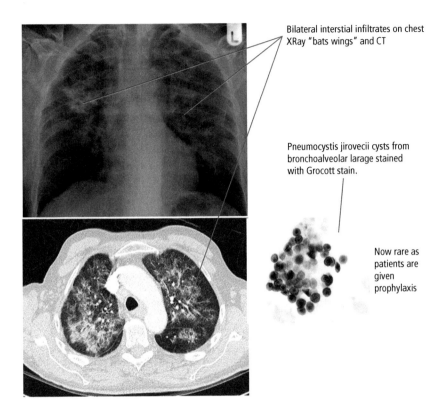

Bilateral interstial infiltrates on chest XRay "bats wings" and CT

Pneumocystis jirovecii cysts from bronchoalveolar larage stained with Grocott stain.

Now rare as patients are given prophylaxis

Figure 28.11 PCP (now known as *Pneumocystis jirovecii*).

> ## Box 28.1 Infectious complications of stem cell transplantation
>
> ### Common opportunistic infections
>
> Haematopoietic stem cell transplant recipients are vulnerable to opportunistic infections. The risk is the greatest in allogeneic stem cell recipients. Common opportunistic infections include:
>
> - Bacterial (including Mycobacteria)
> - Fungal (Candida, Pneumocystis, Aspergillus) (Figures 28.11, 28.15 and 28.16)
> - Viral [Herpes simplex virus (HSV), Cytomegalo virus (CMV), Varicella zoster virus (VZV)] (Figures 28.12, 28.13, 28.14 and 28.17).
> - Parasitic (Toxoplasmosis) (Figure 28.18)

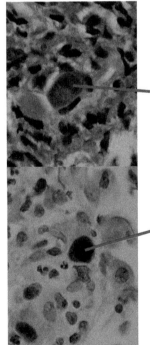

Owl's eye inclusion body in CMV infection (intranuclear collection of viral capsid proteins)

Immunocytochemical stain confirms presence of CMV

Figure 28.12 CMV.

mortality rate (Figure 28.19). New drugs to suppress GVHD have been developed, which include sirolimus, tacrolimus and mycophenolate. Sirolimus, also known as rapamycin, was first discovered as a product of the bacterium *Streptomyces hygroscopicus*

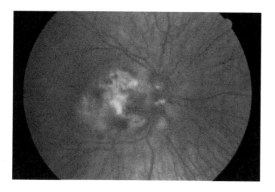

Figure 28.13 CMV retinitis. This appearance has been called "Pizza pie", another food metaphor, as well as "cottage cheese and ketchup".

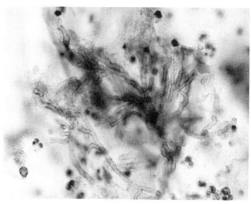

Figure 28.15 *Aspergillus fumigatus* isolated from lungs of a stem cell transplant recipient.

in a soil sample from Rapa Nui, one of the Easter Islands. Both sirolimus and tacrolimus inhibit mTOR (mammalian target of rapamycin), which is a cellular protein kinase that acts as a common step in many signal transduction pathways.

Treatment of recurrent acute leukaemia

Although 50% of patients with good-prognosis acute leukaemia survive, the majority of adults with acute leukaemia still die. Relapse generally occurs within the first 2 years. Patients with acute leukaemias are usually re-treated with chemotherapy, with a 50% chance of re-entering remission and a 10% chance of cure. It is usual in these situations to use a different induction drug regimen, which is frequently more intensive, with a greater risk of treatment complications and death. If remission is achieved allogeneic stem cell transplantation is usually advocated in younger fitter patients, including where necessary matched unrelated donor transplants.

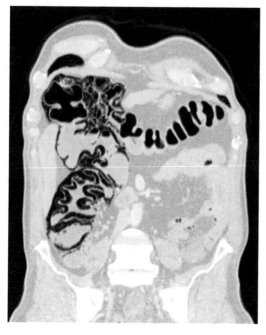

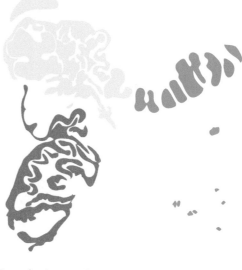

CT scan showing extensive pneumatosis coli of ascending and transverse colon due to CMV. Note the resemblance to Matisse cut-outs of his Jazz period

Figure 28.14 Pneumatosis coli due to CMV. Note how a tracing of the bowel resembles a Matisse cut-out!

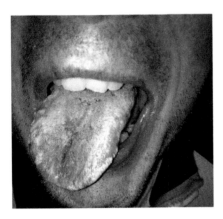

Figure 28.16 Oral *Candida albicans*.

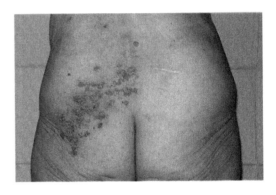

Figure 28.17 Dermatomal Herpes zoster (shingles).

Chronic leukaemia

The management of chronic phase CML has evolved over the years from the use of single-agent alkylating agents, such as busulfan and hydroxyurea, to the use of interferon alpha and then allogeneic stem cell transplantation. Real hopes of cure came with the application of transplant programmes to CML. However, the whole field has changed dramatically over the last decade with the introduction of imatinib (Gleevec), a novel compound that acts to inhibit the tyrosine kinase activity of the BCR–ABL oncoprotein. Imatinib binds to the BCR–ABL protein, inhibiting its kinase activity and effectively controlling disease driven by this kinase. There have been no serious adverse side effects from treatment with this agent, which offers a dramatic improvement over conventional therapy. Remissions in CML are seen with clearance of the Philadelphia chromosome, as shown by cytogenetic analysis. Eighty to ninety per cent of patients respond to imatinib. In about half of these responding patients, a cytogenic response is also seen. Imatinib resistance emerges as a consequence of mutations in the kinase

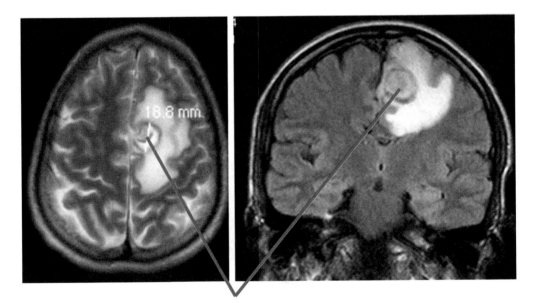

MRI brain scan showing ring enhancing lesion in left frontal lobe with extensive oedema due to cerebral toxoplasmosis

Figure 28.18 Cerebral toxoplasmosis.

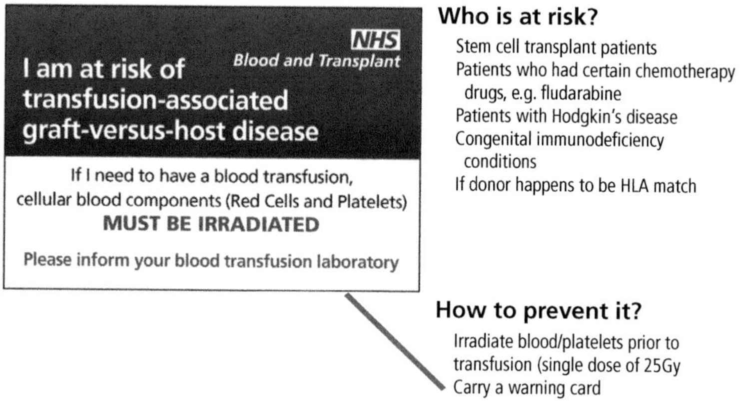

> **I am at risk of transfusion-associated graft-versus-host disease**
>
> **NHS** *Blood and Transplant*
>
> If I need to have a blood transfusion, cellular blood components (Red Cells and Platelets)
> **MUST BE IRRADIATED**
>
> Please inform your blood transfusion laboratory

Who is at risk?

Stem cell transplant patients
Patients who had certain chemotherapy drugs, e.g. fludarabine
Patients with Hodgkin's disease
Congenital immunodeficiency conditions
If donor happens to be HLA match

How to prevent it?

Irradiate blood/platelets prior to transfusion (single dose of 25Gy
Carry a warning card

Figure 28.19
Transfusion-associated graft versus host disease. Warning card reproduced with permission of NHS Blood and Transplant.

domains of BCR–ABL and new inhibitors including dasatinib and nilotinib, which are more potent, may overcome imatinib resistance.

CLL may be an entirely indolent disease with an excellent prognosis, and for many patients treatment may not be necessary. Even when therapy is necessary there is no consensus on what is the ideal first-line treatment. Options include purine analogues such as fludarabine, alkylating agents such as chlorambucil and more recently monoclonal antibodies including rituximab (anti-CD20), ofatumumab (anti-CD20) and altemtuzumab (anti-CD52).

Treatment of recurrent chronic leukaemia

Relapsed CML following imatinib therapy may be treated with second-line tyrosine kinase inhibitor therapy, depending on the resistance mutations in ABL/BCR. Accelerated phase CML may require allogeneic stem cell transplantation if a suitable donor is available, but this is not the practice for CLL where there is no evidence to support intensification of chemotherapy or maintenance therapy.

Leukaemia in young children

Acute lymphocytic leukaemia is the most common childhood leukaemia. Overall, the prospects for cure are very good, with a chance in excess of 80% of a sustained remission. The treatment of acute childhood leukaemia owes a great debt to the MRC-organized trials, which have examined issues such as the duration of therapy both for induction and maintenance, the need for cranial irradiation to prevent central nervous system relapse and the value of the individual drugs within the treatment programmes. Because of the high likelihood of a cure, recent clinical trials have

concentrated on trying to moderate the side effects of treatment, and these are particularly important in limiting neurological toxicity, such as the effects upon intelligence, personality and pituitary function, and the effects on growth and fertility.

 ONLINE RESOURCE

Case Study: The listless infant.

 KEY POINTS

- Leukaemia is the 10th most common cancer in the United Kingdom and is described as either acute or chronic and lymphoid or myeloid, hence ALL, AML, CLL and CML
- Lymphoid leukaemias are derived from lymphocyte precursors and myeloid leukaemias from precursors of erythrocytes, granulocytes, monocytes or megakaryocytes
- The molecular analysis of leukaemias has identified a number of chromosomal translocations and gene mutations that are characteristic of particular subtypes of leukaemia and have been exploited as targets for novel treatments
- Acute leukaemia presents with rapid onset features of anaemia, thrombocytopenia and leucopenia; chronic leukaemia may be diagnosed as an incidental finding, or may present with lymphadenopathy and splenomegaly or anaemia and recurrent infections
- The treatment of leuakaemias with systemic anticancer therapies represents one of the greatest successes of 20th century medicine

29

Hodgkin's lymphoma

Learning objectives

✓ Explain the epidemiology and pathogenesis of Hodgkin's lymphoma
✓ Recognize the common presentation and clinical features of Hodgkin's lymphoma
✓ Describe the treatment strategies and outcomes of Hodgkin's lymphoma

---

Hodgkin's disease or Hodgkin's lymphoma was first named by Samuel Wilks who was Thomas Hodgkin's successor as curator of the medical museum at Guy's Hospital. Hodgkin's original description of seven patients was published in 1832. The physicians in charge of the care of these seven patients included Thomas Addison (who described both Addison's disease of the adrenals and Addison's anaemia, which is better known as pernicious anaemia), Richard Bright (who described Bright's disease of the kidneys) and Robert Carswell (who described multiple sclerosis but failed to get the illness named eponymously after him). As you recall from Chapter 1 only three of the original seven patients actually had Hodgkin's lymphoma.

Epidemiology

Hodgkin's lymphoma is a relatively uncommon tumour, affecting approximately 1845 people in 2011 in the United Kingdom (Table 29.1). Currently, there are 300 deaths annually, including, in 2002, the original Albus Dumbledore actor Richard Harris whose hit record "MacArthur Park" you will all of course remember (although probably as the 1978 Donna Summer version rather than the 1968 original).

Pathogenesis

More men than women develop Hodgkin's disease, and there is a bimodal age distribution with peaks in the third and seventh decades. Little is known of the risk factors for the development of Hodgkin's disease, although there are minor associations with Down's syndrome and smoking. Geographical clustering has been noted, and there have been a few familial cases of Hodgkin's disease. The Epstein–Barr virus (EBV) genome may be found incorporated within Reed–Sternberg (RS) cells, and about half of the cases of Hodgkin's lymphoma in the United Kingdom are linked to EBV. The Reed–Sternberg cell is pathognomonic for the diagnosis and is thought to originate from lymphocytes affected by EBV. There is significant interest in the origins of the Reed–Sternberg cells, which are large cells with multinucleated or bilobed nuclei that according to histopathologists look like owl's eyes (Figure 29.1). Reed–Sternberg cells have a specific immunophenotype, expressing CD15 and CD30, but not expressing CD20 or CD45. Immunoglobulin gene expression is mutated within Reed–Sternberg cells, and there are functional rearrangements that lead to abnormal immune function.

Oncology: Lecture Notes, Third Edition. Mark Bower and Jonathan Waxman.
© 2015 by John Wiley & Sons, Ltd. Published 2015 by John Wiley & Sons, Ltd.
Companion Website: www.lecturenoteseries.com/oncology

Table 29.1 UK registrations for Hodgkin lymphoma cancer 2010

	Percentage of all cancer registrations		Rank of registration		Lifetime risk of cancer		Change in ASR (2000–2010)		5-year overall survival	
	Female	Male	Female	Male	Female	Male	Female	Male	Female	Male
Leukaemia	0.6	0.6	>20th	>20th	1 in 500	1 in 500	+21%	+11%	84%	83%

This leads to defective apoptosis, prolonged B-cell survival and, ultimately, to the development of Hodgkin's disease. EBV proteins remain present in about 40–50% of Reed–Sternberg cells and there is a threefold increased risk of Hodgkin's disease, following infectious mononucleosis (glandular fever). This possibly suggests that EBV is a future target for immunotherapy. There is a 10-fold increase in Hodgkin's disease in people living with HIV, but only a twofold to fourfold increase in allograft transplant recipients. Hodgkin's disease is also associated with various autoimmune diseases including:

- Rheumatoid arthritis (twofold to threefold increased risk)
- Systematic lupus erythematosus (threefold to fivefold increased risk)
- Sjögren's syndrome (fourfold increased risk)
- Sarcoidosis (nearly fourfold increased risk)
- Coeliac disease (twofold increased risk)

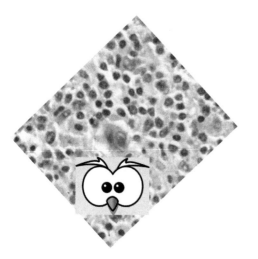

Figure 29.1 Owl's eyes. Histopathological sample demonstrating a Reed–Sternberg cell (a large binucleated cell with prominent nucleoli surrounded by a clear space or lacunae) diagnostic of Hodgkin's disease.

Presentation

The presentation of Hodgkin's disease is usually with enlarged lymph nodes. This is generally painless and may be accompanied by constitutional symptoms that include profound night sweating, sufficient to drench bedclothes, fevers greater than 38°C and weight loss exceeding 10% of body mass. These constitutional symptoms are prognostically important and designated as B symptoms. There are other non-specific symptoms relating to the presentation of Hodgkin's disease, including alcohol-related pain and skin itching. These B symptoms are thought to be generated by cytokine release.

Investigations

In clinic, a careful history should be obtained and an examination made. Investigations will be organized which include a full blood count and erythrocyte sedimentation rate (ESR), liver and renal function tests, a chest X-ray, CT scan of the chest and abdomen and bone marrow aspiration and trephine biopsy. The patient will be reviewed in outpatients with the results of these tests. Admission will then be organized for a biopsy of the lymph glands. The purpose of these investigations is to define the clinical stage of the disease and that of biopsy to make a histological diagnosis. The examination of bone marrow is commonly undertaken during the investigation of patients with Hodgkin's disease. Less than 5% of men and women with Hodgkin's disease have bone marrow involvement, however, and this is generally only present in patients with advanced tumours of stages greater than IIB. There are strong arguments against carrying out this assessment except in advanced-stage patients and with increasing use of PET–CT in staging, marrow assessment is being phased out in most centres.

Mediastinal mass

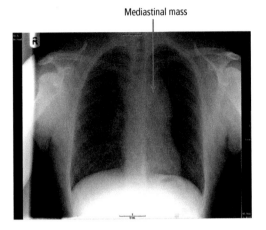

Figure 29.2 Hodgkin's disease with a mediastinal mass. This chest X-ray of a 20-year-old male student shows infilling of the aortopulmonary window and a wide left paratracheal stripe due to mediastinal lymph node enlargement from Hodgkin's disease.

The investigation of Hodgkin's disease is a recapitulation of the history of imaging in the United Kingdom. Plain X-rays (Figure 29.2) remain helpful, but approaches such as lymphography and staging laparotomy with splenectomy have been replaced by CT and MRI, whilst marrow examinations are being replaced by PET-CT scanning.

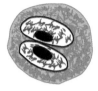

Reed–Sternberg cells are large cells with big dark nucleoli. Classic RS cells have two nuclei.

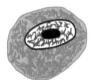

Mononuclear Hodgkin cells have a single nucleus.

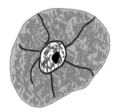

Lacunar cells have a central shrunken nucleus surrounded by a clear space crossed by thin pink strands.

Figure 29.3 The cells of Hodgkin's lymphoma.

Nodular lymphocyte predominant Hodgkin's lymphoma has the immunophenotype of B-lymphocytes (CD20+ve, CD15−ve, CD30−ve) and few if any Reed–Sternberg cells.

Pathology

Two forms of Hodgkin's lymphoma are recognized: classical and nodular lymphocyte predominant Hodgkin's lymphoma (Figure 29.4).

Four different histological variants of classical Hodgkin's disease are described (see also Figure 29.3):

- Nodular sclerosing (70%, nodules of tumour in a background of reactive cells with fibrosis or sclerosis)
- Mixed cellularity (20%, classical Reed–Sternberg cells combined with inflammatory reactive cells, usually EBV associated)
- Lymphocyte-predominant (5%, most favourable prognosis, may be confused with B-cell non-Hodgkin lymphoma (NHL))
- Lymphocyte-depleted (1%, may be confused with diffuse large B-cell lymphoma (DLBCL) and anaplastic large cell lymphoma)

Staging

The results of the staging investigations will help the clinician to determine the clinical stage of the Hodgkin's disease, and this in turn defines treatment. In stage I Hodgkin's disease, one lymph node or two contiguous lymph node groups are affected. In stage II disease, two non-contiguous lymph node groups on the same side of the diaphragm are affected. In stage III Hodgkin's disease, lymph node groups on both sides of the diaphragm are affected. In stage IV disease, there is extranodal spread to the liver, lung or bone but rarely to other sites (see Box 3.1). The tumour is further classified as A or B. "A" defines a lack of constitutional symptoms and "B" indicates the presence of the constitutional symptoms of Hodgkin's disease. Finally, the staging is defined by use of the subscript "S", which indicates splenic involvement, or "E", which defines extension to involve extranodal tissue in direct apposition to an enlarged lymph node group (Figure 29.5).

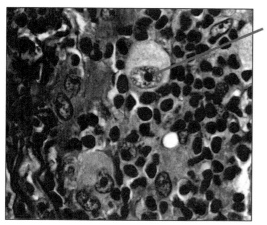

Mononuclear
Reed–Sternberg cell

Figure 29.4 Hodgkin lymphoma.

Treatment and side effects

The purpose of staging is to define treatment groups. Since most patients will be cured of Hodgkin's lymphoma, mortality from treatment-related toxicities has become a major determinant of treatment strategies. Patients with early stage disease (stages I and II) are usually treated with a combination of chemotherapy and radiotherapy, the amounts depend on whether the patient has favourable or unfavourable prognosis disease. This is determined by a combination of age, disease sites, ESR and B symptoms. Patients with advanced stage disease (stages III and IV) are treated with combination chemotherapy.

Radiation

In the past, radiation treatment was generally given according to two well-defined treatment plans. Lymphadenopathy above the diaphragm was treated with mantle radiation which includes the lymph node groups in the neck, axillae and chest to a total dosage of 3500 cGy given over a period of 4-6 weeks. Infradiaphragmatic radiation is generally given in the inverted Y distribution that includes the para-aortic and iliac nodal groups. Treatment is given to a total dosage of 3500 cGy over a 4–6-week period.

Mantle radiotherapy may be complicated by radiation pneumonitis, which is characterized by a period of breathlessness and fever and responds to steroids. It is invariably accompanied by loss of saliva

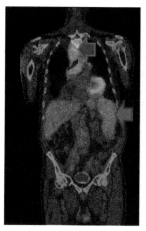
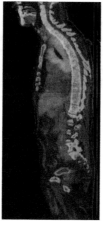
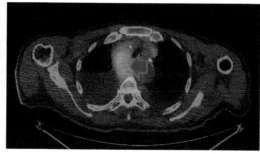

Figure 29.5 FDG–PET images of a patient with mediastinal lymph nodes and splenic involvement by Hodgkin's lymphoma. He had significant weight loss and night sweats (stage IIIB).

production and oesophagitis. Infradiaphragmatic radiotherapy may be complicated by some minor bowel disturbance but generally is well tolerated. Radiation is usually avoided in children and adolescents as it may lead to gross growth disturbance. Infradiaphragmatic radiation may cause sterility.

In view of the toxicity of radiotherapy, current practice is initial treatment with two to four cycles of chemotherapy followed by radiotherapy restricted to the involved field site of initial disease.

Chemotherapy

Combination chemotherapy for Hodgkin's disease was introduced in the mid-1960s. The original treatment regimen, which has the acronym MOPP, combined mustine, vincristine (Oncovin), prednisone and procarbazine. These drugs are given intravenously and orally for 2 weeks and repeated every 4 weeks. Six cycles are administered. Treatment is associated with acute nausea and vomiting, sterility in 90% of males and 50% of females, and the development of second tumours in approximately 5% of patients.

Chemotherapy treatments have been modified over the years in order to reduce side effects. Six is a "magic number" in oncology, and it is possible that in some cases fewer cycles of therapy are as effective as six cycles. The most frequently used current programme is called ABVD which combines adriamycin (doxorubicin), bleomycin, vinblastine and dacarbazine. The efficacy of this regimen was initially disputed as it was described by Italians but proven in an excellent clinical trial based at Harvard. These drugs cause neither sterility nor second malignancies and are of obvious advantage in a disease where there is a high expectation of cure. The initial randomized trial has been followed by further trials which have shown an equivalence of ABVD to standard therapy with MOPP and to hybrid therapies such as the higher dose but shorter duration Stanford V.

Haemopoietic stem cell transplantation

High-dosage chemotherapy with peripheral blood stem cell support is the standard treatment for relapsed Hodgkin's disease. The most commonly applied current programme in the United Kingdom uses "mini-BEAM" or BEAM (carmustine (BCNU), etoposide, cytarabine, melphalan) chemotherapy. Since this chemotherapy wipes out bone marrow reserves, these must be replenished with stem cell infusions. These stem cells are normally autologous blood progenitors harvested prior to the procedure and frozen until needed. Autologous stem cell transplantation in centres of excellence has treatment-related mortality rates of 1–2%. Long-term remissions occur in up to 40% of patients. The evidence base for any benefit for high dose chemotherapy with autologous stem cell rescue in this situation is scant and the side effects of transplantation significant. A Cochrane analysis published in 2013 found that there were only three randomized trials of this approach which involved a total of just 398 patients. The meta-analysis concluded that there probably was a progression-free survival advantage to intensive therapy, but recommended more studies to prove the benefit of this treatment. In patients who are unsuitable for stem cell transplantation, an alternative approach for drug-resistant Hodgkin's disease uses a novel immunoconjugate, Brentuximab vedotin. Brentuximab is a monoclonal antibody to CD30 that is linked to a cytotoxic antitubulin agent. So it delivers this toxin directly to the Hodgkin's cells that it targets because they express CD30.

Prognosis

The results of treatment of Hodgkin's disease are considered to be one of the miracles of modern oncology, in that approximately 90% of patients with small-volume, early-stage disease are curable with radiation and between 40% and 60% of patients with advanced disease are curable with chemotherapy. A poorer prognosis results from the presence of bulk disease, constitutional symptoms or poor-prognosis histology. The patient who is "cured" as a result of treatment is unfortunately at risk from late relapse; this may occur 15–30 years after diagnosis. This risk of a late relapse is small and largely confined to lymphocyte-predominant Hodgkin's disease.

Complications of chemotherapy

Hodgkin's disease is a tumour with significant cure rates, occurring in young people with an expectation of prolonged survival. This leads to a significant onus for providing a therapy that is without major long-term toxicity. Conventional chemotherapy and radiotherapy for Hodgkin's disease using alkylating agents is associated with the development of second tumours. The incidence of second tumours reaches approximately 5%, with staggering increases in the rates of acute leukaemias and lymphomas. The leukaemias present early, 2–4 years after the completion of chemotherapy. The solid tumours, such as breast, colorectal and lung cancer, occur late, sometimes 15–20 years after diagnosis. Sterility is also an important consequence of treatment with any alkylating agent-containing regimen, reaching up to 80% in males and 50% in females. This is a very serious consideration in the design of future treatment programmes to improve upon cure rates in this condition.

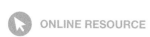 **ONLINE RESOURCE**

Case Study: The medical student.

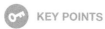 **KEY POINTS**

- Hodgkin's lymphoma is an uncommon cancer with a bimodal age distribution
- Patients present with enlarged lymph nodes which may be more painful after an alcoholic drink
- Staging of Hodgkin's lymphoma depends on the sites of disease and the presence or absence of B symptoms (profound night sweating sufficient to drench bedclothes, fevers greater than 38°C and weight loss exceeding 10% of body mass)
- Treatment usually achieves a cure and involves combination chemotherapy with the addition of radiotherapy if the disease is localized
- Much current research focuses on reducing the long-term side effects of treatment including the risk of secondary cancers and infertility to improve the quality of the cure

30

Non-Hodgkin's lymphoma

Learning objectives

✓ Explain the epidemiology and pathogenesis of non-Hodgkin's lymphoma

✓ Recognize the common presentation and clinical features of non-Hodgkin's lymphoma

✓ Describe the treatment strategies and outcomes of non-Hodgkin's lymphoma

Epidemiology

Non-Hodgkin's lymphoma (NHL) is relatively common (Table 30.1). In the United Kingdom in 2011 there were 12,783 diagnoses and 4646 deaths attributable to NHL. There have been many descriptions of the pathological classification of this disease. Rather than achieving clarity, however, most have tended to confuse the situation further because of their complexity. The current WHO classification lists over 80 different forms of lymphomas! They divide the lymphomas into four groups:

- mature B-cell neoplasms
- mature T cell and natural killer (NK) cell neoplasms
- Hodgkin lymphoma
- immunodeficiency-associated lymphoproliferative disorders

In terms of clinical practice, the most significant divisions are into high- and low-grade lymphoma (Table 30.2). High-grade lymphoma is 3–4 times more common than low-grade lymphoma. About 4000 people are diagnosed in the United Kingdom with low-grade lymphoma each year. Slightly more men are affected than women. Lymphomas arise from lymphoid organs or lymphatic tissue associated with other systems that contain lymphatic tissue. The latter, the so-called extranodal lymphomas, constitute up to 30% of all NHL.

Pathogenesis

There have been extraordinary advances in the molecular biology of lymphoma, and from this we have begun to understand some of the aetiological features involved in this condition. The most prominent factors in the pathogenesis are infections and immune suppression. Viral infection with HIV, EBV, HHV8, HCV and HTLV are all associated with NHL (Table 30.3). *Helicobacter* infection in the stomach leads to a proliferation of gastric lymphoid tissue and the development of low-grade, mucosa-associated tumours. Such tumours may respond to *H. pylori* eradication treatment, but unfortunately they may still evolve into classical lymphoma despite eradication.

In addition to infection, immunosuppression increases the risk of lymphoma including HIV infection which increases the risk of NHL by 60 times. By comparison the risk of lung cancer is increased 17 times in smokers. Similarly allograft transplant recipients, who are prescribed immunosuppressants to prevent graft rejection, are also at greatly increased risk of

Oncology: Lecture Notes, Third Edition. Mark Bower and Jonathan Waxman.
© 2015 by John Wiley & Sons, Ltd. Published 2015 by John Wiley & Sons, Ltd.
Companion Website: www.lecturenoteseries.com/oncology

Table 30.1 UK registrations for non-Hodgkin lymphoma cancer 2010

	Percentage of all cancer registrations		Rank of registration		Lifetime risk of cancer		Change in ASR (2000–2010)		5-year overall survival	
	Female	Male	Female	Male	Female	Male	Female	Male	Female	Male
NHL	4	4	7th	5th	1 in 61	1 in 51	+15%	+14%	66%	62%

lymphoma. Various autoimmune diseases also raise the risk of lymphoma:

- Sjögren's syndrome (19-fold increased risk)
- systematic lupus erythematosus (sevenfold increased risk)
- rheumatoid arthritis (twofold to fourfold increased risk)
- coeliac disease (increased risk of enteropathy-associated T-cell lymphoma)

Presentation

Patients present with nodal enlargement which may be accompanied by constitutional symptoms including weight loss, sweating and fever (Figures 30.1 and 30.2). These symptoms – where weight loss is in excess of 10% of pre-morbid weight, sweating is sufficient to drench night clothes and fever exceeds 38°C – are

Table 30.2 The most common pathological subtypes of non-Hodgkin lymphoma

Pathological subtype	Grade	Percentage of NHL diagnoses
Diffuse large B-cell lymphoma (DLBL)	High grade	31
Follicular lymphoma (FL)	Low grade	22
Marginal zone lymphoma (MZ)	Low grade	8
T-cell lymphoma (TCL)	Low or high grade	7
Small lymphocytic lymphoma	Low or high grade	6
Mantle cell lymphoma (MCL)	High grade	6
Burkitt lymphoma (BL)	High grade	3

Table 30.3 Infections associated with lymphoma

Infection	Lymphoma subtype
Virus	
Epstein barr virus (EBV)	African (endemic) Burkitt lymphoma
	Primary cerebral lymphoma
	Hodgkin's lymphoma
	Diffuse large B-cell lymphoma
	Post-transplant lymphoproliferative disease
	Nasal T/NK non-Hodgkin lymphoma
	Primary effusion lymphoma (with HHV8)
Human herpesvirus8 (HHV8)	Primary effusion lymphoma (with EBV)
Hepatitis C virus	Splenic lymphoma with villous lymphocytes
Human T-lymphotropic virus, type I (HTLV-I)	Adult T-cell leukemia-lymphoma
Bacteria	
Helicobacter pylori	Gastric mucosa associated lymphoma (MALT)
Campylobacter jejuni	Immunoproliferative small intestinal disease (IPSID) – a variant of extranodal marginal zone lymphoma

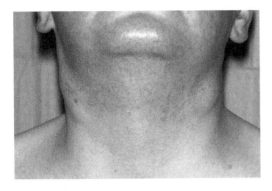

Figure 30.1 Bilateral cervical lymphadenopathy in a man with stage IV follicular lymphoma.

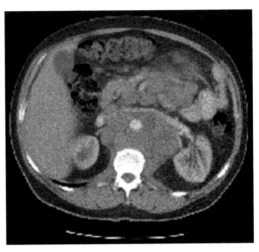

Figure 30.3 CT scan showing massive para-aortic lymphadenopathy to diffuse large B-cell non-Hodgkin's lymphoma.

described as "B" symptoms. "B" symptoms are less common in high-grade lymphoma than low-grade malignancies. Patients with such symptoms should be referred to specialist centres where the chance for survival and the quality of survival are significantly better than in peripheral non-specialist centres. The care of patients with lymphoma should be by oncologists or haematologists, depending upon the specialist interests of the clinicians.

Staging and grading

In outpatients, a careful history is obtained from the patient who is then examined. The investigations organized should include a blood count, renal and hepatic function tests, chest X-ray, bone marrow aspiration and trephine, and PET–CT scan of body (Figures 30.3, 30.4, 30.5, 30.6 and 30.7). These investigations are done in order to define the extent of the disease. From these investigations the clinical staging is obtained (Figure 30.8). This is defined as follows:

- Stage I: disease confined to one lymph node or two contiguous lymph node groups
- Stage II: disease on one side of the diaphragm in lymph node groups that are separate
- Stage III: disease on both sides of the diaphragm
- Stage IV: extranodal spread of the lymphoma

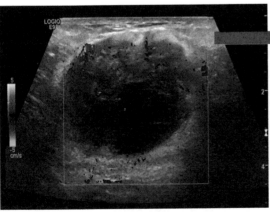
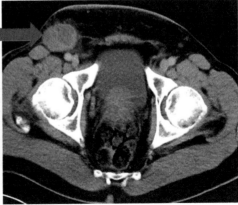

Figure 30.2 Right inguinal lymph node with vascular rim on colour Doppler ultrasound. Core biopsy of lymph node confirmed a diagnosis of diffuse large B-cell non-Hodgkin's lymphoma.

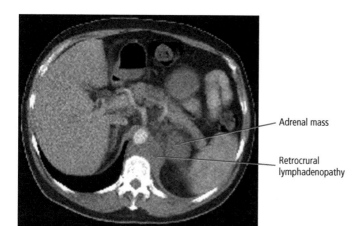

Adrenal mass

Retrocrural lymphadenopathy

Figure 30.4 CT scan showing extensive left retrocrural adenopathy and a left adrenal mass due to high-grade B-cell non-Hodgkin's lymphoma.

Extradural mass displacing and compressing spinal cord

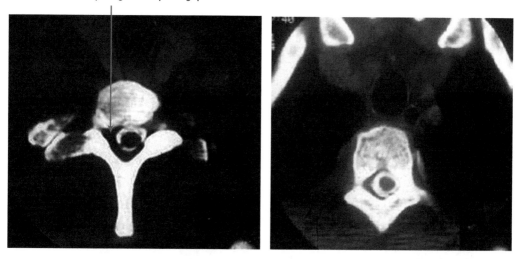

Figure 30.5 Spinal cord compression at T1 by an extradural mass of high-grade non-Hodgkin's lymphoma.

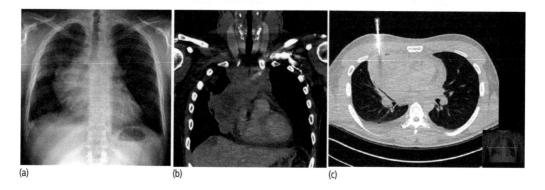

(a)   (b)   (c)

Figure 30.6 Mediastinal mass. A 35-year-old man was presented with a large anterior mediastinal mass (a, b). A diagnosis of non-Hodgkin's lymphoma (mediastinal large B-cell) was established by a CT guided biopsy (c). He was treated with six cycles of R-CHOP and remains in remission 2 years later.

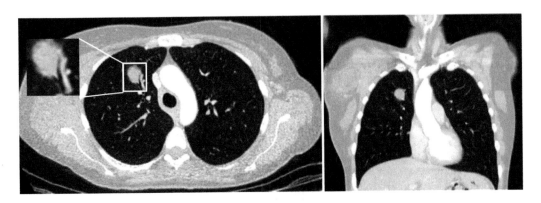

Figure 30.7 Lung opacity with air bronchogram. A branching linear lucency within an opacity in the lung is known as an "air bronchogram", seen most often with consolidation and pulmonary oedema. It is rare in primary lung cancer but is seen in lymphoma of the lung (as here).

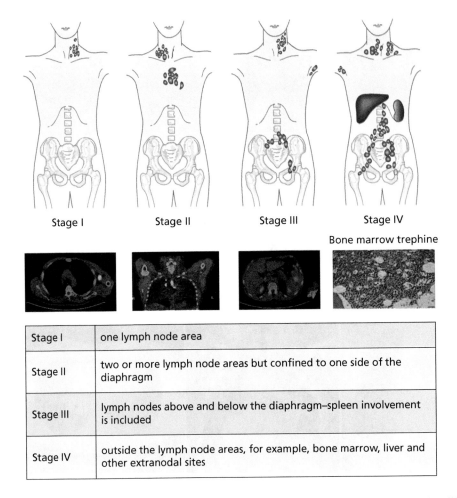

Stage I	one lymph node area
Stage II	two or more lymph node areas but confined to one side of the diaphragm
Stage III	lymph nodes above and below the diaphragm–spleen involvement is included
Stage IV	outside the lymph node areas, for example, bone marrow, liver and other extranodal sites

Figure 30.8 Lymphoma staging. A = without symptoms; B = with symptoms including unexplained weight loss (10% in 6 months prior to diagnosis), unexplained fever and drenching night sweats.

Preliminary investigations having been organized, the patient should then proceed to a lymph node biopsy. Lymph node biopsies used to be required to describe the architectural arrangement of the tumour. In modern times, they are no longer always considered to be necessary. Sufficient material can often be obtained from core needle biopsies to define the pathological diagnosis. There are many classification systems for NHL, which include the WHO classification (Table 30.4), the Kiel classification, the Working Formulation and the Revised European and American Lymphoma Classification (REAL).

For the purposes of defining treatment, the most practical classification, however, is to describe the tumour as being low or high grade. A low-grade tumour tends to have a follicular nature and to contain relatively inactive cells. A high-grade tumour contains cells that have a high index of mitotic activity, meaning that many of the cells are actively proliferating, and there is no follicular structure to the lymph node. There are variant lymphomas, such as mantle cell and Burkitt's lymphomas, which are clinical entities with poor prognosis.

Many modern techniques have been applied to the pathological diagnosis of lymphoma. Immunophenotyping using monoclonal antibodies is the most helpful, firstly, in initially distinguishing between a lymphoma or a carcinoma by using antibodies to the leukocyte common antigen (CD45), and secondly, in defining the lymphoma by using antibodies that are specific for B or T lymphocytes, such as CD20 or CD4, CD2 and CD3. T-cell receptor and immunoglobulin gene rearrangement studies are also carried out, and are helpful in describing tumour clonality. Fluorescent *in situ* hybridization (FISH) is also useful. This is because the observed cytogenetic abnormalities are relatively specific for subtypes NHL. Some of these are outlined in Table 30.5.

Treatment

Low-grade non-Hodgkin's lymphoma

Low-grade tumours are generally disseminated at diagnosis. If they are localized, that is stage I, small bulk, peripheral and without B symptoms, the treatment should be radiotherapy. For stages II–IV disease, treatment is chemotherapy with oral alkylating agents such as chlorambucil or with an intravenous chemotherapy programme known as CVP which uses cyclophosphamide, vincristine and prednisone.

Table 30.4 World Health Organization (WHO) classification of lymphomas

Mature B-cell neoplasms
Chronic lymphocytic leukemia/Small lymphocytic lymphoma
B-cell prolymphocytic leukemia
Lymphoplasmacytic lymphoma (such as Waldenström macroglobulinemia)
Splenic marginal zone lymphoma
Plasma cell neoplasms
  Plasma cell myeloma
  Plasmacytoma
  Monoclonal immunoglobulin deposition diseases
  Heavy chain diseases
Extranodal marginal zone B-cell lymphoma, also called MALT lymphoma
Nodal marginal zone B-cell lymphoma
Follicular lymphoma
Mantle cell lymphoma
Diffuse large B-cell lymphoma
Mediastinal (thymic) large B-cell lymphoma
Intravascular large B-cell lymphoma
Primary effusion lymphoma
Burkitt lymphoma/leukemia

Mature T-cell and natural killer (NK) cell neoplasms
T-cell prolymphocytic leukemia
T-cell large granular lymphocytic leukemia
Aggressive NK cell leukemia
Adult T-cell leukemia/lymphoma
Extranodal NK/T-cell lymphoma, nasal type
Enteropathy-type T-cell lymphoma
Hepatosplenic T-cell lymphoma
Blastic NK cell lymphoma
Mycosis fungoides/Sézary syndrome
Primary cutaneous CD30-positive T-cell lymphoproliferative disorders
  Primary cutaneous anaplastic large cell lymphoma
  Lymphomatoid papulosis
Angioimmunoblastic T-cell lymphoma
Peripheral T-cell lymphoma, unspecified
Anaplastic large cell lymphoma

Hodgkin Lymphoma
Classical Hodgkin lymphomas
  Nodular sclerosis
  Mixed cellularity
  Lymphocyte-rich
  Lymphocyte depleted or not depleted
Nodular lymphocyte-predominant Hodgkin lymphoma

Immunodeficiency-associated lymphoproliferative disorders
Associated with a primary immune disorder
Associated with the HIV
Post-transplant
Associated with methotrexate therapy
Primary central nervous system lymphoma in immuno-compromised patients

Table 30.5 Recurrent chromosomal translocations in non-Hodgkin's lymphoma subtypes, resulting in oncogene dysregulation

Histology	Translocation	Alteration of gene function	Mechanism/features of translocation	Frequency
Follicular lymphoma	t(14;18)(q32;21)	Upregulation of BCL2 (inhibitor of apoptosis)	BCL2 relocates to IgH locus. Error in physiological IgH rearrangement. Seen rarely in normal B-cells	80%
Burkitt's lymphoma	t(8;14)(q24;q32); t(2;8)(p12;q24); t(8;22)(q24;q11)	Upregulation of c-MYC (transcription factor for cell cycle progression/proliferation)	c-MYC relocates to IgH locus or to one of the light chain gene loci (IgL or IgK)	100%
Mantle cell lymphoma	t(11;14)(q13;q32)	Upregulation of cyclin D1 (G1 cyclin)	Cyclin D1 relocates to IgH	>90%
Diffuse large B-cell lymphoma*	t(3;14)(q27;32) and several others involving 3q27	Deregulation of BCL6 (zinc finger transcription factor)	BCL6 relocates to IgH, IgL, IgK or one of many other non-Ig loci	30–40%
Extranodal marginal zone lymphoma (MALT)	t(11;18)(q21;q21)	Gene fusion of AP12 and MLT/MALT1 genes (AP12 is inhibitor of apoptosis)	Gene fusion	20–35%
Extranodal marginal zone lymphoma (MALT)	t(1;14)(q22;q32)	Deregulation of BCL10 (apoptosis regulatory protein)	BCL10 relocates to IgH locus	<5%
Lymphoplasmacytic lymphoma	t(9;14)(q13;q32)	Deregulation of PAX5 (paired homeobox transcription factor)	PAX5 relocates to IgH locus	50%
Anaplastic large cell lymphoma	t(2;5)(p23;q35) and others involving 2p23	Gene fusion of ALK (anaplastic lymphoma kinase, a receptor tyrosine kinase) and NPM (located at 5q35) or other gene malignant transforming capacity *in vitro* and *in vivo*	Gene fusion	ALK-NPM, 50% Others, 15%

Ig, immunoglobulin; MALT, mucosa-associated lymphoid tissue.
*BCL2 (30%) and c-MYC (10%) rearrangements are also seen in diffuse large B-cell non-Hodgkin's lymphoma.

Chlorambucil has very little early toxicity but at high total dosages causes sterility, secondary myelodysplasia (MDS) and acute myeloid leukaemia (AML). CVP leads to hair loss, but apart from this it is without significant morbidity. Both regimens may be associated with marrow toxicity which results in admissions with neutropenic sepsis or with thrombocytopenic bleeding. The monoclonal antibody rituximab is frequently added to these cytotoxic agents. Rituximab is directed against CD20 and usually has very little toxicity apart from the possibility of a hypersensitivity reaction.

Patients with stage I NHL have a 70–95% chance of cure with radiotherapy. The patient with disseminated low-grade lymphoma is not cured by treatment. Although 85% of patients achieve a complete response

to therapy, this response is transient. After a median period of 18 months, the patient relapses and requires re-treatment. The average patient has four such episodes of response and relapse. Finally after a median period of 7.5 years, there is transformation to high-grade lymphoma.

Because treatment for disseminated low-grade lymphoma is not curative, there have been trials of the benefit of more intensive therapy administered with curative intent in this condition. A 2012 Cochrane meta-analysis unearthed five randomized controlled trials of high-dose chemotherapy and autologous stem cell rescue in patients with low-grade follicular NHL. The meta-analysis found a "strong" benefit for this approach in terms of progression-free survival.

High-grade non-Hodgkin's lymphoma

Paradoxically, high-grade lymphomas are more likely to be confined to one lymph node group than low-grade tumours and are curable. Stage I disease may be treated with abbreviated chemotherapy (usually three cycles of R-CHOP) followed by radiotherapy. Patients with small bulk stage I NHL have a 95% chance of cure. Treatment for those with more advanced disease is with the R-CHOP regimen, and there is little evidence that more complex regimens add to the chance of cure. Seventy to eighty per cent of all patients enter remission, which is sustained in about 40–60% of cases. CHOP consists of cyclophosphamide, doxorubicin (hydroxydaunorubicin), vincristine (oncovin) and prednisolone and was introduced in the 1970s. It has remained the gold standard therapy for many high-grade lymphomas ever since with the addition of rituximab for CD20-expressing lymphomas in the late 1990s. In 1993 a pivotal trial compared CHOP with several newer chemotherapy regimens with less memorable but more exotic names (e.g. m-BACOD, ProMACE-CytaBOM and MACOP-B); CHOP emerged as the regimen with the least toxicity but similar efficacy. The addition of rituximab has resulted in RCHOP becoming the gold standard for diffuse large B-cell lymphoma (DLBL). Some higher grade lymphomas such as Burkitt lymphoma require more aggressive alternating combination chemotherapy regimens.

High-dose therapy

Patients with poor-prognosis lymphomas at presentation or with recurrent high-grade lymphomas may be considered for high-dose chemotherapy with autologous or allogeneic haematogenous stem cell support. These cells are usually harvested by leucophoresis following colony stimulating factor administration, or from umbilical cord blood from neonates. Stem cell transplantation programmes may be linked with attempts to purge the stem cells of specific cell populations. Immunosuppression is required for patients receiving allografts and depends on the closeness of the HLA matching of the donor and host. HLA are the human leukocyte antigen genes of the major histocompatibility complex (MHC). Prognosis depends on a number of risk factors. There is an associated mortality rate to these procedures, which is as little as 1–2% for autologous transplants and exceeds 10% for matched unrelated donor allografting.

Nevertheless, it is unlikely that ever higher doses of cytotoxic chemotherapy will improve outcomes particularly as any marginal benefit is likely to be more than offset by greater treatment-related mortality. The future is more likely to lie with scientific advances leading to rational drug design and novel therapies. For example, there are three new promising approaches to mantle cell lymphoma: bortezomib, a proteosome inhibitor; lenalidomide, a thalidomide analogue that acts as an immunomodulator; and idelalisib, a phosphoinoside-3 (PI3) kinase inhibitor.

 ONLINE RESOURCE

Case Study: The Eritrean woman with a swollen jaw.

 KEY POINTS

- NHL are a large collection of cancers with different biology, natural history, treatment and outcomes that derive from lymphoid organs or lymphatic tissue
- NHL are divided into the more common high-grade NHLs and rarer low-grade NHLs
- NHL usually present with enlarged lymph nodes which may be accompanied by constitutional B symptoms (weight loss, sweating and fever)
- High-grade NHL are aggressive cancers that frequently grow rapidly and are treated with combination chemotherapy with curative intent
- Low-grade NHL are generally disseminated at diagnosis and usually indolent; they respond to chemotherapy but relapse following therapy which is therefore not curative

31

Myeloma

Learning objectives

✓ Explain the epidemiology and pathogenesis of myeloma

✓ Recognize the common presentation and clinical features of myeloma

✓ Describe the treatment strategies and outcomes of myeloma

Epidemiology

Myeloma is a relatively common haematological malignancy; 4792 people were diagnosed and 2693 died of myeloma in the United Kingdom in 2011. There is an equal sex distribution and an increasing incidence with age (Table 31.1). Risk factors for myeloma are remarkably absent. There are minor increases in risk with family history, pernicious anaemia, HIV infection and organ transplantation, although none of these associations are very strong.

Pathogenesis

Multiple myeloma is a B-cell neoplasm characterized by the proliferation of plasma cells that synthesize and secrete monoclonal immunoglobulins or fragments thereof. It is believed to evolve from an asymptomatic pre-malignant clonal condition of plasma cells known as monoclonal gammopathy of undetermined significance (MGUS). MGUS affects 3% of the population over 50 years of age and progresses to myeloma at a rate of 1% per year. MGUS is commonly associated with chromosomal translocations of the immunoglobulin heavy chain genes often with cyclin D genes. Those MGUS that lack IgH translocations often have chromosomal trisomy. The subsequent transformation from MGUS to myeloma is associated with further genetic alterations that are less uniform. Amongst these, second hit random alterations are mutations of Ras and p53 genes and methylation of p16 and cyclin D kinase inhibitor genes. T-lymphocytes secrete the cytokine interleukin 6 (IL-6), which appears to be an essential growth factor for myeloma cells in culture. Excessive secretion of IL-6 occurs in myeloma from stromal cells and this may be a primary cause for the condition.

Fashions in molecular biology change their focus with time and the current vogue includes micro RNAs (miRNAs) as a means of regulating gene function. miRs are small 22 nucleotide non-coding RNAs that regulate gene function by base pair binding complementary messenger RNA (mRNA) and hence preventing its translation by ribosomes into proteins. The human genome is thought to encode over 1000 miRs. In myeloma, miR-21 and miR-106b are thought to be overexpressed and by regulating the tumour suppressor p53, interleukin-6 (IL6) and its downstream JAK-STAT signalling lead to deregulation of complex pathways. Similarly, angiogenesis in myeloma is postulated as being affected by changes in miR-16 which targets vascular endothelium growth factor (VEGF).

The destructive bone lesions that are seen in myeloma are thought to be due to dysregulation of the osteoprotegerin Rankl (receptor activator of nuclear factor kappa B ligand) system. Rankl is the ligand for osteoprotegerin and is released in myeloma by the malignant plasma cells and bone marrow stroma, leading to osteoclast activation and hence osteolysis. The osteolytic bone lesions of myeloma are best

---

Oncology: Lecture Notes, Third Edition. Mark Bower and Jonathan Waxman.

© 2015 by John Wiley & Sons, Ltd. Published 2015 by John Wiley & Sons, Ltd.

Companion Website: www.lecturenoteseries.com/oncology

Table 31.1 UK registrations for myeloma cancer 2010

	Percentage of all cancer registrations		Rank of registration		Lifetime risk of cancer		Change in ASR (2000–2010)		5-year overall survival	
	Female	Male	Female	Male	Female	Male	Female	Male	Female	Male
Myeloma	1	2	17th	15th	1 in 155	1 in 120	+8%	+13%	37%	37%

seen on plain X-rays rather than bone scans as they generally lack osteoblastic activity. They appear as punched-out lesions, including the classical "pepper pot" appearance of the skull X-ray (Figure 31.2), and the bone breakdown releases calcium and may cause hypercalcaemia.

Marrow infiltration with an excess of plasma cells leads to a decrease in numbers of other marrow constituents, causing anaemia, thrombocytopenia and neutropenia. This in turn has consequences for both the presentation and the clinical features of the disease as it evolves.

Presentation

In addition to the local effects of myeloma on bone, patients with myeloma may present with hypercalcaemia, renal failure, bone marrow failure or rarely the effects of excess immunoglobulin levels in the blood. Patients with myeloma most often present with significant bone pain due to the lytic lesions that characterize this disease. Vertebral collapse is often a feature of presentation and this may lead in a dramatic fashion to cord compression.

Patients with myeloma may present with symptoms of hypercalcaemia, which every medical student reading this chapter should be able to describe. Renal failure is a common feature of myeloma and may arise through a number of mechanisms. Hypercalcaemia can be one of the precipitating factors for renal failure. The other causes include amyloidosis (AL) (amyloid containing immunoglobulin light chains), precipitation of Bence–Jones protein (urinary free light chain paraprotein) and direct infiltration and infection.

An excess of immunoglobulin may cause the hyperviscosity syndrome, which is more common with an IgG myeloma than an IgM myeloma. This is explained by the fact that a far greater proportion of patients have IgG than IgM myelomas, which represents just 0.5% of all myeloma cases. The symptoms of hyperviscosity include spontaneous bleeding, retinopathy and neurological symptoms ranging from headache to coma. Hyperviscosity can also occur with high blood cell counts in leukaemia and polycythemia. The raised paraprotein levels may cause other problems, including peripheral neuropathy.

Investigations

The investigation of myeloma is relatively simple. It requires the examination of the peripheral blood, paraprotein levels (serum electrophoresis and immunofixation and serum-free light chain assays) (Figure 31.1), blood count, β_2-microglobulin levels, renal function and calcium levels (see Figures 31.3 and 31.4), assessment of the bone marrow, examination of the urine for Bence–Jones protein urea and a skeletal survey (Table 31.2). Bone scanning is of low diagnostic value in myeloma. Myeloma is staged and the staging has prognostic value. Two systems are used, that of Durie and Salmon and the simpler International Staging System (ISS) (Tables 31.3 and 31.4).

Treatment

Before treatment is contemplated the diagnosis of multiple myeloma must be established and differentiated from MGUS and smouldering myeloma (Table 31.2) which do not require therapy. The initial treatment of myeloma requires stabilization of the patient and correction of renal function abnormalities and hypercalcaemia (Table 37.4). The patient is started on allopurinol and may require hydration or transfusion. Hypercalcaemia is treated with bisphosphonates, steroids and by rehydration. Where there is significant bone pain, which is poorly responsive to opiates, radiotherapy may be required. A single fraction treatment will alleviate bone pain in approximately 80% of patients. Anaemia may require

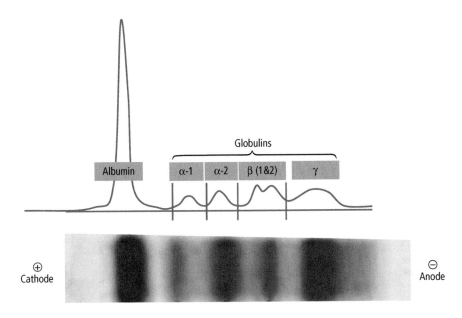

Figure 31.1 Normal serum protein electrophoresis.

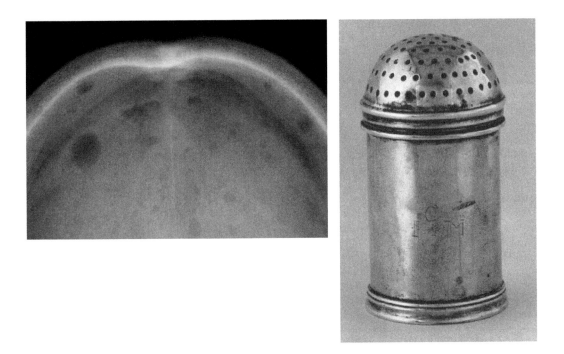

Figure 31.2 The pepper pot skull medical metaphors: (cf. Figures 5.5, 11.1 and 28.13). Skull radiograph of a 52-year-old man with multiple myeloma showing multiple, well-defined lucencies that are fairly uniform in size, unlike bone metastases which usually vary in size.

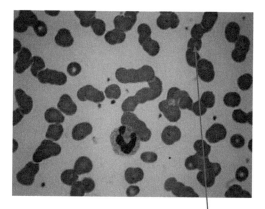

Figure 31.3 Peripheral blood film showing rouleaux formation with erythrocytes stacked up on each other and a single neutrophil. Rouleaux are found at high levels in the blood of proteins such as fibrinogen or γ-globulin. They are particularly prominent in diseases that cause a very high erythrocyte sedimentation rate (ESR), such as multiple myeloma, cancers, chronic infections (e.g. TB) and connective tissue diseases.

Table 31.2 Diagnostic criteria for plasma cell proliferations
Multiple myeloma (all three criteria must be met)
Presence of a serum or urinary monoclonal protein
Presence of clonal plasma cells in the bone marrow or a plasmacytoma
Presence of end organ damage felt to be related to the plasma cell dyscrasia • Increased serum calcium • Lytic bone lesions • Anaemia • Renal failure
Smoldering multiple myeloma (SMM) (both criteria must be met)
Serum monoclonal protein >3 g/dL and/or >10% to <60% bone marrow clonal plasma cells
No end organ damage related to the plasma cell dyscrasia
Monoclonal gammopathy of undetermined significance (MGUS) (all three criteria must be met)
Serum monoclonal protein <3 g/dL
Bone marrow plasma cells <10%
No end organ damage related to plasma cell dyscrasia

transfusion and significant hyperviscosity needs treatment by plasmaphoresis. Plasmaphoresis involves taking blood, removing abnormal proteins from the plasma by extracorporeal filtration and then returning the blood to the patient on a continuous circuit. Plasmaphoresis provides transient reductions in paraprotein levels, allowing relief of acute medical complications of the paraproteinaemia as drug treatment takes effect.

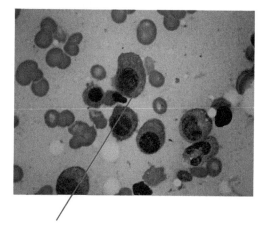

Figure 31.4 Bone marrow aspirate of myeloma showing plasma cells with large eccentric nuclei and basophilic cytoplasm.

Chemotherapy for myeloma has a 50-year history, beginning with the use of alkylating agents such as melphalan and cyclosphosphamide. Nowadays, the initial treatment of multiple myeloma depends on a risk stratification into high-risk, intermediate-risk and low-risk disease based on cytogenetics or gene expression profiling signatures. High-dose chemotherapy with hematopoietic stem cell transplantation has become the preferred treatment for patients under the age of 65. Prior to stem cell transplantation, these patients receive an initial course of induction chemotherapy. The most common induction regimens used are thalidomide–dexamethasone, bortezomib-based regimens and lenalidomide–dexamethasone. Unfortunately, many patients are older and frailer and are not eligible for transplantation; here the standard of care has been chemotherapy with melphalan and prednisone, bortezomib containing regimes or lenalidomide and dexamethasone. Bortezomib inhibits proteosomes, the cellular organelles that identify tagged proteins in the cytoplasm and break them down. It is not quite clear how thalidomide and lenalidomide work but they seem to have both immunomodulatory and

Table 31.3 Durie and Salmon staging system for myeloma

Cell mass category: requirements		High (stage III): one of A, B, C or D	Low (stage I): all of A, B, C and D	Intermediate (stage II)
Haemoglobin (pre-transfusion)	A	<85 g/L	>100 g/L	Neither I or III
Serum calcium	B	>3 μmol/L	Normal	
M component	C	IgG >7 g/dL or IgA >5 g/dL	IgG <5 g/dL or IgA <3 g/dL	
Urinary monoclonal protein (Bence–Jones protein)	D	Urine monoclonal protein excretion >12 g/day	Urine monoclonal protein excretion <4 g/day	
Bone lesion on skeletal survey	E	Advanced lytic disease	None/solitary lesion	

Table 31.4 International staging system

Stage	Criteria
Stage I	Beta-2 microglobulin <3.5 mg/L and serum albumin >35 g/L
Stage II	Neither stage I nor stage III
Stage III	Beta-2 microglobulin >5.5 mg/L

anti-angiogenic actions. Both are potent teratogens and it is essential that they are not prescribed to women who could become pregnant.

All myeloma patients are at risk of pathological bone fractures and should modify their lifestyles to avoid this risk. Patients with skeletal lesions or osteopenia should be given bisphosphonates which reduce the risk of skeletal bone events (Figure 31.5).

There has been recent progress in the development of new treatments for myeloma that have gone beyond thalidomide analogues and proteasome inhibitors. These developments are in the area of the "Ab's" rather than the "Ib's". Daratumumab, a humanized antibody to CD38, has been investigated in both phase 1 and phase 2 drug development trials. This drug was granted breakthrough drug status by the FDA in 2014 because of the benefits seen in myeloma patients in reducing M band levels and bone marrow infiltration with plasma cells. This rapid approval process in the United States will no doubt contrast with UK approval processes, or should we more accurately write,

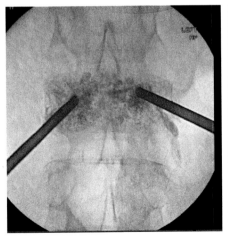 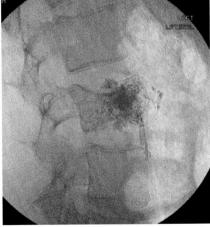

Figure 31.5 Vertebroplasty. Myeloma patients with painful compression fractures of vertebral bodies may have bone cement injected percutaneously. This procedure is only safe when there is no epidural disease or retropulsion of bone fragments into the spinal cord.

"disapproval processes"? We fear, from past experience, that NICE will turn down this drug for approval on the basis of some spurious cost–benefit analysis, after prolonged delays, whilst myeloma patients die waiting. Siltuximab is a chimeric monoclonal antibody to IL6, which is an effective new treatment for Castleman's disease that offers hope in myeloma where it reduces M band levels and is undergoing assessment in this condition currently. It is to be hoped that these new treatments for myeloma will continue to build on to the near doubling of survival in myeloma that has already come with advances in drug treatment. It is the authors' ambition to see the blunderbuss of high-dose chemotherapy and bone marrow transplantation replaced by treatment targeting the molecular biology of this disease.

 ONLINE RESOURCE

Case Study: The pensioner who found washing up painful.

 KEY POINTS

- Myeloma is a relatively common haematological malignancy whose risk increases with age
- Myeloma is thought to evolve from MGUS, an asymptomatic pre-malignant clonal proliferation of plasma cells that affects 3% of the population over 50 years of age and progresses to myeloma at a rate of 1% per year
- Myeloma present with painful destructive bone lesions, hypercalcaemia, renal failure, bone marrow failure or rarely the effects of excess immunoglobulin levels in the blood leading to hyperviscosity
- The diagnosis of myeloma is established by the presence of a monoclonal protein in the serum or urine, clonal plasma cells in the bone marrow and evidence of end organ damage (bone lesions, renal failure, anaemia or hypercalcaemia)
- The current management of myeloma includes treatment of hypercalcaemia and palliation of bone lesions along with chemotherapy but only a third of patients live 5 years

32

Non-melanoma skin tumours

Learning objectives

✓ Explain the epidemiology and pathogenesis of non-melanoma skin tumours

✓ Recognize the common presentation and clinical features of non-melanoma skin tumours

✓ Describe the treatment strategies and outcomes of non-melanoma skin tumours

---

Cinema has wide-ranging influence on fashion trends and one of the most striking examples was the mid-20th century passion for sun tanning. The fashion of the Victorian era was sun avoidance; the upper classes stayed pale in part to distinguish themselves from lower class workers who had to toil in the sun. Yet by the 1950s, the beach culture of southern California spread worldwide via the movies. The ill effects of chronic exposure to ultraviolet radiation on skin ageing are well demonstrated by Clint Eastwood. The carcinogenic effects of sunlight led to the removal of a basal cell carcinoma (BCC) from the former actor, US President Ronald Reagan, whilst his eldest daughter Maureen Reagan died of melanoma.

Epidemiology

Non-melanoma skin cancers (NMSC) probably comprise more than one-third of all cancers in the United Kingdom and have been described as a worldwide epidemic. The term includes two major types: BCC and squamous cell carcinoma (SCC). In the United Kingdom, 74% are BCC and 23% SCC. Other less common NMSC include Kaposi's sarcoma, cutaneous lymphoma and Merkel cell carcinoma. In 2010, there were about 100,000 registered cases of NMSC and only 558 deaths from NMSC in the United Kingdom. However, it is estimated that 30–50% of BCC and 30% of SCC are not recorded. The incidence of NMSC has risen over the last decade by 32% in women and 36% in men, although some of this may be due to better registration of cases.

Pathogenesis

BCC is four times more common than SCC. Sun damage is the major cause of both cancers, especially the ultraviolet B (UVB) spectrum (290–320 nm wavelength). The UV radiation produces DNA mutations, particularly thymidine dimers in the p53 tumour suppressor gene. The incidence of skin cancer rises with latitudes approaching the equator. Light-exposed areas of the body are the most frequent sites for tumours, and occupations with high sun exposure like farming have an increased incidence of BCC and SCC. Ozone absorbs UVB and the ozone layer of the lower stratosphere which lies 20–30 km above ground absorbs 98% of sun-derived medium-frequency UV

Oncology: Lecture Notes, Third Edition. Mark Bower and Jonathan Waxman.
© 2015 by John Wiley & Sons, Ltd. Published 2015 by John Wiley & Sons, Ltd.
Companion Website: www.lecturenoteseries.com/oncology

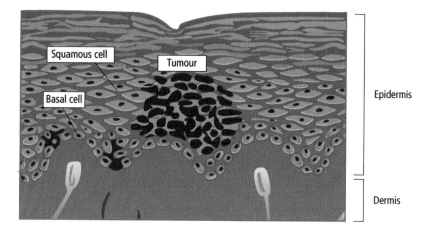

Figure 32.1 Location of non-melanoma skin tumours in skin.

light that would potentially damage all exposed life forms on the surface of our planet. The progressive depletion of the ozone layer by fluorinated hydrocarbons especially chlorofluorocarbons (CFC) may lead to increased UVB exposure and higher NMSC rates. Melanin absorbs UV light, and the lower levels of melanocytes in white people accounts for the higher incidence of skin cancers in white people. The benefits of melanin in areas of high UV exposure are offset against the reduced production of vitamin D3, which requires UV light; so in regions of low sunlight, black people are prone to rickets. This delicately balanced system of biological geodiversity has been abused to justify some of the most barbaric human behaviour.

Inherited genetic predispositions to skin cancers include

- xeroderma pigmentosum
- Gorlin's basal cell nevus syndrome

Patients with xeroderma pigmentosa are unable to repair UV-induced DNA damage because of defective nucleotide excision repair and develop both BCC and SCC under the age of 10 years. Gorlin's basal cell naevus syndrome patients develop BCC in their teens and brain tumours later in life; it is caused by a mutation of a patched gene involved in the Hedgehog pathway signal transduction. The gene name *Hedgehog* was originally coined because mutations lead to spikes on *Drosophila* fruit flies. Humans have three homologues of the gene named after the two common varieties of hedgehogs, "Indian" and "Desert". The third human gene was named *Sonic* after Sega's game character.

Chemical carcinogens, including arsenic, are associated with SCC. Sir Percivall Pott's description in 1775

of scrotal cancers in chimney sweeps is thought to be due to industrial exposure to coal tar. Radiation is associated with an increased incidence of SCC, BCC and Bowen's disease (SCC *in situ*). Allogeneic organ transplant recipients are at greatly increased risk of SCC, with as many as 80% having SCC within 20 years of the graft. This may be related to the finding of genotypes 5 and 8 of human papillomavirus in some skin SCC.

Presentation

BCC begins in the basal cell layer of the epidermis (Figures 32.1 and 32.2), usually develops on chronically sun-exposed areas of the skin, rarely metastasizes and is generally slow growing. If left untreated, however, BCC may spread locally to the bone or other tissues beneath the skin. BCC starts as painless, translucent, pearly nodules with telangiectasia on sun-exposed skin. As they enlarge, they ulcerate and bleed and develop a rolled shiny edge sometimes referred to as a "rodent ulcer", a misleading term because they were thought to originate from mouse or rat bites (Figure 32.3). BCC may progress slowly over many months to years, but less than 0.1% metastasize to regional lymph nodes. They occur mostly on the face, especially the nose, nasolabial fold and inner canthus, usually in elderly people and are more common in men than in women.

SCC arises from more superficial layers of the epidermis and tends to be more aggressive. SCC can invade tissues beneath the skin and 1–2% spread to the

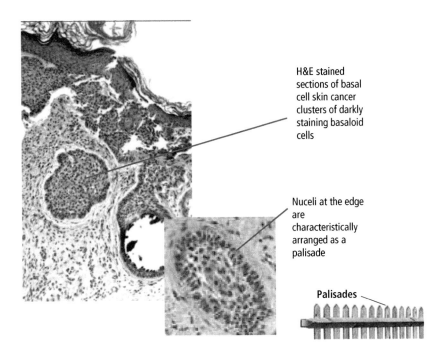

H&E stained sections of basal cell skin cancer clusters of darkly staining basaloid cells

Nuceli at the edge are characteristically arranged as a palisade

Palisades

Figure 32.2 Basal cell carcinoma (BCC).

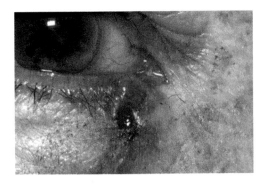

Figure 32.3 A pearly edged, ulcerated lesion characteristic of a basal cell carcinoma of the skin.

lymph nodes (Figures 1.12(b) and 32.4). These cancers typically appear on sun-exposed areas of the body, such as the face, ears, neck, lips and backs of the hands (Figure 32.5). Marjolin ulcers are SCCs arising in long-standing, benign ulcers, such as venous ulcers or scars, such as old burns. SCCs are irregular, red hyperkeratotic tumours that ulcerate and crust. Unlike BCCs, SCCs grow more rapidly over months rather than years and occasionally bleed. Precursors to SCC include actinic keratosis, which are also called solar or senile keratoses, and SCC *in situ*, which is also called Bowens disease. SCC *in situ* is a full-thickness malignant transformation of the epidermis that, by definition, has not invaded the dermis.

Merkel cell carcinoma is a rare but highly malignant tumour in the basal layer of the epidermis, most commonly found in elderly, white patients. It consists of rapidly growing, painless and shiny purple nodules that may occur anywhere on the body. These tumours are thought to arise from neuroendocrine cells and are positive for neuron-specific enolase staining. They resemble small cell lung cancer in their clinical course. In 2008, a polyomavirus (Merkel cell polyomavirus, MCV) was identified in most of these tumours and represents the first of a new class of human oncogenic viruses. Max Perutz, who won the Nobel Prize for his work on crystallography and who was Watson and Crick's PhD supervisor whilst they were discovering the structure of DNA, died of Merkel cell tumour. Merkel cell tumours share the treatment programmes used in small cell lung cancer. Distant metastases are common, and treatment is with combination chemotherapy, although relapses are frequent and the prognosis is poor.

Other uncommon NMSC include Kaposi's sarcoma, which usually starts within the dermis but can also develop in internal organs. This cancer, once extremely rare, has become more common due to its

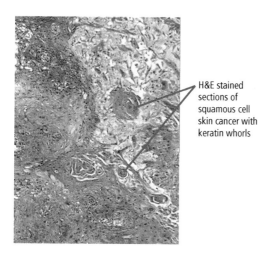

H&E stained
sections of
squamous cell
skin cancer with
keratin whorls

Figure 32.4 Squamous cell carcinoma (SCC).

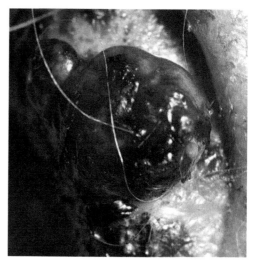

Figure 32.5 A large, raised, bleeding skin lesion on the pinna, a common site for squamous cell cancers of the skin. These tumours are related to UV exposure and may be preceded by actinic or solar keratoses.

association with HIV/AIDS and organ transplantation. It is caused by infection with an oncogenic herpesvirus, human herpesvirus 8 (HHV8). Primary cutaneous lymphoma or mycosis fungoides is a low-grade lymphoma that primarily affects the skin. Generally, it has a slow course and often remains confined to the skin, but progression of the tumour to a more aggressive, life-threatening stage is more likely the longer it has been present. Adnexal tumours, which start in the hair follicles or sweat glands, are extremely rare and usually benign.

Treatment

The goal of treatment for BCC and SCC is to eradicate local disease and achieve the best cosmetic appearance. For BCC, a complete skin examination is indicated because of the increased risk of actinic keratosis or cancers located at other skin sites in persons presenting with a suspicious lesion. For SCC, regional lymph nodes should also be examined. The main options include:

(i) Surgery, which offers a single brief procedure and histological confirmation of completeness of excision.
(ii) Curettage, which is suitable for small, nodular lesions of less than 1 cm and yields good cosmesis.
(iii) Cryotherapy, which can be used for lesions of less than 2 cm but may leave an area of depigmentation, and radiotherapy.

Mohs' micrographic surgery is a specialized form of excisional surgery that provides 100% microscopically controlled histological margins (Figure 32.6). The technique involves tumour excision, mapping of the removed tissue and immediate microscopic assessment of the surgical specimen. If occult tumour extension is detected microscopically, the process is repeated until a tumour-free margin is attained. Frederic Mohs developed this surgical approach whilst still a medical student and, according to at least one of our surgical colleagues, treatment is analogous to peeling rather than chopping a vegetable. Mohs' surgery is curative for 99% of primary BCCs and for 97% of primary SCCs, the highest documented cure rates.

Radiotherapy has the advantages of no pain, no hospitalization and no keloids or contracture; it preserves uninvolved tissue and produces smaller defects. It does, however, require multiple visits and results in depigmentation and loss of hair follicles and sweat glands at the treated site. The decision between surgery and radiotherapy is based on size and site, histology, age of patient, recurrence rates and anticipated cosmetic results.

Topical 5-fluorouracil chemotherapy may be used for actinic keratosis and small, superficial, non-invasive tumours. Side effects include progressive inflammation, erythema, erosions and contact dermatitis. Systemic chemotherapy is reserved for treating locally advanced and metastatic disease. The most

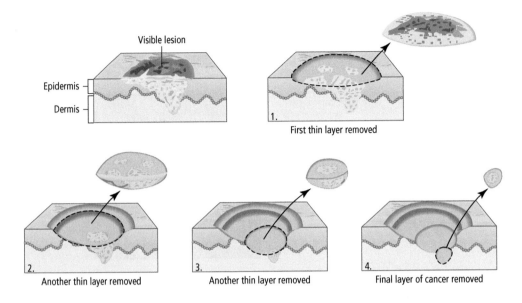

Figure 32.6 Mohs' micrographic surgical technique.

Table 32.1 Skin phototypes

Skin phototype	Features	Tanning ability
Type I	Tend to have freckles, red or fair hair and blue or green eyes	Often burn, rarely tan
Type II	Tend to have light hair, blue or brown eyes	Usually burn, sometimes tan
Type III	Tend to have brown hair and eyes	Sometimes burn, usually tan
Type IV	Tend to have dark brown hair and eyes	Rarely burn, often tan
Type V	Naturally black–brown skin. Often have dark brown eyes and hair	
Type VI	Naturally black–brown skin. Usually have black–brown eyes and hair	

widely used regimens include cisplatin in combination with 5-fluorouracil or doxorubicin.

Prevention remains the most important aspect of the management of skin cancers and requires campaigns to increase public awareness. Children should not get sunburnt and white-skinned people should limit their total cumulative sun exposure. The public should be encouraged to look out for new skin lesions and those that are not obviously benign should be seen and removed in their entirety for pathological examination within 4 weeks. Sunbed use increases the risk of both melanoma and NMSC and since 2012 the use of sunbeds has become illegal for those under 18 years old in the United Kingdom. People with light skin phototypes (Table 32.1), with lots of naevi or freckles, with frequent childhood sunburn, sun damaged skin or pre-malignant skin conditions should all avoid sunbeds.

Prognosis

The prognosis of 5-year survival for patients with non-melanoma skin tumours is given in Table 32.2.

Table 32.2 A prognosis of 5-year survival for patients with non-melanoma skin tumours

Tumour	5-year survival
Basal cell carcinoma	95–100%
Squamous cell carcinoma	92–99%

ONLINE RESOURCE

Case Study: The grateful politician.

KEY POINTS

- Non-melanoma skin cancers (NMSC) probably account for over one-third of all cancers in the United Kingdom but are usually not recorded accurately in cancer registries
- Three quarters of NMSC are BCC and a quarter SCC, the remainder are a mixture of rare tumours such as Kaposi's sarcoma, cutaneous lymphoma and Merkel cell carcinoma
- Ultraviolet light (UVB) exposure is the main risk factor, although genetic deficiencies of DNA damage repair enzymes, immunodeficiency and chemical carcinogens such as arsenic and coal tar contribute
- BCC starts as painless, translucent, pearly nodules with telangiectasia on sun-exposed skin that may enlarge, ulcerate, bleed and develop a rolled shiny edge sometimes referred to as a "rodent ulcer"
- SCC are irregular, red hyperkeratotic tumours on sun-exposed skin that ulcerate and crust and may be preceded by actinic keratoses (solar or senile keratoses) and Bowen's disease (SCC *in situ*)
- Surgical excision cures most BCC and SCC, although the rarer NMSC generally require more aggressive systemic therapy

33

Melanoma

Learning objectives

✓ Explain the epidemiology and pathogenesis of melanoma

✓ Recognize the common presentation and clinical features of melanoma

✓ Describe the treatment strategies and outcomes of melanoma

Epidemiology

Melanoma is a tumour of melanocytes, the pigmented cells of the skin. The incidence of melanoma has increased by a factor of 4 since 1971. In 2011, in the United Kingdom 13,348 people were diagnosed with melanoma and 2209 died of it. The primary cause is thought to be an increase in exposure to sunlight. One hopes that with all the publicity, the risks of exposure to sun are at last entering into the public consciousness. The general public's view of melanoma is that it has a poor outlook based on the outcomes in metastatic disease. However, as can be seen from Table 33.1, the overall outcome is generally better than for most tumour groups.

Pathogenesis

Melanocytes produce two types of melanin:

- eumelanin, a brown–black pigment
- pheomelanin, a pink–red pigment

They are present in different proportions in people with different skin colours and at different parts of the body. This is under the influence of various pigment genes. Melanocortin 1 receptor (MC1R) is the main gene that determines whether pheomelanin or eumelanin is produced. MC1R appears to have undergone mutation and strong selection in archaic hominids in Africa about 1.2 million years ago when body hair became sparser and skin colour darker compared to chimpanzees. In populations living in regions with lower UV exposure, the benefits of reduced UV-induced DNA damage in the skin is offset by the reduced UV-induced hydroxylation of vitamin D, resulting in vitamin D deficiency. Polymorphisms of MC1R and a number of other pigment-related genes lead to paler skin hues and hence greater susceptibility to melanoma. In the United Kingdom, 80% of gingers have MC1R mutations.

The risk of melanoma is dominated by a combination of skin pigment content which relates to skin, eye and hair colour (see Table 32.1) and UV exposure from the sun or sunbeds, with protection by sunscreen and enhancement by sunburn. Another risk for the development of melanoma is the presence of dysplastic or atypical moles. Most skin moles are genetically determined and appear during childhood, although sun exposure may increase their numbers. Large, unusually shaped, variegated moles with poorly defined edges are designated atypical naevi and have a 4–10 times increased risk of melanoma.

This risk is even greater in people with familial atypical multiple mole–melanoma syndrome (FAMMM), although less than 5% of all melanoma cases are familial. They inherit mutations in one of two genes: cyclin-dependent kinase inhibitor gene CDKN2 (also known as p16) on chromosome 9p21 and cyclin-dependent kinase gene CDK4 on chromosome 12q13. Both are implicated in insensitivity to cell cycle checkpoints.

Oncology: Lecture Notes, Third Edition. Mark Bower and Jonathan Waxman.
© 2015 by John Wiley & Sons, Ltd. Published 2015 by John Wiley & Sons, Ltd.
Companion Website: www.lecturenoteseries.com/oncology

Table 33.1 UK registrations for melanoma cancer 2010

	Percentage of all cancer registrations		Rank of registration		Lifetime risk of cancer		Change in ASR (2000–2010)		5 year overall survival	
	Female	Male	Female	Male	Female	Male	Female	Male	Female	Male
Melanoma	4	4	6th	6th	1 in 56	1 in 55	+39%	+57%	92%	84%

Presentation

Public awareness campaigns to encourage people with suspicious skin lesions to seek advice have been based on a simple mnemonic (ABCDE) (Figure 33.1):

- **A**symmetry
- **B**orders (irregular)
- **C**olour (variegated)
- **D**iameter (greater than 6 mm, about the size of a pencil top rubber)
- **E**volving over time

Patients with malignant melanoma generally present with a history of a growing mole, which may bleed or itch (see Figures 33.2 and 33.3). Because of the public awareness of melanoma, generally there is quite rapid self-referral to GPs with these symptoms. Specialist referral to plastic surgery or dermatology is also quick, and many hospitals now offer walk-in skin lesion clinics. In clinic, the specialist will seek to confirm the diagnosis on initial examination (Figure 33.4). If there is no evidence for metastases, he will make arrangements to excise the primary lesion. This procedure requires specialist surgery with wide excision of the surrounding normal tissue. The reasons for this are, firstly, concerns about the incidence of local recurrence following inadequate resection and, secondly, the need for good cosmesis. Although wide excision is common, no evidence from a randomized trial supports this practice.

Staging and grading

There are four main clinical descriptions of melanoma and these are the superficial spreading, nodular, lentigo maligna and acral lentiginous subtypes (Table 33.2).

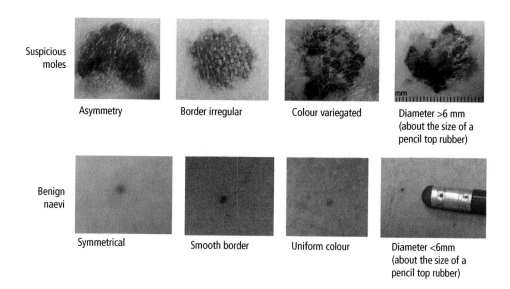

Figure 33.1 Suspicious moles and benign naevi.

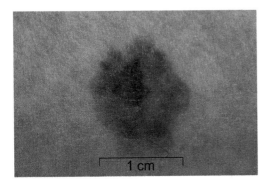

Figure 33.2 Atypical or dysplastic naevi are large naevi (moles) with irregular borders and varied pigmentation. Atypical naevi are the precursors of melanomas.

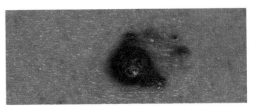

Figure 33.3 A pigmented nodular lesion with an irregular edge and adjacent satellite lesions. This was a nodular melanoma.

Following excision and confirmation of the diagnosis histologically, staging investigations, which should include CT scanning, should be performed. As a result of surgery and staging procedures, the clinical stage can be defined as follows:

- Stage Ia: localized melanoma < 0.75 mm thick
- Stage Ib: localized melanoma 0.76–1.5 mm thick
- Stage IIa: localized melanoma 1.6–4 mm thick
- Stage IIb: localized melanoma > 4 mm thick
- Stage III: limited nodal metastases involving only one regional lymph node group
- Stage IV: advanced regional metastases or distant metastases

There are additional widely practised staging systems which are not included in this book. For prognostic purposes, however, pathological staging is significant and includes the Breslow thickness and Clark's levels:

- Clark's level I: melanoma confined to the epidermis
- Clark's level II: penetration into the papillary dermis
- Clark's level III: extension to the reticular dermis
- Clark's level IV: extension into the deep reticular dermis
- Clark's level V: invasion of the subcutaneous fat

Breslow's staging system measures the vertical thickness of the primary tumour, grouping melanomas into "Breslow's thickness", as <0.75 mm, 0.76–1.5 mm, 1.51–3.99 mm and >4 mm. Breslow thickness is more relevant to prognosis than Clark's level.

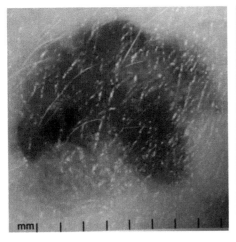

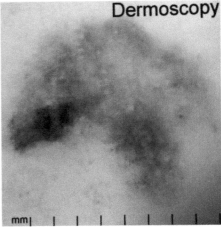

Figure 33.4 Dermatoscopy (also known as dermoscopy or epiluminescence microscopy). Dermoscopy combines a magnifying glass and polarized light to cancel out skin surface reflections. It increases the accuracy of melanoma clinical diagnosis by dermatologists about 20%.

Table 33.2 Clinicopathological features of four common forms of melanoma

Type	Location	Age (median)	Gender and race	Edge	Colour	Frequency
Superficial spreading	All body surfaces, especially legs	56 years	White females	Palpable, irregular	Brown, black, grey or pink; central or halo depigmentation	50%
Nodular	All body surfaces	49 years	White males	Palpable	Uniform bluish black	30%
Lentigo maligna	Sun exposed, areas, especially head and neck	70 years	White females	Flat, irregular	Shades of brown or black, hypopigmentation	15%
Acral lentigenous	Palms, soles and mucous membranes	61 years	Black males	Palpable, irregular nodule	Black, irregularly coloured	5%

Treatment

Adjuvant therapy

Most patients who have had a definitive resection of melanoma do well, but a subset of tumours recur. Many clinical trials have addressed the role of adjuvant immunotherapy to reduce the risk of recurrence. For patients with higher recurrence risks based on tumour size, the presence of ulceration or lymph node involvement and the mitotic rate of the tumour, adjuvant interferon prolongs progression-free survival. This approach should be reserved for patients with a good performance status and no co-morbidities as interferon alpha is associated with frequent and serious toxicities including:

- fatigue
- fever
- myalgia
- nausea
- vomiting
- myelosuppression
- depression, neuropsychiatric and neuropsychological disorders

Management of local skin metastases and nodal disease

Locoregional metastasis in melanoma includes local recurrence, satellite, in-transit and regional lymph node metastases. Satellite metastases are skin or subcutaneous lesions within 2 cm of the primary and are thought to represent intralymphatic extensions of the primary tumour (Figure 33.5). In-transit

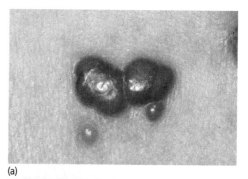
(a)

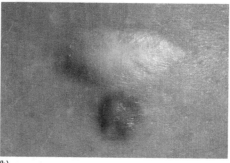
(b)

Figure 33.5 (a) Satellite metastases are skin or subcutaneous lesions within 2 cm of the primary and are thought to represent intralymphatic extensions of the primary tumour. (b) In-transit metastases arise in lymphatics more distant from the primary site but still before reaching the regional lymph nodes.

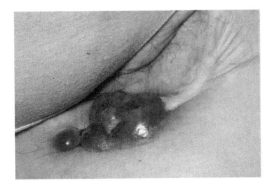

Figure 33.6 Fungating inguinal lymph node melanoma metastasis.

metastases arise in lymphatics more distant from the primary site but still before reaching the regional lymph nodes (Figures 33.6 and 33.7).

The treatment of these patterns of relapse is primarily surgical. Localized recurrence is excised and nodal metastases are managed by radical lymph node dissection. There are advocates of regional infusional programmes (isolated limb perfusion using cytotoxic chemotherapy such as melphalan) but the value of this is contentious. Radiotherapy may be used where localized disease is inoperable or as an adjuvant to surgery, reducing the bulk of disease prior to definitive surgery.

Treatment of metastatic melanoma

The outlook for patients with metastatic melanoma is poor. Patients generally have disease in multiple sites, and the median survival is approximately 6 months (Figure 33.8). Treatment depends upon the patient, on his or her fitness and on the disease site. Patients with metastatic melanoma who have only a single or very limited number of metastases may be considered for surgical metastasectomy.

These have been exciting times for melanoma oncologists with the development of treatment targeting molecular changes in this condition, but cost-benefit analyses have dampened the excitement. Recent advances in the management of advanced melanoma have altered the algorithm of care and produced modest but nonetheless genuine improvements in survival. Initial systemic treatments depend upon the molecular biology of the tumour and the performance status of the patient. The options are immunotherapy with high-dose interleukin-2 (IL-2) or ipilimumab, an anti-CTLA-4 monoclonal antibody or targeted therapy chiefly with inhibitors of BRAF, a signal transduction protein kinase.

Patients whose tumours have the V600 mutations of the BRAF gene are candidates for treatment with the BRAF inhibitors vemurafenib and dabrafenib. If the tumour has wild-type BRAF, treatment with ipilimumab is appropriate. Ipilimumab targets CTLA-4, which normally limits the activation of cytotoxic T-lymphocytes presented with an antigen by dendritic cells. Thus imilimumab takes off this brake and allows host immune cells to destroy melanoma cells. These new approaches have been shown to have profound effects on survival in melanoma. A similar immunotherapeutic approach to melanoma is developed based on the PD-1 (programmed cell death) protein that is expressed on the surface of dying exhausted cytotoxic T-cells. Monoclonal antibodies that block PD-1 and hence rejuvenate the T-cells have shown promise in melanoma as well as other malignancies. Currently there is interest in the potential benefits of the combination of vemurafenib and ipilimumab. However, regard must be given to the

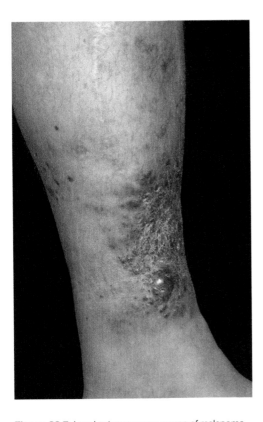

Figure 33.7 Local cutaneous recurrence of melanoma.

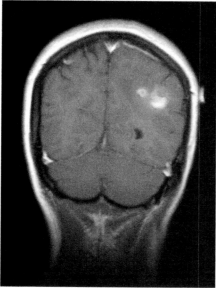
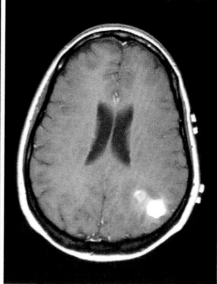

Figure 33.8 Intracerebral metastases of melanoma.

potential toxicities of this combination particularly on the liver and the NHS purse.

Prognosis

On the basis of records of 25,000 patients with localized stage I/II melanoma, two online tools are available that predicts prognosis (http://www.melanomaprognosis.org and http://www.lifemath.net) which interrogates the American SEER (Surveillance, Epidemiology and End Results) database. The most important prognostic factor remains clinical stage, and the depth of tumour invasion is the most important prognostic factor for localized melanoma. This can be described according to Clark's stage and Breslow's thickness. Ten-year survival for a lesion less than 0.75 mm thick or for a Clark's level I melanoma is 90%, for a lesion 0.75–1.5 mm thick or Clark's level II is 80%, for a lesion 1.6–2.49 mm thick or Clark's level III is 60%, for a lesion 2.5–3.99 mm thick or Clark's level IV is 50%, and for a lesion greater than 4 mm or Clark's level V is approximately 30%.

Approximately 90% of stage I patients, 60% of stage II patients and 30% of stage III patients survive for 10 years. The survival of stage IV patients depends upon the metastatic site, survival is better if metastases are confined to the skin or lymph nodes than if there is visceral involvement.

Other important survival factors have been described from multifactorial analyses. They include the type of initial surgical management, pathological stage, ulceration, presence of satellite nodules, a peripheral anatomical location and, to a much lesser extent, the patient's gender, age and tumour diameter.

The American Joint Committee on Cancer, in a study involving 60,000 patients, has provided recent information on survival. This ranges from over 90% survival at 10 years for stage I disease to, as might be expected, the usual miserable outlook of only 15% survival at 5 years for metastatic disease.

 ONLINE RESOURCE

Case Study: The Chelsea pensioner with a leg ulcer.

 KEY POINTS

- Melanoma incidence has risen dramatically in recent decades to become the sixth most common cancer in the United Kingdom chiefly due to increased exposure to UVB in sunlight
- Chief amongst the strategies to combat melanoma is public health prevention

programmes to reduce UV exposure from the sun or sunbeds and encourage use of sunscreens

- Melanomas generally present with a history of a growing mole, which may bleed or itch, suspicious lesions should be evaluated based on the ABCDE mnemonic (Asymmetry, Boarder irregular, Colour variegated, Diameter >6 mm, Evolution over time)

- Treatment of primary melanoma, satellite metastases, metastases in-transit and nodal metastases is surgical excision

- The management of metastatic melanoma is determined by the molecular prolife; tumours with BRAF V600 mutations are candidates for treatment with the BRAF inhibitors (vemurafenib and dabrafenib), tumours with wild-type BRAF are treated with immunotherapy (ipilimumab or high-dose IL-2)

- Whilst overall 5-year survival is about 90%, this falls to 15% for patients with metastatic disease

34

Paediatric solid tumours

Learning objectives

✓ Explain the epidemiology and pathogenesis of paediatric solid tumours

✓ Recognize the common presentation and clinical features of paediatric solid tumours

✓ Describe the treatment strategies and outcomes of paediatric solid tumours

---

Epidemiology

Cancer is a leading cause of death in children in England and Wales, second only to accidental injury. It is responsible for around 10% of deaths in childhood. In 2010, 1603 children were diagnosed with cancer in the United Kingdom and 252 died from cancer. Cancer in children is nonetheless relatively rare, affecting 1 in 600 children and includes a different spectrum of cancers than adults (Tables 1.1 and 34.1). Whilst leukaemias account for 30% of cancers in childhood, the solid tumours encountered in childhood are often embryonal in origin, and many are associated with an inherited predisposition. There are few areas of medicine that can rival the advances made in paediatric oncology in the second half of the 20th century. Eight in ten children with cancer are now cured, compared with fewer than three in ten in the 1960s. It was estimated that in 2012, 33,000 young adults in Britain aged 16–40 years are survivors of childhood cancer.

Pathogenesis

Many paediatric tumours are associated with recognized familial predispositions that are due to inherited mutations of tumour suppressor genes and therefore are inherited as autosomal dominant traits. Examples are hereditary retinoblastoma (mutations of the RB gene on chromosome 13q14) and familial Wilms' tumours (mutations of the WT1 gene on chromosome 11p13). In contrast, environmental oncogenic factors have been less readily identified for paediatric solid tumours; one example, however, is the excess of papillary thyroid cancers in children following the nuclear explosion at Chernobyl (see Chapter 2). There are a few examples of viral infections contributing to the pathogenesis of childhood solid cancers including the association between Epstein–Barr virus and endemic Burkitt's lymphoma and Hodgkin's lymphoma.

Presentation and management of paediatric solid tumours

Many solid cancers of childhood differ notably from tumours of adulthood even those affecting the same organs, whilst lymphomas and germ cell tumours in children share many features with the same illnesses occurring in adults. Embryonal tumours arise in tissues that are normally only found in the developing

---

Oncology: Lecture Notes, Third Edition. Mark Bower and Jonathan Waxman.
© 2015 by John Wiley & Sons, Ltd. Published 2015 by John Wiley & Sons, Ltd.
Companion Website: www.lecturenoteseries.com/oncology

Table 34.1 Relative frequency and 5-year survival for paediatric cancers

Cancer	Proportion of childhood cancers	5-year overall survival
Leukaemias	30%	83%
Brain and central nervous system tumours	27%	71%
Lymphomas	11%	88%
Soft tissue sarcomas	6%	67%
Sympathetic nervous system tumours (neuroblastomas)	5%	64%
Renal tumours	5%	84%
Carcinomas and melanomas	4%	
Bone tumours	4%	61%
Gonadal and germ cell tumours	3%	92%
Retinoblastomas	3%	100%
Hepatic tumours	1%	66%

Table 34.2 The 5-year survival rates for paediatric CNS tumours

Tumour	5-year survival
Any paediatric CNS tumours	56%
Low-grade glioma	80%
High-grade glioma	25%
Optic glioma	80%
Brainstem glioma	5–50%
Medulloblastoma	60%
Ependymoma	60%
Pineal germinoma	90%
Pineal teratoma	65%
Craniopharyngioma	90%

embryo. There are six main types of embryonal tumours:

- neuroblastoma arising in the sympathetic nervous system
- retinoblastoma arising in the eye
- nephroblastoma (also known as Wilm's tumour) arising in the kidney
- hepatoblastoma arising in the liver
- medulloblastoma arising in the brain
- embryonal rhabdomyosarcoma arising in the connective tissue

Presentation and management of CNS tumours

Tumours in the brain and CNS occur throughout childhood and are the second most common group of cancers in children. The age at diagnosis of these tumours is:

- 15% between birth and 2 years old
- 30% from 2 to 5 years old
- 30% from 5 to 10 years old
- 25% from 11 to 18 years old

In contrast to adult brain tumours, most (60%) are infratentorial and 75% are midline, involving the cerebellum, midbrain, pons and medulla. The most common tumours, accounting for 45%, are astrocytomas of varying grades. They include optic nerve gliomas, which are usually well differentiated tumours. A further 20% are medulloblastomas, a small round cell tumour of childhood of primitive neuroectodermal origin. Medulloblastomas usually arise in the posterior fossa and may seed metastases in the neuraxis by dropping them down the subarachnoid space into the spinal canal. Craniopharyngiomas make up 5–10% of CNS tumours of childhood and cause raised intracranial pressure, visual defects and pituitary dysfunction: usually reduced growth hormone, thyroid-stimulating hormone (TSH), antidiuretic hormone (ADH: diabetes insipidus) or luteinizing hormone/follicle-stimulating hormone (LH/FSH) abnormalities (precocious puberty or delayed secondary sexual characteristics). Suprasellar calcification is a characteristic X-ray finding. A further 1–2% are pineal region tumours that present with Perinaud's syndrome (failure of conjugate upward gaze). Histologically, most pineal tumours are extragonadal germ cell tumours (teratomas and germinomas). Naturally, the management of these children will be determined both by the histological diagnosis and the anatomical location of the tumour and frequently involves surgery, radiotherapy and (occasionally) chemotherapy. The overall 5-year survival rates according to the histology are shown in Table 34.2.

Presentation and management of lymphomas

Lymphomas account for 11% childhood cancers and are twice as common in boys. Hodgkin's lymphoma

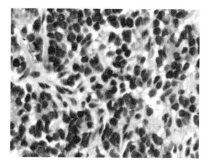

Figure 34.1 Small blue round cell tumours.

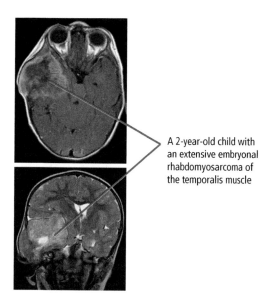

A 2-year-old child with an extensive embryonal rhabdomyosarcoma of the temporalis muscle

accounts for 45% childhood lymphomas and the remainder are mostly high-grade non-Hodgkin's lymphomas including Burkitt's lymphomas. Endemic Burkitt's lymphoma in Africa is always associated with Epstein–Barr virus present within the lymphoma cells and cases are confined to geographic areas where malaria is endemic suggesting a role for chronic immune stimulation by Plasmodium falciparum in the pathogenesis.

Figure 34.2 Embryonal rhabdomyosarcoma.

Presentation and management of soft tissue sarcomas and bone tumours

The paediatric soft tissue sarcomas account for 6% childhood cancers and include in order of frequency: rhabdomyosarcoma, Ewing sarcoma, Askin tumours and peripheral neuroectodermal tumours (PNET) (Figure 34.1). Bone tumours account for a further 4% with some overlap with the soft tissue sarcomas. Osteosarcoma is the most common bone tumour in children.

Rhabdomyosarcoma

Rhabdomyosarcoma is the most common paediatric soft tissue sarcoma, although only 60 children are diagnosed with this tumour in the United Kingdom each year and most are under 10 years old. Rhabdomyosarcoma may be divided into alveolar (25–30%), embryonal (50–60%) and pleomorphic (5%) variants. The embryonal type occurs in the first decade, most often in the head and neck and genitourinary tract (Figure 34.2). The alveolar type occurs in adolescents, in the forearms and trunk. The pleomorphic type

occurs in adults. Consistent chromosomal translocations have been found in a number of soft tissue sarcomas, both benign and malignant. These chromosomal rearrangements may be of help diagnostically; for example, 75% of alveolar rhabdomyosarcomas harbour the t(2:13)(q35:q14) chromosomal translocation that fuses the PAX3 (*Paired box 3*) gene and the FKHR (*forkhead*) gene. The consequence of many of these translocations is the transcription of chimeric mRNA, containing 5′ sequences of one gene and 3′ sequences from another gene, and translation to hybrid proteins. Many of the genes involved with these translocations are themselves transcription factors and it is postulated that the consequence of these translocations is the aberrant expression of a number of downstream genes. Rhabdomyosarcomas present as masses that grow and may become hard and painful. Approximately 15% have metastases at presentation; most frequently in the lungs, bones and lymph nodes. Treatment involves both surgery and chemotherapy but is risk stratified, with radiotherapy reserved for those at higher risk of relapse in order to save those at low risk of recurrence from the late effects of radiotherapy. The 5-year overall survival is 75%.

Ewing's sarcoma

Ewing's sarcoma is named after Dr James Ewing, who described the tumour in the 1920s. Ewing's sarcoma is a childhood bone malignancy of uncertain cellular origin that is associated with the t(11;22) chromosomal translocation that juxtaposes the EWS and Fli-1 genes, resulting in a hybrid transcript from these two transcription factor genes. This same chromosomal translocation occurs in PNETs and Askin lung tumours, suggesting a possible common origin. PNETs are thought to arise from peripheral autonomic nervous system tissue and immunostain for neuron specific enolase (NSE) as well as S-100. Morphologically, all three tumours are small round blue cell tumours – a group that also includes embryonal rhabdomyosarcoma, non-Hodgkin's lymphoma, neuroblastoma and small cell lung cancer. About 30 children each year in the United Kingdom develop Ewing's sarcoma. It most frequently occurs in the teenage years. Ewing's sarcoma is very rare in African and Asian children and is not associated with familial syndromes or prior radiotherapy. It usually starts in a bone at the diaphysis or, less frequently, the metaphysic – most commonly in one of the bones of the hips, upper arm or thigh (see Figures 1.13 and 36.5), although it can also develop in soft tissue. The most common symptom is pain and swelling, but systemic symptoms such as pyrexia, weight loss and night sweats may also occur. X-rays usually demonstrate ill-defined medullary destruction, small areas of new bone formation, periosteal reaction and soft tissue expansion. Approximately a fifth of patients have metastases in their lungs or bones at presentation. Multimodality treatment including surgery, radiotherapy and chemotherapy is a standard practice for Ewing's sarcoma, and the 5-year survival rate is 64%.

Osteosarcoma

The incidence of bone tumours is the highest during adolescence, although they only represent 3% of all childhood cancers. Only about 30 children develop these tumours each year in the United Kingdom. Most tumours occur in areas of rapid growth in the metaphysis near the growth plate, where cellular proliferation and remodelling are the greatest during long bone growth. The most active growth plates are in the distal femur and proximal tibia (see Figure 36.4). These are also the most common sites for primary bone cancers. Known risk factors include hereditary retinoblastoma, Li–Fraumeni syndrome and prior radiotherapy. Most primary bone tumours present as painful swellings that may cause stiffness and effusions in nearby joints. Occasionally, tumours present as pathological fractures. The radiological appearances are a lytic or sclerotic expansile lesion associated with a wide transition zone, cortical destruction, a soft tissue mass, periosteal reaction and calcification. The clinical management of bone tumours requires a specialist multidisciplinary unit including orthopaedic surgeons, plastic surgeons and oncologists. Clinical management should happen in the context of an adolescent oncology unit, since the majority of patients fit into this age group, with all its special needs. Neoadjuvant chemotherapy plays an important role in localized osteosarcoma and Ewing's sarcoma to shrink the tumour and hopefully allow limb sparing surgery without increasing relapse rates. Postoperative adjuvant chemotherapy and radiotherapy are useful in some tumours. The 5-year survival has steadily risen from under 20% in the late 1960s to over 60%.

Presentation and management of neuroblastoma

Neuroblastoma is the most common malignancy in infants under a year old and often is clinically apparent at birth. About 100 new cases of neuroblastoma are diagnosed each year in the United Kingdom. Tumours often have amplification of the n-Myc oncogene on chromosome 1, either as small "double minute" (DM) chromosomes or as "homogenously staining regions" (HSR). They may arise from any site along the craniospinal axis derived from neural crest. The sites include abdominal sites (55%) such as the adrenal medulla (33%), pelvis (25%), thorax (13%) and head and neck (7%). In the case of head and neck neuroblastoma, these occur most commonly in the sympathetic ganglion or olfactory bulb (the latter are more common in adults). The most common finding is a large, firm and irregular abdominal mass that characteristically crosses the midline. Neuroblastomas may present with non-specific symptoms such as weight loss, failure to thrive, fever and pallor, especially if widespread metastases are present. Seventy per cent are disseminated at diagnosis via lymphatic and haematogenous spread. Metastases to bones of the skull are common, and orbital swelling is a frequent presentation. Paraneoplastic opsoclonus (rapid involuntary eye movements) or myoclonus (brief involuntary muscle twitches) is a rare feature. These tumours have the highest spontaneous regression rate of any tumour, usually by maturation to ganglioneuroma. Plain abdominal X-ray may show calcification: this occurs in 70% of neuroblastoma and 15% of Wilms' tumours (Figure 34.3). Other diagnostic investigations include [131]-I-labelled meta-iodobenzyl

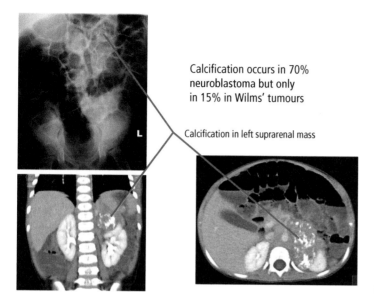

Calcification occurs in 70% neuroblastoma but only in 15% in Wilms' tumours

Calcification in left suprarenal mass

Figure 34.3 Neuroblastoma.

guanidine (MIBG) scan and blood or urinary catecholamines including vanillylmandelic acid (VMA), serum neuron-specific enolase (NSE) and ferritin. Localized disease has a high cure rate with surgery and radiotherapy. On account of the high rate of disseminated disease at presentation, which is 70%, however, the overall 5-year survival rate for neuroblastoma is 64%.

Presentation and management of Wilms' tumours (nephroblastoma)

This highly malignant embryonal tumour of the kidney is the most common malignant lesion of the genitourinary tract in children. It was named after Dr Max Wilms, who first described it, and is also known as nephroblastoma. Most occur in children under 5 years old and some are hereditary. Only about 75 children develop a Wilms' tumour each year in Britain. Wilms' tumours are associated with congenital abnormalities including aniridia (absence of the iris usually affecting both eyes) and the WAGR syndrome (Wilms' tumour, aniridia, gonadoblastoma and mental retardation), Denys–Drash syndrome (Wilms' tumour, male pseudohermaphroditism and diffuse glomerular disease) and Beckwith–Wiedemann syndrome (organomegaly, hemihypertrophy, increased incidence of Wilms' tumour, hepatoblastoma and adrenocortical tumours).

Wilms' tumours present in usually healthy children as abdominal swellings with a smooth, firm, non-tender mass. A quarter has gross haematuria and occasionally children present with hypertension, malaise or fever. Up to 20% have metastases at diagnosis; lungs are the most common sites of metastases. The mainstay of treatment is surgical resection with adjuvant radiotherapy to the tumour bed, reserved for children with a high risk of relapse. The 5-year survival for Wilms' tumours now exceeds 80%, and one of the goals of more recent trials is to reduce the long-term morbidity of treatment.

Presentation and management of retinoblastoma

Retinoblastoma most often occurs in children under 5 years old and in a third of cases is bilateral. There are about 40 new cases of retinoblastoma diagnosed each year in the United Kingdom. Up to 40% are hereditary due to germ line mutations of the retinoblastoma (RB) gene and these children frequently have bilateral retinoblastoma and present at a younger age. Hereditary retinoblastoma was the basis of Knudsen's two-hit model of tumour suppressor genes (Figures 1.3 and 2.14). These tumours present with whitening of the pupil, squint or secondary glaucoma (Figure 34.4). Retinoblastoma is usually confined to the orbit, and hence the cure rate with enucleation is high. Smaller

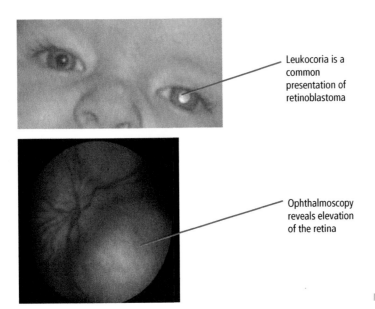

Leukocoria is a common presentation of retinoblastoma

Ophthalmoscopy reveals elevation of the retina

Figure 34.4 Leukocoria (white eye).

tumours may be treated with localized cryotherapy, laser treatment or a radioactive iodine plaque stitched to the outer surface of the eye. Overall, 99% of children with retinoblastoma are cured. Hereditary retinoblastoma, however, is also associated with other malignancies, especially osteosarcoma, soft tissue sarcoma and melanoma. Genetic counselling is an integral part of therapy for retinoblastoma. All siblings should be examined periodically: DNA polymorphism analysis may identify relatives at high risk.

Presentation and management of liver tumours

Fewer than 10 children in the United Kingdom develop liver tumours each year. Liver cancers are divided into hepatoblastoma (80%), which usually occurs before the age of 3 years, and hepatocellular cancers (20%), which occur at any age. Hepatoblastoma occurs as part of the Beckwith–Wiedemann syndrome and is also associated with familial adenomatous polyposis. Hepatoblastoma is the third most common intra-abdominal malignancy in young children – after neuroblastoma and Wilms' tumours. It most frequently affects the right lobe of the liver, and 10% have disseminated disease at presentation with regional lymph node involvement or lung metastases. Hepatocellular carcinoma is associated with hepatitis

B and C infection, tyrosinaemia, biliary cirrhosis and α_1-antitrypsin deficiency. Surgical resection with or without neoadjuvant chemotherapy has dramatically improved the prognosis in hepatoblastoma, where the 5-year overall survival is now 70%. In contrast, the prognosis for hepatocellular carcinoma in children is not greatly different from that for adults with 5-year overall survival rates of around 25%.

Langerhans' cell histiocytosis

Langerhans' cell histiocytosis (LCH), previously known as histiocytosis X, may not strictly be a cancer but may behave in an aggressive fashion and is often treated by oncologists. About 30 children develop LCH in the United Kingdom each year; most of them are under 2 years old. LCH is a proliferation of epidermal histiocytes or Langerhans' cells, which are antigen-presenting dendritic cells named after Paul Langerhans, who first described them in 1868 when he was a 21-year-old medical student in Berlin. LCH comprises three overlapping syndromes:

- unifocal bone disease (solitary eosinophilic granuloma)
- multifocal disease of bone (Hand–Schüller–Christian disease)
- multifocal, multisystem disease (Letterer–Siwe disease)

Letterer–Siwe disease occurs mainly in boys under 2 years old; Hand–Schüller–Christian syndrome has a peak of onset in children aged 2–10 years; whilst

Table 34.3 Small blue round cell tumours.

Paediatric embryonal tumours
  Neuroblastoma
  Medulloblastoma
  Rhabdomyosarcoma
  Wilm's tumour (nephroblastoma)
  Retinoblastoma
  Hepatoblastoma (anaplastic form only)
Teenage young adult tumours
  Ewing's sarcoma/PNET
  Synovial sarcoma
Adult tumours
  Carcinoid tumour
  Small cell lung cancer
  Small cell lymphoma

solitary eosinophilic granuloma occurs in those aged 5–15 years. Solitary eosinophilic granuloma occurs at any site in bones and is usually asymptomatic and frequently an incidental finding. Patients with Hand–Schüller–Christian syndrome often present with recurrent episodes of otitis media and mastoiditis or with polyuria and polydipsia due to diabetes insipidus. Letterer–Siwe disease presents with symptoms suggestive of a systemic infection or malignancy with a generalized skin eruption, anaemia and hepatosplenomegaly and other protean manifestations (Table 34.4). This eponymous classification of LCH has in part been abandoned, and a simpler classification into either restricted LCH (skin or bone lesions) or extensive LCH (visceral organ involvement) has

been introduced. The diagnosis is confirmed histologically; the characteristic cytological features are CD1a surface antigen expression and Birbeck granules that are tennis racket shaped cytoplasmic organelles seen under the electron microscope. Localized bone disease is treated surgically or, less frequently, with radiotherapy, whilst systemic disease requires chemotherapy with cladribine often with desmopressin for the management of the diabetes insipidus. Survival exceeds 95% in unifocal disease and 80% in multifocal bone disease, but is only 50% in patients with systemic multiorgan disease. Bearing in mind the multiple manifestations and rarity of LCH, it comes as no surprise that it is the final diagnosis in an episode of House.

Table 34.4 Clinical manifestations of extensive Langerhans' cell histiocytosis

System	Clinical manifestations
Systemic effects	Pyrexia, weight loss, fatigue
Bone	Painful swelling (skull (50%), femur (17%), ribs (8%), pelvis, vertebrae), associated soft tissue swelling (proptosis, mastoiditis and deafness, gums)
Skin	Scaly, erythematous, seborrhoea-like brown to red papules (behind the ears and in the axillary, inguinal and perineal areas) (50%)
Endocrine glands	Diabetes insipidus (20%) due to involvement of the hypothalamus or pituitary stalk
Bone marrow	Pancytopenia
Lymph nodes	Lymphadenopathy (30%)
Liver and spleen	Hepatosplenomegaly
Gastrointestinal tract	Failure to thrive, malabsorption, diarrhoea, vomiting (5–10%)
Lungs	Dyspnoea, honey-comb lungs, bullae, spontaneous pneumothorax, emphysema (20%)
Central nervous system	Progressive ataxia, dysarthria, intracranial hypertension, cranial nerve palsies (10%)

Complications of childhood treatment of cancer

Although many of the delayed effects of chemotherapy and radiotherapy in children are similar to those in adults, the effects on developing organs also produce unique late side effects, particularly on the skeleton, brain and endocrine systems. These delayed effects of multimodality therapy on the developing child are substantial and the late sequelae cause considerable morbidity in this group of patients where the long-term survival rates are high. Radiotherapy retards bone and cartilage growth and causes intellectual impairment, gonadal toxicity, hypothalamic and thyroid dysfunction as well as pneumonitis, nephrotoxicity and hepatotoxicity.

Proton beam radiotherapy delivers charged protons (p^+), the subatomic particle that is composed of 2 up and 1 down quarks, that forms the nucleus of a hydrogen atom and was discovered by Ernest Rutherford in 1920. Proton therapy offers an advance in the treatment of childhood malignancies particularly in those tumours where the delivery of high-intensity focussed radiation is critical. For example, the treatment of brain tumours using protons allows radiation to be delivered without scatter to neighbouring critical structures such as the optic chiasm in the course of irradiating the pineal gland.

Late consequences of chemotherapy include infertility, anthracycline-related cardiotoxicity, bleomycin-related pulmonary fibrosis and platinum-related nephrotoxicity and neurotoxicity. Up to 5% of children cured of this cancer will develop a second malignancy as a consequence of an inherited cancer predisposition or the late sequelae of cancer treatment. Second malignancies occur most frequently following combined chemotherapy and radiotherapy.

 ONLINE RESOURCE

Case Study: The boy who fell off his bike.

 KEY POINTS

- Cancer in children is rare affecting fewer than 1 in 600 but is the second most common cause of death in childhood after accidental injury
- Leukaemias account for 30% of cancers in childhood, but the solid paediatric tumours encountered in childhood are often embryonal in origin and are often associated with an inherited predisposition
- Many paediatric solid tumours are curable even if they present with advanced disease because they are generally highly chemosensitive cancers.
- Eight in ten children with cancer are cured

35

Cancers in teenagers and young adults

Learning objectives

✓ Explain the epidemiology and pathogenesis of cancers in teenagers and young adults

✓ Recognize the common presentation and clinical features of cancers in teenagers and young adults

✓ Describe the treatment strategies and outcomes of cancers in teenagers and young adults

---

Epidemiology

Teenage and young adults (TYA) refer to people aged between 16 and 24 years. In 2010, 2214 TYA were diagnosed with cancer and 311 died of the disease. The types of cancers that occur in TYA differ from those seen in childhood and adulthood (see Tables 1.1 and 35.1). Survival has steadily improved over recent decades so that over 80% TYA with cancer survive 5 years or more from their cancer diagnosis.

Presentation and management of paediatric solid tumours

The clinical presentation and routes to diagnosis of cancer in TYA differ from those for children and adults. Around a quarter of cancers in TYA are diagnosed via an emergency admission, although this rate varies with tumour type. For example, only 2%

Table 35.1 Frequency and survival for cancers in TYA

Cancer	Proportion of cancers in female TYA	Proportion of cancers in male TYA	Proportion of all cancers in TYA	5-year overall survival
Lymphomas	20%	22%	20%	89%
Carcinoma	31%	9%	19%	81%
Germ cell tumours	3%	27%	15%	96%
Brain and CNS tumours	14%	13%	14%	81%
Melanoma	16%	7%	11%	93%
Leukaemias	7%	10%	9%	62%
Bone tumours	4%	6%	5%	56%
Soft tissue sarcomas	4%	4%	4%	61%

Oncology: Lecture Notes, Third Edition. Mark Bower and Jonathan Waxman.
© 2015 by John Wiley & Sons, Ltd. Published 2015 by John Wiley & Sons, Ltd.
Companion Website: www.lecturenoteseries.com/oncology

melanomas in TYA are diagnosed as an emergency whilst over 50% of leukaemias are diagnosed in an emergency department. In contrast, 54% of children with cancer present as an emergency but only 15% of adults present in this way.

The major difference in the management of cancer in TYA relates to the way the service has been delivered in the United Kingdom since 2008. Treatment of TYA with cancer is confined to designated treatment centres providing age-appropriate facilities. Although the clinical management plans remain with tumour site-specific multi-disciplinary teams (MDTs), this should be in joint collaboration with a TYA MDT based at one of 13 principal treatment centres for TYA with cancer in the United Kingdom.

 ONLINE RESOURCE

Case Study: The fainting dancer.

 KEY POINTS

- Cancers in TYA occur in those aged between 16 and 24 years
- Some cancers in TYA resemble those seen in childhood and some resemble tumours in adults, with an overall survival of 80% at 5 years
- The treatment of cancer in TYA should be in specialist centres and follows patterns established for similar cancers occurring in adults and children

36

Bone and soft tissue sarcomas

Learning objectives

✓ Explain the epidemiology and pathogenesis of bone and soft tissue sarcomas

✓ Recognize the common presentation and clinical features of bone and soft tissue sarcomas

✓ Describe the treatment strategies and outcomes of bone and soft tissue sarcomas

---

Bone tumours are amongst the oldest cancers discovered in humans according to palaeopathological evidence. A Bronze Age woman with bone metastases in her skull has been dated to 1600–1900 BC, whilst Saxon bones from Standlake in Oxfordshire, the United Kingdom, demonstrate features of osteosarcoma in a young adult warrior. St Peregrine, born in 1260 at Forlì, Italy, is the patron saint of cancer sufferers (the feast day is on 4 May). He was due for an amputation for a sarcoma of the leg, but the cancer was cured on the night prior to surgery, following a vision of Christ. He lived a further 20 years and was canonized in 1726.

Epidemiology

Sarcomas are tumours of the connective tissues or mesenchymal cells, which support the body and include bone, muscle, tendon, fat and synovial tissue. Sarcomas are usually divided into bone tumours and soft tissue sarcomas, although some cancers have feet in both camps, such as Ewing's sarcoma which may involve either bone or soft tissues. Sarcomas constitute about 1% of adult tumours and there are as many as 50 different subtypes. The presumed cell of origin of the sarcoma defines the classification (Tables 36.1 and 36.2).

In 2010, 559 people were diagnosed with bone sarcoma and 3272 with soft tissue sarcoma (Table 36.3). The most common bone tumours are osteosarcoma (35% of primary bone tumours) and Ewing's sarcoma (20% of primary bone tumours). The most frequent soft tissue sarcomas are leiomyosarcoma (18% soft tissue sarcomas), fibroblastic sarcomas (14%) and liposarcoma (13%), although the largest group of all are the soft tissue sarcoma "not otherwise specified" (20%)! The epidemiology of the different sarcomas varies. For example, osteosarcomas have a bimodal age distribution with peaks in adolescence and in the over-65-year olds, whilst chondrosarcoma incidence rises steadily after the age of 40 years.

Pathogenesis

Ionizing radiation exposure increases the risk of developing bone sarcomas, including therapeutic radiotherapy. Thus there is an increased risk of second primary bone sarcoma in cancer survivors,

---

Oncology: Lecture Notes, Third Edition. Mark Bower and Jonathan Waxman.
© 2015 by John Wiley & Sons, Ltd. Published 2015 by John Wiley & Sons, Ltd.
Companion Website: www.lecturenoteseries.com/oncology

Table 36.1 Origins of primary bone tumours

Origin	Benign tumour	Malignant tumour
Cartilage	Enchondroma Osteochondroma	Chondrosarcoma
Origin	Benign tumour Chondroblastoma	Malignant tumour
Bone	Osteoid osteoma Osteoblastoma	Osteosarcoma
Unknown origin	Giant cell tumour	Ewing's sarcoma Malignant fibrous histiocytoma

although occasionally this may be a consequence of a shared inherited genetic predisposition. Thus familial hereditary retinoblastoma increases the risk of not only retinoblastoma but also osteosarcoma and leiomyosarcomas. Similarly in people with Li-Fraumeni syndrome there is an increased risk of osteosarcoma and rhabdomyosarcomas and in those with hereditary multiple exostoses, a high risk of chondrosarcoma. Non-hereditary medical conditions also increase the risk of bone sarcomas. Paget's disease, which may affect up to 5% of the population, carries a risk of osteosarcoma, although the risk is small (about 1%). Similarly Ollier's disease is associated with an increased risk of chrondrosarcoma. Kaposi's sarcoma, both the immunosuppression-associated and classical forms are caused by a human herpesvirus, HHV8/KSHV. Finally, Stewart–Treves syndrome is the rare occurrence of angiosarcoma, developing in a limb affected by chronic lymphoedema, including the arm of women treated for ipsilateral breast cancer.

Advances in the molecular biology of sarcomas have resulted in the identification of signature somatic mutations, including chromosomal translocations in subtypes of sarcomas. For example, molecular analysis of Ewing's sarcoma has revealed a specific chromosomal translocation between chromosomes 22 and 11. This translocation is present in a group of small, round, blue cell tumours which include peripheral neuroectodermal tumours (PNETs), classic Ewing's and extraosseous Ewing's sarcoma; these are now grouped together for treatment purposes. In patients with this group of tumours there may be difficulty in obtaining a histopathological diagnosis. Modern advances in molecular biology have led to the identification of the EWS/FLI-1 translocation present

Table 36.2 Clinical features of soft tissue sarcomas

Tumour	Age (years)	Commonest sites	Primary therapy	5-year survival
Fibrosarcoma	20–50	Thigh, arm, head and neck	Wide excision and adjuvant radiation	90% (well differentiated) 50% (poorly differentiated)
Liposarcoma	40–60	Thigh, head and neck (rarely arise from lipoma)	Wide excision and adjuvant radiation	66% (myxoid) 10% (pleomorphic)
Embryonal rhabdomyosarcoma	0–10	Head and neck, genitourinary (botyroid)	Neoadjuvant chemoradiation and surgery	40%
Alveolar rhabdomyosarcoma	10–20	Thigh	Neoadjuvant chemoradiation and surgery	60%
Pleomorphic rhabdomyosarcoma	40–70	Thigh, upper arm	Wide excision and adjuvant radiation	10%
Synovial sarcoma	20–40	Leg	Wide excision and adjuvant radiation	40%
Angiosarcoma	50–70	Skin, superficial soft tissues	Wide excision and adjuvant radiation	15%
Leiomyosarcoma	45–65	Retroperitoneal, uterine	Wide excision and adjuvant radiation	40%

Table 36.3 UK registrations for sarcomas cancer 2010

	Percentage of all cancer registrations		Change in ASR (2000–2010)		5-year overall survival	
	Female	Male	Female	Male	Female	Male
Bone sarcoma	0.1	0.2	+0%	+0%	54%	58%
Soft tissue sarcoma	1	1	+0%	+17%	56%	56%

in patients with Ewing's sarcoma. The presence of this translocation is identifiable by fluorescence *in situ* hybridization (FISH) and this aids diagnosis.

Presentation

Most soft tissue sarcomas occur in the limbs and patients present to their GPs with localized swelling. Patients with bone and soft tissue sarcomas generally present with pain, and the diagnosis usually comes as a result of the classic X-ray appearances of these tumours. Fractures are common and nerve palsies

may be seen where there is a cranial presentation. Patients may also present with metastases. Because of the rarity of these tumours and the requirement for a multidisciplinary specialist approach, patients with a suspected diagnosis of sarcoma should be referred on to specialist centres, where results have been shown to be vastly superior to those achieved by peripheral clinics. These tumours are usually diagnosed after a significant delay which ranges from 3 to 6 months from the development of symptoms to diagnosis.

Tables 36.4–36.6 list the clinical features of the different types of bone cancers and sarcomas, some of which are illustrated in Figures 36.1, 36.2, 36.3, 36.4 and 36.5.

Table 36.4 Clinical features of cartilage-derived bone tumours

	Enchondroma	Osteochondroma (exostosis)	Chondroblastoma	Chondrosarcoma
Age	10–50 years	10–20 years	5–20 years	30–60 years
Site	Hands, wrist	Knee, shoulder, pelvis	Knee, shoulder, ribs	Knee, shoulder, pelvis
	Diaphysis	Metaphysis	Epiphysis prior to fusion	Metaphysis or diaphysis
X-ray	Well-defined lucency, thin sclerotic rim, calcification	Eccentric protrusion from bone, calcification	Well-defined lucency, thin sclerotic rim, calcification	Expansile lucency, sclerotic margin, cortical destruction, soft tissue mass
Notes	Ollier's disease = multiple enchondromas	1% transform to chondrosarcoma		

Table 36.5 Clinical features of osteoid-derived bone tumours

	Osteoid osteoma	Osteoblastoma	Osteosarcoma
Age	10–30 years	10–20 years	10–25 years and >60 years
Site	Knee	Vertebra	Knee, shoulder, pelvis
	Diaphysis	Metaphysis	Metaphysis
X-ray	<1 cm central lucency, surrounding bone sclerosis, periosteal reaction	Well-defined lucency, sclerotic rim, cortex preserved, calcification	Lytic/sclerotic expansile lesion, wide transition zone, cortical destruction, soft tissue mass, periosteal reaction, calcification

Table 36.6 Clinical features of bone tumours of uncertain origins

	Giant cell tumour	Ewing's sarcoma	Malignant fibrous histiocytoma
Age	20–40 years	5–15 years	10–20 years and >60 years
Site	Long bones, knee	Knee, shoulder, pelvis	Knee, pelvis, shoulder
	Epiphysis and metaphysis post closure	Diaphysis, less often metaphysis	Metaphysis
X-ray	Lucency with ill-defined endosteal margin, cortical destruction, soft tissue mass, eccentric expansion bone/lung metastases	Ill-defined medullary destruction, small areas of new bone formation, periosteal reaction, soft tissue expansion	Cortical destruction, periosteal reaction, soft tissue mass

Investigations and management of bone sarcomas

In a patient where a diagnosis of soft tissue sarcoma is suspected, an initial biopsy should be carried out by the surgeon who is to perform definitive surgery. Fine-needle aspiration cytology, core needle biopsy and incisional biopsies are all techniques that are considered by the surgeon, and for those patients with rare abdominal or thoracic soft tissue sarcomas, CT-guided biopsies may be required. The surface entry point of the biopsy needle is tattooed to allow the biopsy tract to be identified and excised at the time of definitive surgery. After the pathological

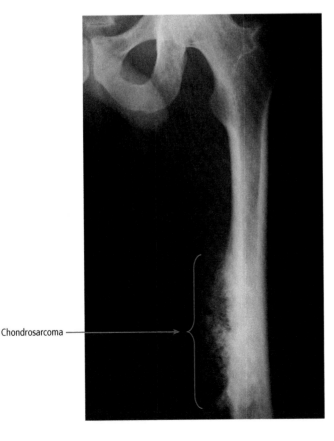

Chondrosarcoma

Figure 36.1 Femur chondrosarcoma showing an expansile lesion with sclerotic margin, cortical destruction and punctuate internal calcification and an associated soft tissue mass. These tumours are most common in middle age and occur around the knee, shoulder or pelvis.

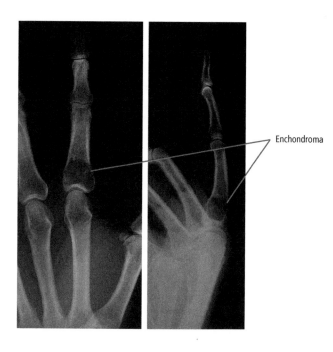

Enchondroma

Figure 36.2 Enchondroma of the ring finger proximal phalynx showing well-defined lucency and a thin sclerotic rim with preserved cortex. These cartilage-derived tumours occur in 10–50-year-olds most frequently in the diaphyses of the hand or wrist. Multiple enchondromas occur in Ollier's disease, a non-hereditary condition that is associated with an increased risk of chondrosarcoma.

diagnosis has been established, definitive surgery can be planned. This requires a multidisciplinary approach that takes place in the context of magnetic resonance (MR) staging of the local tumour and CT definition of the metastatic sites. The surgical approach requires the removal of the muscle compartment to include the fascia. This limits the risk of local relapse.

In those patients with Ewing's sarcoma and osteosarcoma, initial staging will include CT assessment of the chest, abdomen and pelvis, and MR imaging of

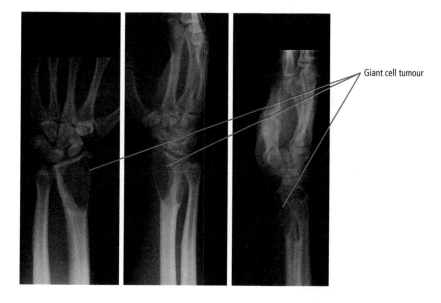

Giant cell tumour

Figure 36.3 Giant cell tumour of the distal radius showing expansion and lucency with cortical destruction giving a multiloculated appearance. These tumours occur most commonly in 20–40-year-olds in long bones at the epiphyses and metaphyses after closure.

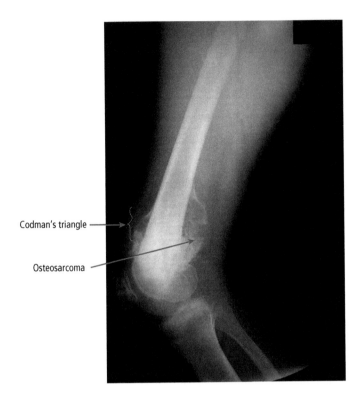

Codman's triangle

Osteosarcoma

Figure 36.4 Osteosarcoma of the distal femur showing an expansile soft tissue mass with internal calcification and cortical destruction. There is a marked periosteal reaction with lifting of the periosteum that is described as Codman's triangle, which is almost always due to an aggressive malignant bone tumour extending into adjacent soft tissues.

the primary tumour site. The initial management option for Ewing's sarcoma includes the consideration of either primary surgery or radiotherapy to control the local lesion. If the lesion is small and it is possible to have substantial resection margins, surgery is the best option with immediate endoprosthetic replacement.

For the majority of patients, however, radiotherapy remains the most important treatment modality for the control of local disease.

Osteosarcomas are rare and for this reason also best managed in specialist centres. This is particularly important for teenage patients with sarcomas. For these

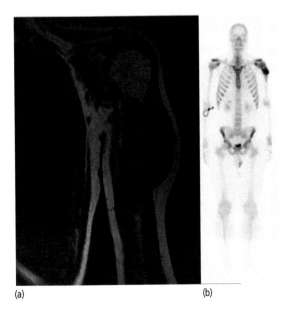

(a)

(b)

Figure 36.5 Ewing's sarcoma of proximal left humerus on (a) MRI and (b) isotope bone scan.

patients, chemotherapy, radiation, surgery and counselling all have a significant role in management. Patients with osteosarcomas are generally managed well because of the excellent results achieved using multidisciplinary specialist approaches. In osteosarcoma, bone scanning as well as CT and MR scanning are essential in the initial work-up of a patient. Biopsy of the tumour is required with the open approach preferred. Surgical advances have meant that bone tumours are managed much better than they were, with the aim of limb-sparing prosthetic surgery.

Treatment of Ewing's sarcomas

For patients with Ewing's tumours, the last 20 or 30 years have seen a significant evolution of treatment protocols. One type of management generally consists of treatment with induction chemotherapy, followed by local treatment to the primary site with either surgery or radiotherapy or both. This will be followed by further consolidation chemotherapy.

Treatment of osteosarcomas

Similarly in sarcomas, primary chemotherapy to debulk the tumour is followed by surgery. Both chemotherapy and surgery are complex and highly specialized, requiring immense technical skill and input from many areas of medical and paramedical expertise. Patients with metastatic osteosarcoma can be cured, and, once more, surgery is enormously important. Surgical excision of pulmonary metastases is considered and may be curative in a limited number of patients.

Investigations and management of soft tissue sarcomas

Pathology

The most helpful classification of soft tissue sarcomas is into tumours of fibrous tissue, adipose tissue tumours, tumours of muscle, tumours of blood vessels, tumours of lymph vessels, tumours of synovium, tumours of peripheral nerves, tumours of cartilage and bone-forming tissue, tumours of pleuripotential mesochyme, tumours of uncertain histogenesis and unclassified soft tissue tumours. This latter tumour group is extremely diverse, with at least 50 different subtypes. A simplified classification of the more common adult soft tissue sarcomas is shown in Table 36.7.

These groups may in turn be divided into benign and malignant conditions. Benign tumours do not generally metastasize and microscopic examination shows a low mitotic rate. Malignant tumours have a high mitotic rate and do tend to metastasize. Approximately one-third of tumours are low grade and two-thirds are high grade.

Treatment of soft tissue sarcomas

The clinical features of soft tissue sarcomas are listed in Table 36.2, along with the primary therapy.

Table 36.7 Tissue origins and common sites of soft tissue sarcomas

Tissue of origin	Cancer	Usual site in body
Fibrous tissue	Fibroblastic sarcoma	Arms, legs, trunk
	Malignant fibrous histiocytoma	Legs
	Dermatofibrosarcoma	Trunk
Fat	Liposarcoma	Arms, legs, trunk
Striated muscle	Rhabdomyosarcoma	Arms, legs
Smooth muscle	Leiomyosarcoma	Uterus, GI tract
Blood vessels	Haemangiosarcoma	Arms, legs, trunk
	Kaposi's sarcoma	Legs, trunk
Lymph vessels	Lymphangiosarcoma	Arms
Synovial tissues of joints	Synovial sarcoma	Legs
Peripheral nerves	Malignant peripheral nerve sheath tumour	Arms, legs, trunk

Treatment of the primary tumour

There is considerable discussion as to the appropriate management of a soft tissue sarcoma. Low-grade tumours, which by definition should not spread, should be treated by surgical excision alone. Local control should result in 85–100% recovery in these patients. The situation is different for those patients with high-grade tumours, and there is debate as to whether surgery alone, surgery combined with radiation, or surgery, radiation and chemotherapy in combination is the correct approach.

Surgery

There is little argument that surgery is necessary, and the operation of first choice should be one that allows a reasonably wide margin of normal tissue to be excised with the tumour. If a "good" procedure is carried out, such as muscle compartmental excision, the local failure rate is 7–18%. If less radical procedures such as excision biopsy are performed, then the local failure rate is approximately 50%. More radical procedures such as amputation have a lower local recurrence rate of approximately 5%. Over the last decade, there has been a trend towards radical compartmental excision with limb-sparing procedures.

Adjuvant chemotherapy and radiation

After definitive surgery has been performed, the need for radiation and chemotherapy is assessed. Radiation is not given for low-grade tumours. In high-grade tumours, radiotherapy to the tumour bed has an advantage in terms of reduced local recurrence rates in extremity lesions where effective dosages can be given without risking vital structures. Local radiation has no effect upon the progression of distant metastases. Because patients with high-grade sarcomas are at great risk from the progression of their cancer to a metastatic state, adjuvant chemotherapy has been investigated in a number of trials. The original studies, which were non-randomized, showed an advantage to combination chemotherapy. This result has not held up and the consensus view now is that adjuvant chemotherapy has no advantage in terms of 5-year survival. This remains very much a subject for debate, however, and in many centres adjuvant chemotherapy is still administered.

Treatment of metastatic sarcoma

The treatment of metastatic soft tissue sarcoma requires the use of chemotherapy. The most effective single-agent treatments lead to responses in 15–35% of patients. Attempts are made to capitalize on this by the use of combination chemotherapy programmes. A slight increase in response rates has been found by some groups of clinicians. This supposed advantage is, however, much debated. Many cancer doctors would advocate the administration of single-agent chemotherapy to their patients simply because combination therapies maximize toxicities and do not provide a significant advantage. There have been advances in treatment that have progressed beyond the use of standard cytotoxic chemotherapy drugs. Imatinib is effective in dermatofibrosarcoma protuberans, pazopanib in non-adipocytic soft tissue sarcomas and sunitinib in alveolar soft part sarcoma and extraskeletal chondrosarcoma.

Prognosis

The prognosis of bone and soft tissue sarcomas vary depending on the stage and the tumour subtype. For bone sarcomas, the 5-year overall survival is 56% but varies from 42% in osteosarcoma to 68% in chondrosarcoma. Similarly, but more markedly, for soft tissue sarcomas the overall 5-year survival is 56% but varies from 30% in angiosarcoma to 99% in dermatofibrosarcoma.

 ONLINE RESOURCE

Case Study: The council worker who slipped.

 KEY POINTS

- Sarcomas are tumours of the connective tissues, including bone, muscle, tendon, fat and synovial tissue and are usually separated into bone tumours and soft tissue sarcomas
- Sarcomas account for 1% cancers in adults and germ line hereditary familial syndromes, radiation exposure and viral infection are all implicated in the pathogenesis of sarcomas
- Soft tissue and bone sarcomas in the limbs present with localized swelling and pain or less frequently with metastases
- The mainstay of treatment is highly specialized surgery working within a multidisciplinary team with rehabilitation and prosthetic experts
- More than half of all patients survive 5 years

37

Cancer of unknown primary

Learning objectives

✓ Explain the epidemiology and pathogenesis of cancer of unknown primary

✓ Recognize the common presentation and clinical features of cancer of unknown primary

✓ Describe the treatment strategies and outcomes of cancer of unknown primary

Epidemiology and pathogenesis

For most patients who present with metastatic disease, routine examination and investigation will quickly disclose the underlying primary tumour. Occasionally, the primary tumour may be more elusive, and a number of clinical, histopathological and serological clues may help to establish its site. For 3–5% of patients, however, the primary site remains undisclosed because it is too small to be detected or has regressed. The usual histological diagnosis in these patients with a cancer of unknown primary (CUP) site is adenocarcinoma or poorly differentiated carcinoma. The benefits of establishing the primary site include:

- diagnosing treatable disease (Table 37.1)
- avoiding overtreating unresponsive disease and hence iatrogenic morbidity in resistant disease
- preventing complications that relate to occult primary disease, such as bowel obstruction
- clarifying the prognosis

In 2010, a total of 9762 people were diagnosed with CUP and 10,812 people died of CUP. That more people died of CUP than were diagnosed with it is chiefly a consequence of the vagaries of data recording. Although CUP accounts for 3% of cancers diagnosed in the United Kingdom, it causes nearly 7% of cancer deaths. Over the last decade, the incidence of CUP has declined markedly – by 34% in women and 39% in men. This probably, in part, reflects improvements in imaging and immunohistochemical staining to establish a primary tumour site. The incidence of CUP rises with age and whilst it accounts for 3% of cancers overall, 7% of cancers in those over 85 years old are CUP.

Clinical sites of metastatic spread

Different tumours follow different patterns of metastatic spread. This may be related to chemokine and chemokine receptor expression by tumours and stromal cells (see Box 1.4 and Box 2.2). The most common sites of metastases are shown in Table 37.2 and Figure 37.1.

Table 37.1 Treatable unknown primary diagnoses

Chemosensitive tumours	Hormone-sensitive tumours
Non-Hodgkin's lymphoma	Breast cancer
Germ cell tumours	Prostate cancer
Neuroendocrine tumours (including small cell lung cancer)	Endometrial cancer
Ovarian cancer	Thyroid cancer

Table 37.2 Table of most common sites of cancer metastases

Site	First metastatic location incidence	Incidence of involvement at presentation
Lymph node	26%	41%
Lung	17%	27%
Bone	15%	29%
Liver	11%	34%
Brain	8%	6%
Pleura	7%	11%
Skin	5%	4%
Peritoneum	4%	9%
Adrenal gland	–	6%
Bone marrow	–	3%

Brain and meningeal metastases

Up to a quarter of solid tumours develop parenchymal brain metastases. Parenchymal brain secondaries that may occur with any solid tumour are usually treated with whole-brain radiotherapy, although surgery may be considered for patients with solitary brain metastases and limited systemic disease (Figures 13.8, 33.8 and 37.1). Carcinomatous meningitis is less common and presents with multiple, anatomically distant, cranial and spinal root neuropathies. The diagnosis may be confirmed by finding malignant cells in the cerebrospinal fluid. Treatment usually involves a combination of intrathecal chemotherapy and craniospinal radiotherapy. Carcinomatous meningitis most frequently occurs with leukaemias and lymphomas and occasionally with breast cancer.

Bone metastases

Bone metastases are a major source of morbidity in patients with cancer and often have a prolonged course. Bone metastases cause pain, reduced mobility, pathological fractures, hypercalcaemia, myelosuppression and nerve compression syndromes. The tumours that commonly metastasize to bone are lung, breast, prostate, renal and thyroid tumours and sarcomas. Metastases usually occur in the axial skeleton,

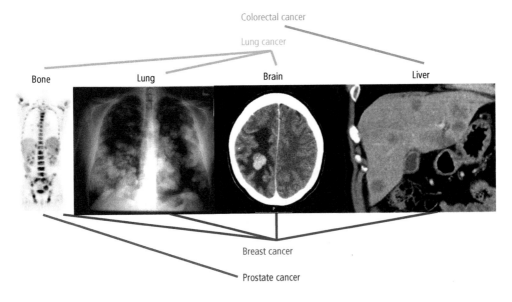

Figure 37.1 Common patterns of metastatic spread for the four most frequent cancers.

Table 37.3 Differential diagnosis of bone metastases

Diagnosis	Pain	Site	Age	X-ray	Bone scan, CT/MRI	Biochemistry
Metastases	Common	Axial skeleton	Any	Discrete lesions, pathological fracture, loss of vertebral pedicles	Soft tissue extension on MRI/CT	Raised ALP and Ca
Degenerative disease	Common	Limbs	Old	Symmetrical	Symmetrical uptake on bone scan	Normal
Osteoporosis	Painless (unless pathological fracture)	Vertebrae	Old (female)	Osteopenia	Normal bone scan/MRI	Normal
Paget's disease	Painless	Skull (often)	Old	Expanded sclerotic bones	Diffusely hot bone scan	Raised ALP and urinary hydroxyproline
Traumatic fracture	Always	Ribs	Any	Fracture	Intense linear uptake on bone scan	Normal

ALP, alkaline phosphatase; Ca, calcium; CT, computed tomography; MRI, magnetic resonance imaging.

femur or humerus. If they are found elsewhere, then renal cancer and melanoma should be considered as possible primary tumour sites. Most bone metastases are lucent, lytic lesions; occasionally dense, sclerotic deposits are seen in prostate, breast, carcinoid tumours and Hodgkin's disease. The diagnosis of bone metastases is rarely complicated. The differential diagnosis is outlined in Table 37.3 (Figures 3.4, 3.6, 5.6, 7.3, 12.1, 14.3, 14.4, 14.5, 26.4, 31.2, 31.5, 37.1, 40.6d, 40.7, 40.8 and 40.9).

Lung metastases

The lungs are the second most common site for metastases via haematogenous spread. Lung, breast, renal, thyroid, sarcoma and germ cell tumours commonly metastasize to the lung. Surgical resection of pulmonary metastases is occasionally undertaken where the primary site is controlled and the lungs are the sole site of metastasis (see Figures 15.1 and 37.1).

Liver metastases

Of all patients with liver metastases

- 60% have a colorectal primary tumour
- 20% have melanoma
- 15% lung cancer
- 5% breast cancer

Hepatic resection for patients with up to three metastases from colorectal cancer results in 5-year survivals of 30% and is the best treatment available for selected patients (see Figures 9.1, 23.2 and 37.1).

Malignant effusions

Eighty per cent of malignant pleural effusions are due to lung and breast cancers, lymphoma and leukaemia. Malignant pericardial effusion is rarer than pleural effusions; breast and lung cancers account for 75%. Metastases to the heart and pericardium are 40 times more common than primary tumours at these sites, but only 15% will develop tamponade. Malignant ascites is a common complication of ovarian, pancreatic, colorectal and gastric cancers and lymphoma. Measures for long-term control of malignant effusions include sclerosis with talc, bleomycin or tetracycline for pleural effusions, drainage by pericardial window for pericardial effusions and peritoneovenous shunts for malignant ascites (see Figure 40.20 and 40.21).

Clinical CUP syndromes

Five highly treatable subsets of unknown primary sites have been identified, which have more favourable outcomes and require distinct management:

1. Women with isolated axillary lymphadenopathy (adenocarcinoma or undifferentiated carcinoma) usually have an occult breast primary and should be managed as stage II breast cancer. They have a similar prognosis (5-year survival is 70%).
2. Women with peritoneal carcinomatosis (often papillary carcinoma with elevated serum CA-125) should be managed as stage III ovarian cancer.
3. Men with extragonadal germ cell syndrome or atypical teratoma present with features reminiscent of gonadal germ cell tumours. They occur predominantly in young men with pulmonary or lymph node metastases. Germ cell tumour markers (α-foetoprotein (AFP) and human chorionic gonadotrophin (HCG)) may be detected in the serum and in tissue by immunocytochemistry. Cytogenetic analysis for isochromosome 12p (see Box 1.4) is positive in 90% of cases. Empirical chemotherapy with cisplatin-based combinations yields response rates of over 50% and up to 30% long-term survival.
4. Patients with neuroendocrine carcinoma of an unknown primary site overlap with extrapulmonary small cell carcinoma, anaplastic islet cell carcinoma, Merkel cell tumours and paragangliomas. Immunocytochemical staining for chromogranin,

neuron-specific enolase, synaptophysin and epithelial antigens (cytokeratins and epithelial membrane antigen) is usually positive. Patients often present with bone metastases and diffuse liver involvement. These tumours are frequently responsive to platinum-based combination chemotherapy. Patients with neuroendocrine cancers may have prolonged survival and their tumours mistakenly identified as adenocarcinomas.

5. Patients with high cervical lymphadenopathy containing squamous cell carcinoma may have occult head and neck tumours of the nasopharynx, oropharynx or hypopharynx. Radical neck dissection followed by extended field radiotherapy that includes these possible primary sites may yield 5-year survival rates of 30%. Adenocarcinoma in high cervical nodes and lower cervical adenopathy containing either histology, however, have a much worse prognosis and should not be treated in this aggressive fashion.

Unfortunately, the majority of unknown primary tumours do not fit into any of these subsets and the response rates to chemotherapy are below 20%. These responses are usually of brief duration, with limited impact on overall survival. The median survival is under 12 months. The exception to this rule is in the group of patients who are under 45 years old. In this group, treatment with BEP (bleomycin, etoposide and cisplatin) or a taxane combination is worthwhile. For this group of patients, 50% survive in excess of 2 years despite the fact that the tumours do not have the characteristics of germ cell cancers and do not stain positively for HCG or AFP.

Table 37.4 Immunohistochemical staining profiles in CUP that suggest a primary tumour site

Primary tumour site	Immunohistochemical profile
Lung (adenocarcinoma, large cell)	CK7+, CK20–, TTF-1+
Lung neuroendocrine (small cell)	Chromogranin+, synaptophysin+, TTF-1+
Colorectal	CK7–, CK20+, CDX-2+
Breast	CK7+, ER+, GCDFP-15+, mammoglobulin+
Prostate	CK7–, CK20–, PSA+
Ovary	CK7+, ER+, WT-1+
Melanoma	S100+. melan-A+, HMB45+
Renal	RCC+, vimentin+, CD10+, PAX-8+
Liver	Hepar+, CD10+, CD13+
Germ cell	PLAP+, OCT-4+
Adrenal	Alpha-inhibin+, melan-A+
Thyroid (follicular, papillary)	TTF-1+, thyroglobuin+

CK, cytokeratin; TTF, thyroid transcription factor; CDX, caudal type homeobox; ER, estrogen receptor; GCDFP, gross cystic disease fluid protein; PSA, prostate-specific antigen; WT, Wilms' tumour; HMB, human melanoma black; RCC, renal cell carcinoma; CD, cluster differentiation; PAX, paired box; PLAP, placental alkaline phosphatase; OCT, octamer binding transcription factor.

Table 37.5 The most common serum tumour markers and their uses

Name	Natural occurrence	Tumour	Comments	Screening	Diagnosis	Prognosis	Follow-up
Carcino embryonic antigen (CEA)	Glycoprotein found in intestinal mucosa during embryonic and foetal life	Colorectal cancer (especially liver metastases), gastric, breast and lung cancers	Elevated in smokers' cirrhosis, chronic hepatitis, UC, Crohn's, pneumonia and TB (usually <10 ng/mL)	No	Yes	Yes	Yes
Alpha-foetoprotein (AFP)	Glycoprotein found in yolk sac and foetal liver	Germ cell tumours (GCTs) (80% non-seminomatous GCTs), hepatocellular cancer (50%), neural tube defects, Down's pregnancies	Role in screening in pregnancy not cancer Only prognostic for GCT not HCC Transient increase in liver diseases	No	Yes	Yes	Yes
Prostate-specific antigen (PSA)	Glycoprotein member of human kallikrein gene family; PSA is a serine protease that liquefies semen in excretory ducts of prostate	Prostate cancer (95%), also benign prostatic hypertrophy and prostatitis (usually <10 ng/mL)	Tissue specific but not tumour specific, although a level of >10 ng/mL is 90% specific for cancer	*	Yes	No	Yes
Cancer antigen 125 (CA-125)	Differentiation antigen of coelomic epithelium (Muller's duct)	Ovarian epithelial cancer (75%), also gastrointestinal, lung and breast cancers	Raised in cirrhosis, chronic pancreatitis, autoimmune diseases and any cause of ascites	*	Yes	No	Yes
Human chorionic gondadotrophin (HCG)	Glycoprotein hormone, 14 kD α subunit and 24 kD β subunit from placental syncytiotrophoblasts	Choriocarcinoma (100%), hydatidiform moles (97%), non-seminomatous GCT (50–80%), seminoma (15%)	Screening post-hydatidiform mole for trophoblastic tumours, also used to follow pregnancies and diagnose ectopic pregnancies	Yes	Yes	Yes	Yes
Calcitonin	32 amino acid peptide from C cells of thyroid	Medullary cell carcinoma of thyroid	Screening test in MEN 2	Yes	Yes	Yes	Yes
Beta-2-microglobulin	Part of HLA common fragment present on surface of lymphocytes, macrophages and some epithelial cells	Non-Hodgkin's lymphoma, myeloma	Elevated in autoimmune disease, renal glomerular disease	No	No	Yes	Yes
Thyroglobulin	Matrix protein for thyroid hormone synthesis in normal thyroid follicles	Papillary and follicular thyroid cancer		No	Yes	No	Yes
Placental alkaline phosphatase (PLAP)	Isoenzyme of alkaline phosphatase	Seminoma and ovarian dysgerminoma (50%)		No	Yes	No	Yes

*See Part 3.
HCC, hepatocellular carcinoma; HLA, human leucocyte antigen; TB, tuberculosis; UC, ulcerative colitis; MEN, multiple endocrine neoplasia.

Histopathological characterization

The histopathological characterization of unknown primaries to establish their origin includes a number of techniques: light microscopy, immunocytochemical staining (Table 37.4), immunophenotyping, electron microscopy, cytogenetics and molecular analysis. These are described in detail in Chapter 3. There are numerous studies investigating the role of molecular diagnostics, including microarray-based gene expression profiling of CUP tumours.

Use of tumour markers

Tumour markers are proteins produced by cancers that are detectable in the blood of patients. Ideally, serum tumour markers should be quick and cheap to measure, have high sensitivity (of more than 50%) and specificity (over 95%) and yield a high predictive value of positive (PPV) and negative (NPV) results. Under these circumstances, tumour markers may be used for population screening, diagnosis, as prognostic factors, for monitoring treatment, diagnosing remission and detecting relapse and for imaging metastases. A large number of serum tumour markers are available, and each may be valuable for any of screening, diagnosis, prognostication and monitoring treatment (Table 37.5).

Approach to investigation of metastatic disease to establish primary site

There is a worrying tendency to over-investigate patients with unknown primary cancer while at the same time ignoring their palliative care needs. So often the greater the eminence and number of consultants whose advice is sought, the larger the number of esoteric investigations ordered, and the less well the patient and their family are informed. Investigations should be restricted to those that will alter clinical management. It is estimated that in the absence of a localizing symptom, extensive radiological investigation leads to the identification of a primary site in less than 5% of all patients. The prognosis is generally poor, with a median survival of 3–4 months. Less than 25% of patients survive to 1 year and less than 10% are alive after 5 years. The site of the primary is usually on the same side of the diaphragm as the metastases, and 75% of tumours are infradiaphragmatic; of the 25% that arise above the diaphragm, nearly all arise from the lung. Where identified, the most common primary sites, in order of frequency, are lung, pancreas, liver, colorectal, stomach, kidney, prostate, ovary, breast, lymphoid and testis. A good performance status is the most important predictor of survival, while extensive weight loss and older age are adverse prognostic factors. With the exception of the five clinical syndromes listed above, treatment other than symptom palliation is rarely appropriate.

 ONLINE RESOURCE

Case Study: A tired retired engineer.

 KEY POINTS

- Cancer of unknown primary is common, accounting for 3% adult cancers
- Whilst histopathological examination frequently identifies a likely primary tumour site, further extensive investigations rarely do
- Frequently the treatment of CUP is palliative, but good responses and occasional long-term survival are seen in younger men and when CUP was a misdiagnosed neuroendocrine tumour
- Tumour markers have important roles in the screening, diagnosis, prognosis and follow-up of cancers and students should be aware of the value of AFP, CA-125, CEA, HCG and PSA as tumour markers

38

Immunodeficiency-related cancers

Learning objectives

✓ Explain the epidemiology and pathogenesis of immunodeficiency-related cancers

✓ Recognize the common presentation and clinical features of immunodeficiency-related cancers

✓ Describe the treatment strategies and outcomes of immunodeficiency-related cancers

---

Two forms of acquired immunodeficiency dominated the last quarter of the 20th century and are responsible for the majority of cancers in the immunosuppressed. Both human immunodeficiency virus (HIV) and iatrogenic immunosuppression following allogenic transplantation are associated with cancers that are linked with oncogenic viruses. The first renal transplant was performed between identical twins by Joseph Murray at Boston's Brigham Hospital in 1953. The development of azathioprine by George Hitchings and Gertrude Elion 10 years later enabled successful allogeneic transplantation and began an era of transplantation medicine dependent upon iatrogenic immunosuppression. The allogeneic organ transplant recipients who received immunosuppressant therapy were found to be prone to post-transplantation lymphoproliferative diseases (PTLDs) and other tumours. The emergence of post-transplant tumours is widely quoted as evidence to support Burnet's immune surveillance theory that states that the immune system acts to remove abnormal clones of cells. In 1949, Frank Macfarlane Burnet described a theory of acquired immunological tolerance, proposing that lymphocytes that were able to respond to self-antigens were deleted in prenatal life. This hypothesis was confirmed experimentally by Peter Medawar who shared the Nobel Prize with Burnet in 1960. Peter Medawar also wrote several wonderful books and collections of essays and I would encourage anyone who is thinking of doing scientific research to read *Advice to a Young Scientist*. In the 1960s, however, in a *volte face* that signalled a paradigm shift, Burnet began to champion the view that a major function of the immune system is to eliminate malignant cells. This was based upon evidence that animals can be immunized against syngeneic transplantable tumours. This theory of immune surveillance led to the identification of tumour antigens and of immunotherapy strategies to treat tumours.

Hereditary or primary immunodeficiency

In addition to these acquired, secondary forms of immunodeficiency, hereditary primary immunodeficiencies, although rare, also predispose to malignancy.

Oncology: Lecture Notes, Third Edition. Mark Bower and Jonathan Waxman.
© 2015 by John Wiley & Sons, Ltd. Published 2015 by John Wiley & Sons, Ltd.
Companion Website: www.lecturenoteseries.com/oncology

Primary immunodeficiencies are mainly single-gene inherited disorders that present in early childhood. They include nearly 100 syndromes, three-quarters of which have been characterized genetically. One important exception is common variable immunodeficiency (CVID), a complex, polygenic disease that often manifests first in early adulthood. Classically, primary immunodeficiency disorders are classified into B-lymphocyte, T-lymphocyte, phagocytic cell and complement deficiencies. This classification is useful, as it helps us establish the clinical manifestations. For example, B-cell deficiencies usually present after the age of 6 months, when maternal antibodies are exhausted, and the most common pathogens are encapsulated bacteria (like *Streptococcus* and *Haemophillus*), fungi (such as *Giardia* and *Cryptosporidia*) and enteroviruses. In contrast, primary T-cell deficiencies usually present within the first 6 months of life, with opportunistic infections, such as *Mycobacterium*, *Candida*, *Pneumocystis jiroveci* and cytomegalovirus. Both B-cell and T-cell primary immunodeficiency may be associated with an increased risk of malignancy (Table 38.1). An increased risk of cancer has not been found with complement deficiencies or phagocyte abnormalities.

Acquired or secondary immunodeficiency

Tumours in allograft recipients

The risk of cancer following an organ transplant varies with the organ that has been transplanted, and the type and duration of the immunosuppressive regimen used post-transplant. Physicians involved in transplantation tend to continue with immunosuppression of their patients for very long periods; however, the duration of immunosuppression required has not been established and the longer the treatment continues the more significant is the risk of malignancy developing. The greatest risk of cancer is with heart and heart–lung transplants because they require more aggressive immunosuppression, but overall more cancers occur in renal transplant recipients as many more renal transplants are performed.

In addition to PTLD that is caused by the Epstein–Barr virus (EBV), the risks of Kaposi's sarcoma (caused by Kaposi sarcoma herpesvirus (KSHV) which is also known as Human Herpesvirus 8 (HHV8)), cervical cancer (caused by human papillomavirus (HPV)) and non-melanoma skin cancers are most dramatically increased. In the case of PTLD and post-transplantation Kaposi's sarcoma, reducing the immunosuppression may sometimes lead to regression of the tumours at an early point in their development when they are still under viral influence but this of course increases the risk of graft rejection. EBV infection generally antedates transplantation occurring in childhood or adolescence. EBV establishes lifelong latent infection in memory lymphocytes following primary infection. Immunosuppression leads to reactivation of latent EBV that drives tumourigenesis. There are stages in the development of EBV-related malignancy that reflect the degree of autonomy of the tumour from its viral master. The risk of cancers after a stem cell transplant in childhood for haematological malignancy is 9%, 20-fold greater than that expected in a non-leukaemic age-matched population. There is a similar increased risk in renal transplantation that is twofold greater than expected in an age-matched population.

Tumours in HIV patients

Studies by the World Health Organization (WHO) estimated that by December 2012, over 30 million people had died of acquired immune deficiency syndrome (AIDS) and 35.3 million people were living with the virus. The number of people newly infected with HIV worldwide is approximately 2.3 million per year and 1.6 million die due to HIV/AIDS. On the brighter side, 9.7 million people living with HIV are on combination antiretroviral therapy (cART) in middle and low income countries where the cost of these drugs is now just $140 per person per year. Along with opportunistic infections, tumours are a major feature of HIV infection. The most frequent tumours in this population are Kaposi's sarcoma (KS), non-Hodgkin's lymphoma and cervical cancer and these three are AIDS-defining illnesses. The management of cancer in the immunodeficient host requires careful attention to the balance between antitumour effects and the toxicity associated with treatment. Combination antiretroviral treatment has both dramatically reduced the incidence of opportunistic infections and prolonged the survival of people with HIV infection. In addition, this highly active cART has reduced the incidence of AIDS-defining malignancies and improved their prognosis. However, although the use of cART reduces the incidence of AIDS-defining cancers, a number of other malignancies occur more frequently in people living with HIV and are not falling with wider use of cART.

Table 38.1 Description of primary immunodeficiency syndromes

Syndrome	Inheritance and incidence	Genetic defect	Immunological defect	Clinical manifestations	Cancer risk
B-cell/antibody deficiency					
X-linked (Bruton's) agammaglobulinemia (XLA)	X-linked recessive (1 in 200,000 male live births)	Defect of Btk Bruton's (B-cell progenitor tyrosine kinase) intracellular signalling path involved in pre-B-cell development. Less often, the mutation is of the mu heavy chain gene	There are virtually no immunoglobulins present in the serum and the number of residual B lymphocytes in blood is very low	Recurrent pyogenic bacterial infections starting aged 6 months after maternal IgG is exhausted. Chronic sinusitis and bronchiectasis may follow	Small increased risk of lymphoma
Common variable immunodeficiency (CVID)	Polygenic, most common primary immunodeficiency (1 in 30,000)		Characterized by variably decreased concentrations of all immunoglobulin classes	Recurrent bacterial infections of the respiratory tract. These disorders are also associated with autoimmune diseases (e.g. Crohn's)	Increased risk of lymphomas and gastrointestinal cancers
Selective IgA deficiency	(1 in 700 live births)	Mapped to chromosome 6p21	No secreted IgA but surface IgA present on B-cells	Common mild onset in childhood. Sinusitis and recurrent lung infections	No increased risk
Hyper IgM syndrome (HIM)	X-linked (CD40 ligand = CD154; <1 in 1,000,000 male live births), autosomal recessive (CD40 or activation-induced deaminase)	Three defects causing lack of isotype class switching from IgM to IgG, IgA and IgE	Excess IgM production but no IgG, IgA or IgE	Prone to opportunistic infections particularly *Pneumocystis carinii* and *Cryptosporidium parvum*. The latter may progress to sclerosing cholangitis and cirrhosis	Liver cancer in X-linked HIM
Hyper IgE syndrome (HIE)	Autosomal dominant	Gene not identified yet. Mapped to chromosome 4q	Elevated IgE, defective neutrophil chemotaxis, impaired lymphocyte response to *Candida* antigen	Recurrent bacterial skin and lung infections, chronic mucocutaneous candidiasis, craniofacial abnormalities, scoliosis and bone fractures	No increased risk
X-linked lymphoproliferative syndrome (XLPS; Duncan's syndrome)	X-linked signalling lymphocyte-activating molecule (SLAM)-associated protein (SAP) (<1 in 1,000,000 male live births)	SLAM activates cytotoxic T-cells and this action is regulated by SAP	Overproduction of polyclonal CD8 + cytotoxic T-cells in response to EBV infection	EBV-induced T-cell proliferation causes severe organ damage, and hypogammaglobulinaemia	Increased risk of EBV-associated lymphomas

(continued)

Table 38.1 (*Continued*)

Syndrome	Inheritance and incidence	Genetic defect	Immunological defect	Clinical manifestations	Cancer risk
T-cell deficiency					
DiGeorge syndrome (thymic aplasia)	Most have deletions of 22q11; 1 in 3500 live births	The third and fourth branchial pouches fail to form properly	Moderate to severe lack of T-cells	Tetany and cardiac malformations just after birth. Lack of T-cells may lead to fungal, viral or other infection in infancy. Increased risk of autoimmune diseases (e.g. thyroiditis)	No increased risk
Severe combined immunodeficiency (SCID) syndromes	Nine genetic (8 autosomal recessive, 1 X-linked) defects of T-cell maturation; 1 in 30,000 live births	Genetic defects affect purine metabolism (e.g. adenosine deaminase), VDJ recombination (e.g. recombinase activating genes) and lymphocyte signalling (e.g. common γ chain of interleukin receptors)	A variety of profound deficiencies of both T-cell and B-cell function	Failure to thrive and repeated infections caused by opportunistic infections by 6 months old. Protracted diarrhoea and death by 2 years in the absence of treatment	None known
DNA-repair defects (see Chapter 2)					
Ataxia telangiectasia (AT; Louis–Bar syndrome)	Autosomal recessive ataxia-telangiectasia mutated (ATM), a protein kinase that reacts to DNA damage and affects the accumulation of p53 (1 in 60,000 live births)	Chromosomal instability due to defective DNA repair may interfere with immunoglobulin and T-cell receptor gene rearrangement	Most have IgA deficiency. Other hypoimmunoglobulinaemia and T-cell function deficits occur	Progressive cerebellar ataxia, skin telangiectasia. Most die in third decade of respiratory infections or tumours	Increased risk of acute leukaemias and lymphomas
Nijmegen breakage syndrome	Autosomal recessive	Chromosomal instability due to defective DNA repair may interfere with immunoglobulin and T-cell receptor gene rearrangement	Lymphopenia	As for AT but in addition have progressive microcephaly (bird-like face)	Increased risk of acute leukaemias and lymphomas
Other					
Wiskott–Aldrich syndrome	X-linked recessive	Defective gene for WASP (Wiskott–Aldrich syndrome protein) involved in cytoskeleton reorganization following activation of platelets and T-cells	Low IgM and raised IgE levels	Thrombocytopenia, eczema and increased autoimmune diseases (including vasculitis). Usually die by age 10 years	Increased risk of EBV-associated lymphomas

Tumours in primary immunodeficiency

The cancers that occur with primary immunodeficiency syndromes are rare and as a consequence treatment protocols and outcome data are scarce. Most patients succumb to infections and these continue to pose a major threat to life during the treatment of associated tumours.

Management of immunodeficiency-associated malignancies

The incidence of congenital immunodeficiency-associated tumours is sufficiently low for there to be little consensus upon their clinical management. In contrast, the incidence of both PTLD and KS has risen dramatically in recent years with the spread of the HIV pandemic and the marked increase in transplant surgery. The management of PTLD relies upon enhanced immunity against EBV by reducing immunosuppression and infusing cytotoxic T lymphocytes against EBV. In addition, antiviral agents, low-dose chemotherapy and anti-CD20 monoclonal antibodies may be useful. The introduction of cART has reduced the incidence of HIV-associated KS in established market economies where this treatment is available. Moreover, early-stage KS may be successfully treated with cART alone, leading to regression of KS (Figure 38.1). Visceral KS is usually treated with systemic liposomal anthracycline chemotherapy with concomitant cART. Other tumours that arise in

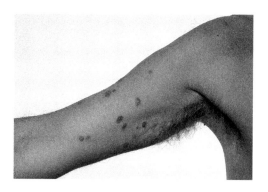

Figure 38.1 Multiple pigmented Kaposi sarcoma skin lesion in a man with HIV infection. Following combination antiretroviral therapy (cART) alone there was a marked regression of these lesions.

immunodeficient individuals are generally treated along conventional lines, with extra attention to the risk of infectious complications of therapy.

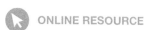 ONLINE RESOURCE

Case Study: The purple spotted geek.

 KEY POINTS

- The risk of cancer in people with immunodeficiency is greatly increased and most immunodeficiency-related cancers have a viral oncogenesis
- The risk of immunodeficiency-related cancer rises with degree of immunodeficiency, so combination antiretroviral therapy for HIV reduces the risk of AIDS-defining cancers

Part 3

The practice of oncology

Paraneoplastic complications of cancer

Paraneoplastic complications of malignancy are remote effects of cancer that occur without local spread. Most of these paraneoplastic syndromes arise due to secretion by tumours of hormones, cytokines and growth factors. Paraneoplastic syndromes also arise when normal cells secrete products in response to the presence of tumour cells. For example, antibodies produced in this fashion are responsible for many paraneoplastic neurological syndromes including cerebellar degeneration, Lambert–Eaton myasthenic syndrome and paraneoplastic retinopathy. Paraneoplastic neurological complications always appear on the list of differential diagnoses. However, just as viewers of *House MD* will know that "it's not lupus", it is rarely paraneoplastic either.

Paraneoplastic endocrine complications

Cushing's syndrome

Cushing's syndrome is a clinical disorder resulting from prolonged exposure to excess glucocorticoids and should not be confused with Cushing's disease which refers exclusively to those cases that arise due to an adrenocorticotrophic hormone (ACTH) secreting pituitary adenoma (Table 39.1). Clinically overt Cushing's syndrome caused by ectopic secretion of ACTH by non-endocrine-derived tumours is

rare. Approximately 20% of cases of Cushing's syndrome are caused by ectopic ACTH secretion by a tumour that is frequently occult at presentation. For this reason the differential diagnosis between pituitary adenoma and ectopic ACTH is important clinically but biochemical overlap often makes this difficult. More than half the cases of ectopic ACTH syndrome are due to small cell lung cancer, with carcinoid tumours and neural crest tumours (phaeochromocytoma, neuroblastoma, medullary cell carcinoma of the thyroid) accounting for a further 15%. The typical presentation is of a middle-aged smoker with features of severe hypercortisolism and hypokalaemic metabolic alkalosis. Patients have muscle weakness or atrophy, oedema, hypertension, mental changes, glucose intolerance and weight loss. When ectopic ACTH production arises from a more benign tumour, for example, bronchial carcinoid or thymoma, the other classic features of Cushing's syndrome may be present including truncal obesity, moon facies and cutaneous striae (Figure 39.1).

The diagnosis of Cushing's syndrome may be confirmed by elevated urinary free cortisol, loss of diurnal variation of plasma cortisol and failure of cortisol suppression in the low-dose dexamethasone (2 mg) test. After establishing the diagnosis, an elevated plasma ACTH supports the diagnosis of pituitary adenoma or ectopic ACTH syndrome. Failure of cortisol suppression following high-dose dexamethasone (2 mg four times daily for 2 days, or 8 mg overnight) and very high levels of ACTH (>200 pg/mL)

Oncology: Lecture Notes, Third Edition. Mark Bower and Jonathan Waxman.
© 2015 by John Wiley & Sons, Ltd. Published 2015 by John Wiley & Sons, Ltd.
Companion Website: www.lecturenoteseries.com/oncology

Table 39.1 Aetiology of Cushing's syndrome

Type	Example
ACTH dependent	Pituitary adenoma (Cushing's disease)
	Ectopic ACTH secretion
	Ectopic CRH secretion (very rare)
ACTH independent	Exogenous glucocorticoid administration
	Adrenal adenoma
	Adrenal carcinoma
	Nodular adrenal hyperplasia

ACTH, adrenocorticotrophic hormone; CRH, corticotrophin-releasing hormone.

suggest an ectopic source of ACTH. In difficult cases, a corticotrophin-releasing hormone (CRH) stimulation test, selective venous catheterization of the inferior petrosal sinus with ACTH estimations, somatostatin analogue scintigraphy and technetium-99 methoxyisobutylisonitrile (MIBI) imaging may be necessary to determine the source of ACTH.

The mainstay of palliative therapy for Cushing's syndrome due to ectopic ACTH production is inhibition of steroid synthesis, although inhibition of ACTH release and blocking glucocorticoid receptors have also been attempted. Several steroid synthesis inhibitors are available and successful use in these circumstances has been reported with aminoglutethamide, metyrapone, mitotane, ketoconazole and octreotide. On rare occasions laparoscopic bilateral adrenalectomy or adrenal artery embolization may be necessary to control symptoms.

Syndrome of inappropriate antidiuresis

Hyponatraemia is a common finding in association with advanced malignancy and many factors may contribute including cardiac and hepatic failure, hyperglycaemia and diuretics. However, the detection of concentrated urine in conjunction with hypo-osmolar plasma suggests abnormal renal free water excretion and the presence of the syndrome of inappropriate antidiuresis (SIAD). This acronym is

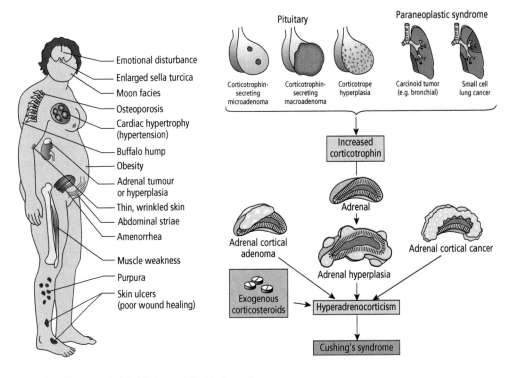

Figure 39.1 Causes and clinical features of Cushing's syndrome.

Table 39.2 Causes of the syndrome of inappropriate diuresis (SIAD)

Source of ADH	Examples
Ectopic ADH production	
Malignancy	Small cell lung cancer
Inappropriate pituitary secretion of ADH	
Malignancy	Lung cancer
	Lymphoma
Inflammatory lung disease	Pneumonia
	Lung abscess
Neurological disease	Meningitis
	Head injury
	Subdural haematoma
	Surgery
Drugs	Antidepressants (tricyclics, SSRIs)
	Carbamazepine
	Chlorpropamide
	Phenothiazines
	Vincristine
	Cyclophosphamide
	Ecstasy*
Postoperative	
Others	Hypothyroidism
	Porphyria
	Addison's disease

ADH, antidiuretic hormone; SSRI, selective serotonin reuptake inhibitor.
*Excessive water consumption may contribute to the development of hyponatraemia with ecstasy.

Table 39.3 Diagnosis of the syndrome of inappropriate diuresis (SIAD)

Essential criteria to establish diagnosis

Plasma hypo-osmolality (plasma osmolality <275 mosmol/kg water and plasma sodium <135 mmol/L)

Concentrated urine (plasma osmolality >100 mosmol/kg water)

Normal plasma/extracellular fluid volume

High urinary sodium on a normal salt and water intake (urine sodium >20 mmol/L)

Exclude (i) hypothyroidism, (ii) hypoadrenalism and (iii) diuretics

Supportive criteria for diagnosis

Abnormal water load test (unable to excrete >90% of a 20 mL/kg water load in 4 hours and/or failure to dilute urine to osmolality <100 mosmol/kg water)

Elevated plasma arginine vasopressin levels

better than the previous term "syndrome of inappropriate antidiuretic hormone" (SIADH), since there is no vasopressin (ADH) secretion in approximately 15% of cases. In malignancy-related SIAD, tumours secrete ectopic arginine vasopressin or vasopressin-like peptides. In many respects SIAD is the opposite of diabetes insipidus; patients with SIAD are waterlogged with low plasma osmolality and sodium and high urine osmolality, whilst patients with diabetes insipidus are dehydrated with high plasma osmolality and sodium and low urine osmolality. SIAD is most frequently associated with small cell lung cancer or carcinoid tumours but has also been described in pancreatic, oesophageal, prostatic and haematological malignancies. Nonetheless many factors may contribute to SIAD (Table 39.2). Ecstasy (MDMA, methylenedioxymethamphetamine) is another cause of SIAD although over-drinking water at raves may contribute to the hyponatraemia too.

Significant symptoms of hyponatraemia appear at plasma sodium levels below 125 mmol/L, with confusion progressing to stupor, coma and seizures as levels fall. Nausea, vomiting and focal neurological deficits may also occur. The clinical features depend on both the levels of plasma sodium and the rate of decline. With gradual falls in sodium, the brain cells are able to compensate against cerebral oedema by secreting potassium and other intracellular solutes. Asymptomatic hyponatraemia therefore suggests chronic SIAD rather than acute SIAD. The division into chronic and acute SIAD is of therapeutic importance as their management differs. The diagnosis of SIAD requires the demonstration of plasma hyponatraemia and hypo-osmolality in the presence of concentrated urine and normal extracellular fluid volume (Table 39.3).

The management of SIAD depends upon the rate of onset of hyponatraemia and the presence of neurological complications. Acute SIAD with an onset over 2–3 days and falls in serum sodium in excess of 0.5 mmol/L per day are associated with neurological sequelae and require prompt correction by intravenous hypertonic saline. However, correcting the plasma sodium too fast can also lead to severe neurological consequences including central pontine myelinolysis, an osmotic demyelination that causes acute paralysis, dysphagia, dysarthria and coma (Figure 39.2). Hyponatraemia should not be corrected faster than 10 mmol/L/24 hours. In contrast, the mainstay of therapy for chronic asymptomatic SIAD is

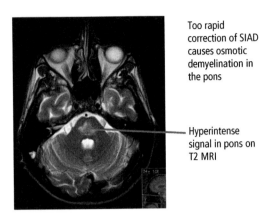

Too rapid correction of SIAD causes osmotic demyelination in the pons

Hyperintense signal in pons on T2 MRI

Figure 39.2 Central pontine myelinolysis.

fluid restriction and inhibition of tubular reabsorption of water with drugs including the tetracycline antibiotic demeclocycline.

Non-islet cell tumour hypoglycaemia

Tumour-related hypoglycaemia is a frequent complication of β-islet cell tumours of the pancreas that secrete insulin (insulinomas), see Chapter 10, but occurs uncommonly with non-islet cell tumours. Most non-islet cell tumours produce hypoglycaemia through increased glucose use or by secreting insulin-like growth factors (IGF1 and IGF2). Non-islet cell tumours associated with hypoglycaemia are usually large retroperitoneal or intrathoracic sarcomas. Unlike other endocrine complications of malignancy, hypoglycaemia is very rarely associated with lung cancer. The clinical manifestations are due to cerebral hypoglycaemia and secondary secretion of catecholamines; they include agitation, stupor, coma and seizures that may follow exercise or fasting. Tumour-related hypoglycaemia should be differentiated from other causes of hypoglycaemia including drugs, for example, sulphonylureas, hypoadrenalism, hypopituitarism and liver failure. In advanced malignancy the most common cause of hypoglycaemia is continued oral hypoglycaemic medication in long-standing diabetics.

Enteropancreatic hormone syndromes

Enteropancreatic hormone production is relatively uncommon in malignant disease. A variety of clinical syndromes occur associated with hormone secretion by endocrine tumours of the pancreas and less frequently tumours arising in other organs (see Chapter 10). The majority of pancreatic islet cell tumours are malignant with the exception of most insulinomas, and metastases are frequently present at diagnosis. For many patients the distressing clinical manifestations arising from excessive secretion of gastrointestinal peptides require palliation and this may be difficult to achieve. These tumours often secrete more than one polypeptide hormone and may switch their hormone production during follow-up.

Carcinoid syndrome

Carcinoid tumours arise from enterochromaffin cells principally in the gastrointestinal tract, pancreas and lungs but occasionally in the thymus and gonads (see Chapter 23). Chromaffin cells stain with or have an affinity for chromium salts, usually because the cells contain catecholamines. One in ten patients with carcinoid tumours develops the carcinoid syndrome after the development of hepatic metastases. This avoids the first pass metabolism of 5-hydroxytryptamine (serotonin, 5HT) and kinins in the liver so that the systemic symptoms occur. The acute symptoms are vasomotor flushing (typically of upper body lasting up to 30 minutes), fever, pruritic wheals, diarrhoea, asthma/wheezing, borborygmi and abdominal pain. Chronic complications include tricuspid regurgitation, arthropathy, pulmonary stenosis, mesenteric fibrosis, cirrhosis, pellagra (due to secondary deficiency of trytophan) and telangiectasia. The diagnostic investigation is 24-hour urinary collection of 5-hydroxyindole-acetic acid (5HIAA), a metabolite of 5HT. Somatostatin analogues are considered by most physicians to be the first-line treatment of choice for patients with carcinoid syndrome and indeed most enteropancreatic hormone syndromes. Palliation of the clinical manifestations of carcinoid syndrome includes symptomatic therapy of diarrhoea with codeine phosphate, loperamide or diphenoxylate, β$_2$-adrenergic agonists for wheezing, and avoiding precipitating factors to reduce flushing such as including alcohol and some foods.

Phaeochromocytoma

Phaeochromocytomas arise from the chromaffin cells of the sympathetic nervous system, most frequently in the adrenal medulla but occasionally from sympathetic ganglia (see Chapter 22). Phaeochromocytomas commonly secrete norepinephrine (noradrenaline) and epinephrine (adrenaline) but in some cases significant quantities of dopamine are also

Box 39.1 Oncological mnemonics

Causes of hypercalcaemia: GRIM FED

Granulomas (TB, sarcoid)

Renal failure

Immobility

Malignancy

Familial (familial hypocalciuric hypercalcaemia)

Endocrine **PATH** (**p**haeochromocytoma, **A**ddison's, **t**hyrotoxicosis, **h**yperparathyroidism)

Drugs (thiazides, lithium, vitamins A and D, milk alkali syndrome)

Causes of SIADH: SIADH

Surgery

Intracranial (infection, head injury, cerebrovascular accident)

Alveolar (pus, cancer)

Drugs **ABCD** (**a**nalgesics: opiates, non-steroidal anti-inflammatory drugs, **b**arbiturates, **c**yclophosphamide/**c**arbamazepine/**c**hlorpromazine, **d**iuretic: thiazides)

Hormonal (hypothyroid, Addison's)

Causes of Cushingoid features: CUSHINGOID

Cataracts

Ulcers

Striae

Hypertension, hirsutism

Infections

Necrosis (avascular necrosis of femoral head)

Glycouria, glycaemia

Osteoporosis, obesity

Immunosuppression

Diabetes

Phaeochromocytoma: rule of 10s

This mnemonic applies to *adults* with phaeochromocytomas.

10% are extra-adrenal

10% are bilateral or multiple

10% are malignant

10% are familial

Phaeochromocytoma symptoms: 5 Hs

Headache

Hypertension

Hypotension (postural)

Heartbeat (palpitations)

Hyperhidrosis (sweating)

Causes of gynaecomastia: GYNAECOMASTIA

Genetic (Kleinfelter's, Kallman's)

Youth (puberty)*

Neonate*

Antifungals (ketoconazole)

Estrogen

Cirrhosis/cimetidine

Old age*

Marijuana

Alcoholism

Spirolonactone/stilboestrol

Tumours (testicular, adrenal)

Isoniazid

Alkylating agents

Causes of clubbing: CLUBBING

Cyanotic congenital heart disease

Lung disease (abscess, bronchiectasis, cystic fibrosis, empyema, fibrosing alveolitis)

Ulcerative colitis/Crohn's disease

Biliary cirrhosis

Birth defect (hereditary pachydermoperiostosis)

Infective endocarditis

Neoplasia (non-small cell lung cancer, mesothelioma, gastrointestinal lymphoma)

Goitre (thyrotoxicosis)

Features of MEN

MEN 1: 3Ps

Pituitary adenoma

Pancreatic islet cell tumours

Parathyroid

MEN 2: 2Cs

Catecholamines (phaeochromocytoma)

Cell carcinoma (medullary) of thyroid

Plus:

MEN 2a: parathyroid tumours

MEN 2b (also known as MEN 3): mucocutaneous neuromas

* Physiological causes

produced. Phaeochromocytomas are associated with a number of familial inherited cancer syndromes including multiple endocrine neoplasia (MEN) 2a, MEN 2b, von Hippel–Lindau syndrome and neurofibromatosis. The catecholamines cause intermittent, episodic or sustained hypertension and other clinical manifestations including anxiety, tremor, palpitations, sweating, flushing, headaches, gastrointestinal disturbances and polyuria. These symptoms are all attributable to excessive adrenergic stimulation.

Plasma or 24-hour urinary collection for urinary free catecholamines (epinephrine, norepinephrine and dopamine) are the most widely employed diagnostic tests although some centres also measure catecholamine metabolites such as metanephrines and vanillylmandelic acid (VMA). The tumour may be localized by radiolabelled meta-iodobenzyl guanidine (MIBG) scintigraphy.

Initial treatment should be α-blockade to control hypertension followed by β-blockade to control tachycardia. This combination will control symptoms in most patients with malignant phaeochromocytoma. If palliation is not achieved, high-dose ^{131}I-MIBG may be used as therapy for phaeochromocytoma and neuroblastoma as it reduces catecholamine synthesis. This may only have a chance of success if the patient has small volume metastases, because ^{131}I-MIBG is β-emitting and β-particles have poor tissue penetration.

Gynaecomastia

Gynaecomastia results from elevation in the oestrogen/androgen ratio, which may be either a consequence of decreased androgen production or activity or increased oestrogen formation, usually by peripheral aromatization of circulating androgens to oestrogens. In men with advanced cancer, gynaecomastia is most often a consequence of drug therapy, either chemotherapy (alkylating agents, vinca alkaloids, nitrosoureas), anti-emetics (metoclopramide, phenothiazines) or anti-androgens (cyproterone acetate, flutamide, bicalutamide). Occasionally other tumour secretion of oestrogens or gonadotrophins may be responsible. Tumours may either secrete oestrogens (Leydig cell testicular tumours and feminizing adrenocortical tumours), promote the conversion of androgens to oestrogens (Sertoli cell testicular tumours and hepatoma) or secrete human chorionic gonadotrophin (HCG) (testicular tumours, non-small cell lung cancers, hepatoma and islet cell tumours of the pancreas).

Paraneoplastic neurological conditions

In contrast to the metabolic and endocrine paraneoplastic conditions where products secreted by the tumours are responsible, most neurological paraneoplastic syndromes are immune mediated. Moreover with neurological paraneoplastic syndromes, the tumour may be asymptomatic or occult. It is thought that antibodies reacting to antigens on the surface of cancer cells cross-react with neural antigens and are the basis of these syndromes. The antibodies may be directed at ion channels, for example, the presynaptic P-type voltage-gated calcium channel in the case of Lambert–Eaton myasthenic syndrome and the nicotinic acetylcholine receptor in myasthenia gravis. Alternatively, antibodies may bind intracellular proteins such as Hu, a neuronal nuclear RNA-binding protein, and Yo, a cytoplasmic protein in Purkinje cells of the cerebellum. The most common paraneoplastic neurological manifestations are described in association with small cell lung cancer (Table 39.4; see also Figure 39.3).

Paraneoplastic dermatological conditions

A number of paraneoplastic dermatological manifestations have been described, and some are listed in Table 39.5 and shown in Figures 39.4 and 39.5. Amongst the most common paraneoplastic dermatological manifestation is finger clubbing (Figure 39.6), a clinical sign beloved of physicians and first described by Hippocrates over 2400 years ago. It is characterized by softening of the nail bed and periungual erythema with loss of the normal 15° angle at the hyponychium. As this advances, bulging of the distal phalynx and curvature of the nail lead to a drumstick end appearance. Clubbing may be associated with hypertrophic osteoarthropathy with new subperiosteal cancellous bone formation at the distal ends of long bones, particularly the radius and ulna or tibia and fibula (Figure 39.7). A hereditary form of clubbing with hypertrophic osteo-arthropathy, Touraine–Solente-Golé syndrome, has recently been shown to be due to germline mutations of the 15-hydroxyprostaglandin dehydrogenase gene that catabolizes prostaglandin E2. Whether paraneoplastic clubbing is due to

Table 39.4 Paraneoplastic neurological manifestations

Condition	Clinical features	Antibodies	Percentages that are paraneoplastic	Underlying malignancy
Dermatomyositis	Erythematous rash, arthralgia	Anti-Jo-1	20	NSCLC, SCLC, lymphoma
Encephalomyelitis	Fluctuating confusion, anxiety, depression, impaired short-term memory	Anti-Hu, anti-CV2	10	SCLC, thymoma
Lambert–Eaton syndrome	Proximal muscle weakness sparing eyes; power increases with repetition	Anti-VGCC	60	SCLC
Myasthenia gravis	Muscle fatigability, ptosis, ophthalmoplegia	Anti-AChR	5	Thymoma
Opsoclonus–myoclonus syndrome	Opsoclonus (irregular, rapid, horizontal and vertical eye movements) and myoclonus (brief, shock-like muscle spasms), intention tremor, unsteady gait	Anti-Hu, anti-Ri	20–50	Neuroblastoma, breast
Polymyositis	Proximal muscle weakness, rash	Anti-Jo-1	10	NSCLC, SCLC, lymphoma
Retinopathy	Night blindness, ring scotomas, photosensitivity	Anti-recoverin		SCLC, melanoma
Sensory neuropathy	Rapid progressive loss of all sensory modalities, especially proprioception	Anti-Hu	10–20	SCLC
Subacute cerebellar degeneration	Ataxia, nystagmus, dysarthria	Anti-Yo, anti-Hu, anti-VGCC, anti-Tr	50	SCLC, ovary, Hodgkin's

NSCLC, non-small cell lung cancer; SCLC, small cell lung cancer.

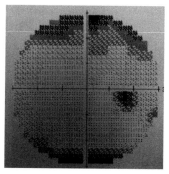
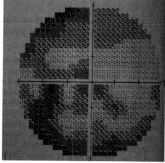

Figure 39.3 Paraneoplastic retinopathy. Cancer-associated paraneoplastic retinopathy in a patient with small cell lung cancer. She experienced both visual loss and flickering of light. The visual field test show bilateral heterogenous visual loss. Anti-recoverin antibodies were present in the plasma.

Table 39.5 Paraneoplastic dermatological conditions

Condition	Clinical features	Underlying malignancy
Acanthosis nigricans	Grey-brown, symmetrical, velvety plaques on neck, axillae and flexor areas	Adenocarcinoma, predominantly gastric
Acquired ichthyosis	Generalized dry, cracking skin; hyperkeratotic palms and soles	Hodgkin's disease, lymphomas, myeloma
Acrokeratosis paraneoplastica (Bazex syndrome)	Symmetrical psoriasiform hyperkeratosis with scales and pruritis on toes, ears and nose; nail dystrophy	Squamous carcinoma of oesophagus, head and neck and lungs
Bullous pemphigoid	Large tense blisters, antibodies to desmoplakin	Lymphomas and others
Cushing's syndrome	Broad purple striae, plethora, telangiectasia, mild hirsutism	Small cell lung cancer, thyroid, testis, ovary and adrenal tumours, pancreatic islet cell tumours, pituitary tumours
Dermatitis herpetiformis	Pleomorphic, symmetrical, subepidermal bullae	Lymphoma and others
Dermatomyositis	Erythema or telangiectasia of knuckles and periorbital regions	Miscellaneous tumours
Erythema annulare centrifugum	Slowly migrating annular red lesions	Prostate tumours, myeloma and others
Erythema gyratum repens	Progressive scaling erythema with pruritis	Lung, breast, uterus and gastrointestinal tumours
Exfoliative dermatitis	Progressive erythema followed by scaling	Cutaneous T-cell lymphoma, Hodgkin's disease and other lymphomas
Flushing	Episodic reddening of face and neck	Carcinoid syndrome, medullary cell carcinoma of the thyroid
Generalized melanosis	Diffuse grey-brown skin pigmentation	Melanoma, ACTH-producing tumours
Hirsutism	Increased hair in male distribution	Adrenal tumours, ovarian tumours
Hypertrichosis lanuginosa	Rapid development of fine, long, silky hair	Lung, colon, bladder, uterus and gallbladder tumours
Muir–Torre syndrome Necrolytic migratory erythema	Sebaceous gland neoplasm Circinate area of blistering and erythema on face, abdomen and limbs	Colon cancer, lymphoma Islet cell tumour of the pancreas (glucagonoma)
Pachydermoperiostosis	Thickening of skin folds, lips and ears; macroglossia; clubbing; excessive sweating	Lung cancer
Paget's disease of the nipple	Red keratotic patch over areola, nipple or accessory breast tissue	Breast cancer
Pemphigus vulgaris	Bullae of skin and oral blisters	Lymphomas, breast cancer
Pruritis	Generalized itching	Lymphoma, leukaemia, myeloma, central nervous system tumours, abdominal tumours
Sign of Leser–Trelat	Sudden onset of large number of seborrhoeic keratoses	Adenocarcinoma of the stomach, lymphoma, breast cancer

(continued)

Table 39.5 Paraneoplastic dermatological conditions (*Continued*)

Condition	Clinical features	Underlying malignancy
Sweet's syndrome	Painful, raised, red plaques; fever; neutrophilia	Leukaemias
Systemic nodular panniculitis (Weber–Christian disease)	Recurrent crops of tender, violaceous, subcutaneous nodules, which may be accompanied by abdominal pain and fat necrosis in bone marrow and lungs	Adenocarcinoma of the pancreas
Tripe palms	Hyperpigmented, velvety, thickened palms with exaggerated ridges	Gastric and lung cancer

ACTH, adrenocorticotrophic hormone.

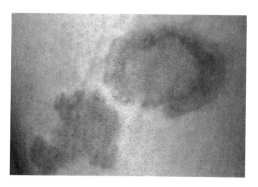

Figure 39.4 Necrolytic migratory erythema. Paraneoplastic rash in a patient with a pancreatic glucagonoma.

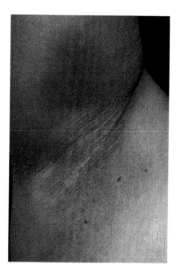

Figure 39.5 Acanthosis nigricans. Velvety axillary pigmentation in a woman with cancer of the gastrooesophageal junction.

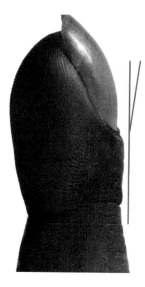

Angle between nail bed and nail fold <15°

Figure 39.6 Finger nail clubbing is characterized by increased longitudinal curving of the nail, loss of the angle between the nail and its bed and bogginess of the nail fold.

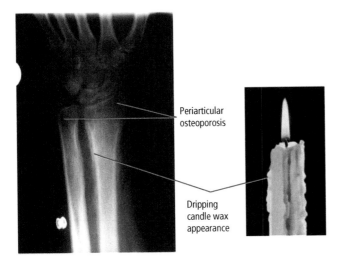

Periarticular osteoporosis

Dripping candle wax appearance

Figure 39.7 Forearm radiograph showing a periosteal reaction in the metaphysis and diaphysis of the radius and ulnar and periarticular osteoporosis due to hypertrophic osteoarthropathy secondary to non-small cell lung cancer (squamous cell).

elevated levels of prostaglandin E2 or tumour-related secretion of growth factors, including PDGF (platelet-derived growth factor) and HGF (hepatocyte growth factor), remains unclear.

Cachexia

Cachexia or severe protein-calorie malnutrition is one of the most debilitating and life-threatening aspects of cancer. This highly distressing symptom severely impairs the quality of life of many patients with cancer but is the focus of relatively little research. The normal balance between hunger and satiety, anorexia and obesity in humans is maintained by the equilibrium between adipose-derived hormones including

leptin and gut-derived hormones including ghrelin. An empty stomach stimulates ghrelin release which acts to promote neuropeptide Y (NPY) and Agouti-related peptide (AgRP) secretion in the hypothalamus, resulting in stimulation of the hunger centre. At the same time, ghrelin inhibits the release of pro-opiomelanocortin (POMC) hormones including α-melanocyte-stimulating hormone (MSH) from the hypothalamus, thus inhibiting the satiety centre and blocking anorexigenic pathways. Leptin, which is produced by fat cells, antagonizes ghrelin's actions on the hypothalamus by inhibiting NPY and AgRP release and stimulating α-MSH secretion (Figure 39.8). Amongst the mechanisms invoked in cancer cachexia is the disruption of this delicate homoeostatic mechanism. In addition, tumour-related secretion of pro-inflammatory cytokines including interleukin-1

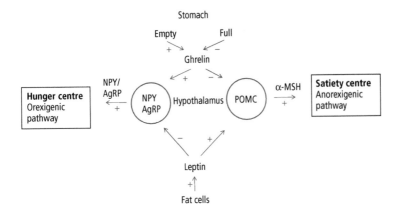

Figure 39.8 Schematic diagram of the hypothalamic control of hunger (see text for abbreviations).

(IL-1) and interleukin-6 (IL-6), interferon gamma (IFN-γ) and tumour necrosis factor alpha (TNF-α) are thought to play a role in the pathogenesis of cancer cachexia. These effects may be mediated partly via the hypothalamic leptin/gherlin axis. Another clue to cancer cachexia has been found with the identification of proteolysis-inducing factor (PIF) and lipid-mobilizing factor (LMF). PIF causes breakdown of muscle proteins in skeletal muscle by activating the ubiquitin proteosome pathway and levels of PIF are raised in cancer patients with wasting. LMF, which is produced by tumour cells, causes lipolysis by raising the levels of the mitochondrial uncoupling proteins that turn brown fat into heat in hibernating animals.

Severe weight loss shortens survival and decreases quality of life substantially, indeed for many malignancies weight loss of >10% body weight is an independent adverse prognostic factor. The two major options for pharmacological therapy that aim to enhance appetite are progestogens, such as megestrol acetate, and corticosteroids. Neither these drugs nor enteral or parenteral nutrition has proved universally beneficial,

and both approaches are associated with appreciable toxicity. This is particularly so for corticosteroids, which, although they stimulate appetite, are catabolic in effect, leading to muscle loss. As the molecular aetiology of cancer cachexia is unveiled, novel therapeutic strategies are emerging.

 KEY POINTS

- Paraneoplastic complications of malignancy are remote effects of cancer attributed to the secretion by tumours of hormones, cytokines and growth factors or when normal cells secrete products in response to the presence of tumour cells
- The most common cancer associated with most paraneoplastic complications is small cell lung cancer, although finger clubbing is most common with squamous cell lung cancer
- Paraneoplastic complications of cancer often regress with successful treatment of the cancer

40

Oncological emergencies

Learning objectives

✓ List the common oncological emergencies

✓ Describe the clinical presentation, investigation and management of the common oncological emergencies

---

Over the last couple of years a new discipline of acute oncology has emerged in the United Kingdom that covers the care of non-elective inpatients with cancer. The role of the multi-disciplinary acute oncology team is to manage patients admitted with the complications of their cancer and its treatment. These emergencies can be divided into tumour- and treatment-related complications (Table 40.1).

Metabolic disorders

Hypercalcaemia

One in ten cancer patients develops hypercalcaemia, and malignancy accounts for about half the cases of hypercalcaemia amongst hospital inpatients. Hypercalcaemia occurs most frequently with myeloma, breast, lung and renal cancers, and 20% of cases occur in the absence of bone metastases. Hypercalcaemia, except in patients with myeloma, carries a poor prognosis and is associated with a median survival of 3 months. Most patients with hypercalcaemia of malignancy have disseminated disease and 80% die within 1 year. Thus hypercalcaemia is usually a complication of advanced disease and its treatment should be directed at palliation as it may produce a number of distressing symptoms (Table 40.2). The treatment of hypercalcaemia of malignancy frequently ameliorates these symptoms, and for this reason the diagnosis should always be sought.

In recent years there have been significant advances in our understanding of the biochemical processes that cause hypercalcaemia in malignancy, such that the factors involved in local osteolysis and in the evolution of humoral hypercalcaemia have now been delineated. A number of different cytokines have been implicated in the development of hypercalcaemia as a result of local osteolysis. The final common pathway of osetolysis at the molecular level involves a triad of osteoprotegerin (OPG), Receptor Activator of NF kappa B (RANK) and Receptor Activator of NF kappa B Ligand (RANKL). Bone destruction in the presence of osteolytic skeletal metastases is not caused directly by tumour cells but by osteoclasts. The tumour cells either directly produce RANKL or stimulate bone stromal cells to produce RANKL. RANKL is an osteoclast-activating factor that stimulates the RANK membrane receptor on osteoclast precursors. In conjunction with macrophage colony-stimulating factor (M-CSF), RANKL causes the differentiation of precursors into osteoclasts and the fusion and activation of osteoclasts into functional multinucleated osteoclasts that mediate bone resorption. OPG is a soluble decoy receptor for RANKL that inhibits RANK by competing for RANKL binding. OPG production is decreased in myeloma and metastatic prostate cancer. This RANKL/RANK/OPG equilibrium is disrupted by cytokines, chemokines and prostaglandins, uncoupling the usual homeostatic balance between osteoclastic bone resorption and osteoblastic bone formation.

Oncology: Lecture Notes, Third Edition. Mark Bower and Jonathan Waxman.
© 2015 by John Wiley & Sons, Ltd. Published 2015 by John Wiley & Sons, Ltd.
Companion Website: www.lecturenoteseries.com/oncology

Table 40.1 Classification of common oncological emergencies

Tumour related	Treatment related
Metabolic disorders	*Metabolic disorders*
Hypercalcaemia	Hyperkalaemia
Hyponatraemia	Hyperuricaemia
Hyperkalaemia	Tumour lysis
Hyperuricaemia	
Hypoglycaemia	
Mechanical disorders	*Haematological disorders*
Superior vena cava	Neutropenia
obstruction	Anaemia
Spinal cord compression	Thrombocytopenia
Intestinal obstruction	Hyperviscosity
Hydrocephalus	Venous catheter
Bronchial obstruction	thrombosis
Urinary obstruction	
Thrombosis	
Effusions	*Infections*
Pericardial effusion	Febrile neutropenia
Ascites	Opportunistic infections
Pleural effusion	

Humoral hypercalcaemia was described in 1941 by Albright but it was only in the late 1980s that the humoral factor causing hypercalcaemia was characterized. In the 1970s hypercalcaemia was thought to result from the ectopic production of parathyroid hormone (PTH), but this hypothesis remained unproven because the use of PTH antisera failed to demonstrate excessive secretion of PTH in patients with humoral hypercalcaemia. In addition, low serum concentrations of 1,25-vitamin D3 and urinary cyclic adenosine monophosphate (AMP) levels failed to reflect excess PTH activity and no PTH mRNA was found in the tumours of patients with humoral hypercalcaemia.

In the late 1980s polyadenylated RNA from a renal carcinoma from a patient with humoral hypercalcaemia was used to construct a cDNA library which was screened with a codon-preference oligonucleotide, synthesized on the basis of a partial N-terminal amino acid sequence from a human tumour-derived peptide and a 2.0-kilobase cDNA was identified. The cDNA encoded a 177 amino acid prohormone, which consisted of a 36 amino acid leader sequence that is cleaved to produce a 141 amino acid, mature peptide and PTH-related peptide. The first 13 amino acids of the mature peptide have a sequence homology with PTH, and the N-terminal sequence is thought to be the PTH receptor-binding region. It turns out that PTH-related peptide is expressed in most normal human tissue, but its role is undetermined. The gene for PTH-related peptide has been mapped to the short arm of chromosome 12 whilst the PTH gene is on the short arm of chromosome 11. The gene for PTH-related peptide is complex and contains a six exon, 12 kilobase, single copy sequence, encoding up to five mRNA species. Exons 2, 3 and 4 are similar to the PTH gene.

A radioimmunoassay for PTH-related peptide was used to screen patients with hypercalcaemia-associated malignancy and the results contrasted with patients who were normocalcaemic and had malignant disease, patients with primary hyperparathyroidism and normal controls. PTH-related peptide was elevated in 19 of 39 (49%) patients with malignant hypercalcaemia, 12 of 74 (16%) normocalcaemic patients with malignancy and 4 of 20 patients (20%) with hyperparathyroidism, but in none of 22 normal controls.

The clinical manifestations of hypercalcaemia are varied (Table 40.2) and many symptoms may be wrongly attributed to the underlying malignancy. A diagnosis of hypercalcaemia can only be made by biochemical investigation, so all symptomatic patients

Table 40.2 Clinical features of hypercalcaemia of malignancy

General	Gastrointestinal	Neurological	Cardiological
Dehydration	Anorexia	Fatigue	Bradycardia
Polydipsia	Weight loss	Lethargy	Atrial arrhythmias
Polyuria	Nausea	Confusion	Ventricular arrhythmias
Pruritis	Vomiting	Myopathy	Prolonged P-R interval
	Constipation	Hyporeflexia	Reduced Q-T interval
	Ileus	Seizures	Wide T waves
		Psychosis	
		Coma	

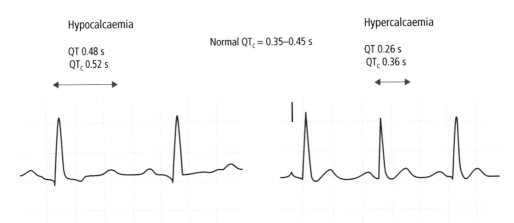

QT interval is measured from the start of the Q wave to the end of the T wave. A lengthened QT interval is a marker for the potential of ventricular tachyarrhythmias like Torsades de pointes and sudden death. Amongst the causes are genetic (long QT syndrome), metabolic (hypocalcaemia, hypothyroidsim) and drugs (antipsycotics, antihistamines, antidepressants and some–nibs such as sunitinib) QT_c is corrected for heart rate.

Figure 40.1 QT interval and serum calcium.

with malignancy should have their corrected serum calcium measured if treatment is likely to be appropriate (Figure 40.1):

$$\text{Corrected calcium} = \text{measured calcium} + [(40 - \text{serum albumin (g/L)}) \times 0.02]$$

The mainstay of therapy is rehydration with large volumes of intravenous fluids followed by the administration of calcium-lowering agents, most commonly bisphosphonates. Low calcium diets are unpalatable, exacerbate malnutrition and have no place in palliative therapy. Drugs promoting hypercalcaemia (e.g. thiazide diuretics, vitamins A and D) should be withdrawn. The cornerstone of the re-establishment of normocalcaemia is treatment with a bisphosphonate. Bisphosphonates have multiple functions in hypercalcaemia. They reduce serum calcium levels by a direct effect on the osteoclast, by stabilizing hydroxyapatite crystals. There are two classes of effect of bisphosphonates. One group of bisphosphonates, which include clodronate and etidronate, acts through their incorporation into non-hydrolyzable analogues of adenosine triphosphate (ATP) that accumulates in osteoclasts and induces apoptosis. Conversely, agents such as pamidronate and zoledronate inhibit an enzyme called farnesyl diphosphate synthase (FPPS) which functions in the cellular metabolic pathway that is known variously as the mevalonate, HMG-CoA reductase or isoprenoid pathway and is necessary for the synthesis of steroids, haem and ubiquinones.

Inhibition of this metabolic path at the FPPS level prevents the formation of metabolites required for protein prenylation that is the linking of small proteins to lipids of the cell membrane.

The bisphosphonates of choice are currently pamidronate, zoledronate and ibandronate. Approximately 80% of patients respond to hydration and bisphosphonate treatment by normalization of serum calcium levels. Calcium levels start to fall within the first 24 hours of treatment with bisphosphonates and usually reach normal levels within 3 days. It is dogma that treatment with bisphosphonates has to be repeated, usually on a 3–4-weekly cycle. However, there is some information that suggests that a single treatment may be sufficient with re-setting of the calcium-stabilizing mechanisms. As well as these actions, bisphosphonates have valuable analgesic activity in patients with metastatic bone pain and reduce skeletal morbidity in patients with breast cancer and myeloma. It may take 7–10 days for the symptoms of hypercalcaemia to resolve following normalization of calcium levels. In 20% of patients with hypercalcaemia, bisphosphonates do not work. Alternative treatments include the use of a somatostatin analogue such as octreotide which acts to reduce serum levels of PTH-related peptide. Other more old-fashioned treatments include calcitonin and mithramycin. Denosumab is a monoclonal antibody to RANKL that is used for postmenopausal osteoporosis and to reduce skeletal events in patients with bone metastases and myeloma. Its value in hypercalcaemia is under investigation.

Tumour lysis syndrome

The acute destruction of a large number of cells is associated with metabolic sequelae and is termed the "tumour lysis syndrome". Cell destruction results in the release of different chemicals into the circulation, some of which may cause profound complications. Electrolyte release may cause transient hypercalcaemia, hyperphosphataemia and hyperkalaemia. The release of calcium and phosphate into the blood stream rarely causes any significant consequences. However, the calcium and phosphate may co-precipitate and cause some impairment of renal function. Hyperkalaemia can be a much more significant problem and may manifest as minor electrocardiograph (ECG) abnormalities which, of course, all students reading this book can describe in intimate detail (Table 40.3). Even more significant, however, are the cardiac arrhythmias which may include ventricular tachycardia or ventricular fibrillation and may lead to the demise of the patient. Nucleic acid breakdown leads to hyperuricaemia and this, unless treated appropriately, can be complicated by renal failure due to the precipitation of uric acid crystals in the renal tubular system. So, of course, it is best that these things do not happen because we do not like our patients dying, least of all because of the complications of the treatment that we give them.

There are certain malignancies whose treatment is associated with a higher than usual risk of tumour lysis syndrome and these include acute promyelocytic leukaemia and high-grade lymphomas. Patients with acute promyelocytic leukaemia can develop the tumour lysis syndrome, following minor trauma, or even infection. This is caused by release of pro-coagulants from blast cells with the risk of a devastating coagulopathy. Patients with high-grade T-cell lymphomas may also be at risk from circumstances where one would not normally expect there to be a problem. For example, if these patients are started on steroids, they may develop tumour lysis because steroids have cytotoxic qualities in lymphoma. In these malignancies the risk of tumour lysis syndrome is pre-empted by a cunning pretreatment plan. Patients are started 2 days prior to chemotherapy or radiation therapy with allopurinol. The day before treatment, intravenous hydration is started and these efforts generally prevent the development of tumour lysis syndrome. Many clinicians advise alkalinization of the urine. However, in practice it is very difficult to achieve an alkaline urine and there are significant dangers inherent in the use of significant amounts of sodium bicarbonate. A proportion of patients will go on to develop tumour lysis syndrome despite these measures. For this reason patients who are treated require careful monitoring with two-hourly measurement of serum potassium levels for the first 8–12 hours of treatment. Many clinicians will also advise ECG monitoring but it is our experience that these monitors are generally not observed to best effect. A new drug has become recently available for the treatment of this condition. Recombinant urate oxidase (rasburicase) converts uric acid, which is insoluble, into allantoin (Figure 40.2). Clinical trials have shown that urate oxidase controls hyperuricaemia faster and more reliably than allopurinol and its use is indicated in children with haematological malignancy.

Mechanical complications
Superior vena cava obstruction

Superior vena cava obstruction (SVCO) restricts the venous return from the upper body resulting in

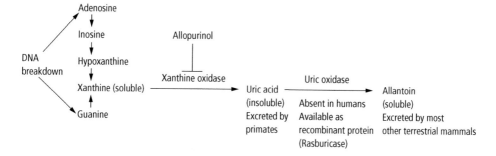

Figure 40.2 Purine catabolism pathway and the therapy of tumour lysis.

Table 40.3 ECGs for oncologists

Oncological emergency	ECG features	Tracings
Hypercalcaemia	Short QT Broad-based, tall, peaked T waves Wide QRS Low R wave Disappearance of P waves	
Pericardial effusion	Sinus tachycardia Low voltage complexes PR segment depression Alternation of the QRS complexes, usually in a 2:1 ratio (electrical alternans)	
Tumour lysis Hyperkalaemia	Peaked T waves Flattened P waves Prolonged PR interval Widened QRS complexes Deep S wave	
Hypocalcaemia	Long QT interval Narrow QRS Reduced PR interval Flat or inverted T waves Prominent U wave Ventricular arrhythmia	

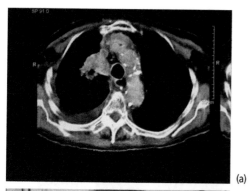

(a)

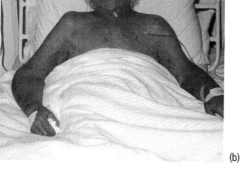

(b)

Figure 40.3 An 80-year-old woman presented with shortness of breath, headaches and swollen arms. (a) The CT scan shows a large right hilar mass that was small cell lung cancer compressing the superior vena cava and collateral circulation. (b) The clinical image also shows dilated veins on the anterior chest wall due to collateral circulation. The flow of blood in these veins will be from above as the blood is bypassing the obstructed superior vena cava to return via the patent inferior vena cava.

oedema of the arms and face, distension of the neck and arm veins, headaches and a dusky blue skin discoloration over the upper chest, arms and face. SVCO is caused by a mediastinal mass compressing the vessel with or without intraluminal thrombus. Collateral circulation via the azygous vein may provide some drainage and over a period of weeks collaterals may form over the chest wall. In this case the flow of blood in these collateral veins will be from above downwards into the inferior vena cava circulation and this may be demonstrated clinically as an aid to confirm the diagnosis.

The presenting symptoms of SVCO include dyspnoea, swelling of the face and arms, headaches, a choking sensation, cough and chest pain (see Figures 40.3 and 40.4). The most important clinical sign is loss of venous pulsations in the distended neck veins. This is usually accompanied by facial oedema, plethora and cyanosis and tachypnoea. The severity of the symptoms is determined by the rate of obstruction and the development of a compensatory collateral circulation. The symptoms may deteriorate when lying flat or bending, which further compromises the obstructed venous return. Careful assessment of the patient's history is frequently suggestive of a long period with minor symptoms of SVCO. In 9 out of 10 cases, the cause of SVCO is a malignancy, most often lung cancer (disproportionately more often small cell lung cancer) (Figures 40.5a and b), lymphoma or metastatic breast or germ cell cancer. Rare non-malignant causes are listed in Table 40.4.

The management of SVCO depends upon the cause and severity, along with the patient's prognosis, and includes relieving symptoms as well as treating the underlying cause. SVCO is an oncological emergency in the presence of airway compromise, and delays whilst histological findings are confirmed may adversely affect the outcome. In such circumstances

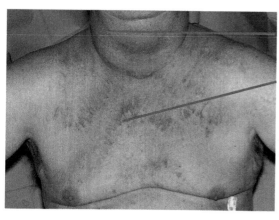

Swollen neck

Dilated anterior chest wall collateral veins (blood flowing downwards)

Figure 40.4 Superior vena cava obstruction (SVCO).

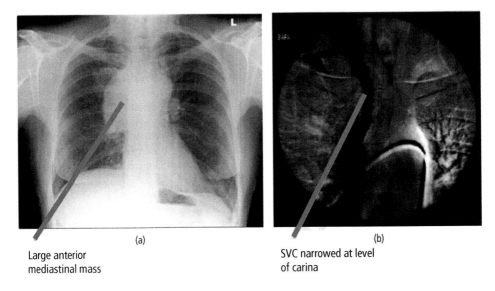

Large anterior
mediastinal mass

(a)

SVC narrowed at level
of carina

(b)

Figure 40.5 Superior vena cava obstruction (SVCO) due to small cell lung cancer.

patients are treated empirically with steroids and radiotherapy. However, when it is safe to do so, it is important to establish the diagnosis as this will determine the optimum treatment and a delay of 1–2 days to obtain a histological diagnosis is often appropriate, particularly in the context of a patient with minor symptoms and a long clinical history. Diagnostic procedures should include a plain chest X-ray (CXR), sputum cytology, bronchoscopy, thoracoscopy or mediastinoscopy, computed tomography scans (Figure 40.6a) or magnetic resonance imaging and venography. A palpable lymph node may be amenable to biopsy, thereby providing a diagnosis.

Patients may respond to being sat upright with oxygen therapy and intravenous corticosteroids should be administered. In the acute setting, insertion of expandable wire stents under radiological guidance can be effective (Figures 40.6b–e). Studies report instantaneous symptomatic relief. In the majority of cases subsequent radiotherapy is the most appropriate treatment modality and relieves symptoms in most patients within a fortnight. Where a diagnosis of lymphoma, small cell lung cancer or germ cell tumour has been obtained, chemotherapy may be the optimal initial treatment. Although relief of the obstruction can be achieved surgically, surgery is usually only reserved for patients with benign causes of SVCO.

Table 40.4 Non-malignant causes of superior vena cava obstruction (SVCO)

Mediastinal fibrosis	Idiopathic
	Histoplasmosis
	Actinomycosis
	Tuberculosis
Vena cava thrombosis	Idiopathic
	Behcet's syndrome
	Polycythemia vera
	Paroxysmal nocturnal haemoglobinuria
	Long-term venous catheters, shunts or pacemakers
Benign mediastinal tumours	Aortic aneurysm
	Dermoid tumour
	Retrosternal goitre
	Sarcoidosis
	Cystic hygroma

Spinal cord compression

Spinal cord compression is a relatively common complication of disseminated cancer and affects 5% of patients with cancer. Spinal cord compression occurs with many tumour types, but is particularly frequent in myeloma and prostate cancer. Up to 30% of these patients will survive for 1 year, so it is essential to be spared paraplegia for this remaining time by making the diagnosis swiftly and instituting treatment quickly. In general, the residual neurological deficit reflects the extent of deficit at the start of treatment, so early treatment leaves less

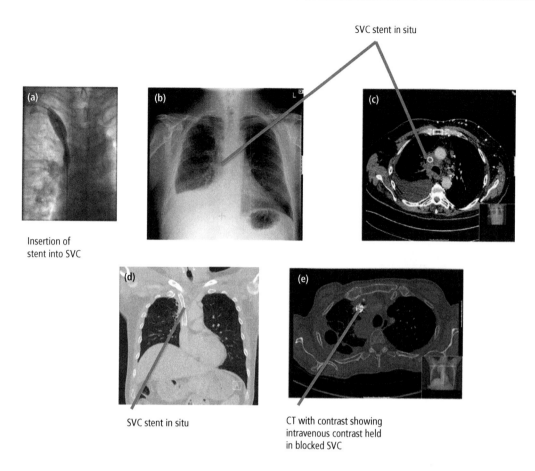

SVC stent in situ

(a)

(b)

(c)

Insertion of
stent into SVC

(d)

(e)

SVC stent in situ

CT with contrast showing
intravenous contrast held
in blocked SVC

Figures 40.6 Superior vena cava obstruction (SVCO) stenting. Metallic vascular stent is introduced radiologically via the right subclavian vein (a). The metallic stent can be seen in place on chest X-ray (b), and transverse (c) and coronal (d) CT scan images. Complications of SVCO stents include blockage due to thrombus occluding the stent lumen as shown in (e).

damage. Neoplastic cord compression is nearly always due to extramedullary, extradural metastases usually from breast, lung, prostate, lymphoma or renal cancers. Commonly compression occurs by posterior expansion of vertebral metastases or extension of paraspinal metastases through the intervertebral foramina. These result in demyelination, arterial compromise, venous occlusion and vasogenic oedema of the spinal cord progressing to ischaemic myopathy; 70% occur in the thoracic spine, 20% in the lumbar spine and 10% in the cervical spine.

The earliest symptom of cord compression is vertebral pain, especially on coughing and lying flat. Subsequent signs include sensory changes one or two dermatomes below the level of compression. A complaint of back pain with focal weakness and bladder or bowel dysfunction with a sensory level requires urgent investigation in a patient with cancer. This will progress to motor weakness distal to the block and finally sphincter disturbance. If spinal cord compres-

sion is missed, or left untreated, patients can develop severe neurological deficits and double incontinence.

Spinal cord compression should be treated as a medical emergency. High-dose intravenous corticosteroids should be initiated on clinical suspicion alone to prevent further evolution of neurological deficit. Plain X-rays of the spine looking for vertebral collapse and MRI of the spinal axis to define the presence and level(s) of spinal cord compression should then be performed (Figures 40.7, 40.8, 40.9 and 40.10). Twenty to thirty per cent of patients have multiple levels of cord compression and imaging of the whole cord is therefore essential. If appropriate, a neurosurgical opinion should be obtained regarding the potential of surgical decompression, especially if there is vertebral instability or if the level of the compression has been previously irradiated. Otherwise, the definitive treatment is urgent local radiotherapy. It is important to provide adequate analgesia. Pretreatment ambulatory function is

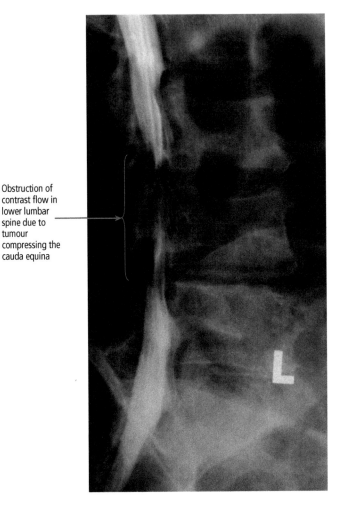

Obstruction of contrast flow in lower lumbar spine due to tumour compressing the cauda equina

Figure 40.7 Myelogram demonstrating cauda equine compression. This invasive technique has been largely replaced by MRI.

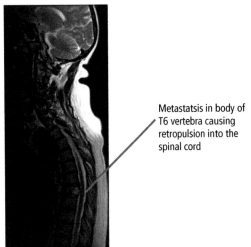

Metastatsis in body of T6 vertebra causing retropulsion into the spinal cord

Figure 40.8 MRI showing spinal cord compression.

the main determinant of post-treatment gait function, thus prompt diagnosis and treatment is the key to gait and continence preservation. In clinical trials it has been shown that surgery using an anterior approach is more effective than steroids and radiotherapy in relieving cord compression. However, it takes a considerable time to recover from such extensive surgery and so surgery is often avoided as patients with cord compression have a median survival of 3 months.

Cancer-related obstruction

Tumours obstruct "tubes" in the body by exerting local pressure on them or occasional growing within them. The most frequently affected tubes include the bowel, urinary tract, bronchi and cerebral ventricular system (Figures 40.11, 40.12, 40.13

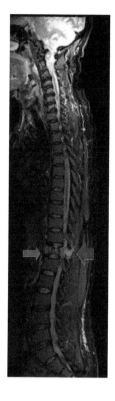
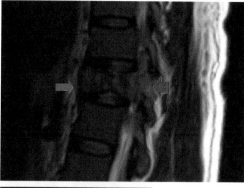
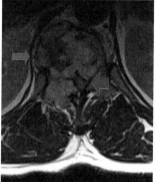

Bone metastasis destroying T9 vertebral body (✱) and causing spinal cord compression (✱)

Figure 40.9 Bone metastasis destroying T9 vertebral body and causing spinal cord compression.

and 40.14). The consequences are intestinal obstruction, hydronephrosis, bronchial obstruction and hydrocephalus. After localizing the obstruction, relief is often achieved by radiological or endoscopic stenting (see Figures 3.5 and 14.2).

Cancer-related thromboses

Patients with cancer have an increased tendency to thrombosis, a problem that was first documented by Trousseau, who sadly went on to develop venous thromboses and died from cancer. Patients with cancer have an increased risk of developing thromboses for two major reasons. The first may be a pressure effect, where the primary tumour mass or secondary nodal masses impinge upon the vasculature, producing venous stasis and thrombosis. The second reason for the increased risk is the release from the tumour of pro-coagulants. A number of tissue pro-coagulants have been described, ranging from factors S and C to the current view that activated factor 10 is released by tumours, which sparks off the clotting cascade.

The incidence of venous thrombosis and thromboembolism in cancer patients is variably reported (Figures 40.15 and 40.16). One study looked at a group of patients presenting to A&E with deep venous thromboses. Screening of these patients showed that almost 30% had a cancer that was most commonly a pelvic malignancy. As always in medicine, there is initial positive reporting and later studies showed the true incidence of previously undetected cancer in patients presenting with venous thrombosis to be in the order of 5%. Once cancer has been diagnosed, thromboembolic events are remarkably common and described in about 10% of all patients. The incidence increases significantly when long lines (Hickman or PICC) are inserted in cancer patients for the purposes of chemotherapy or supportive care. In this group of patients the incidence of thromboembolism increases to 20%. For this reason prophylaxis with low-dose warfarin is recommended and this decreases the risk of subsequent thrombosis to between 2% and 5%. These statistics, however, are considered controversial and are debated endlessly. Because of the high risk of thrombosis in cancer patients it has been suggested

(a)

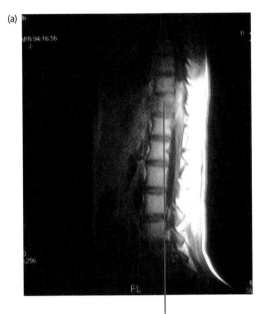

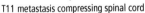

T11 metastasis compressing spinal cord

(b)

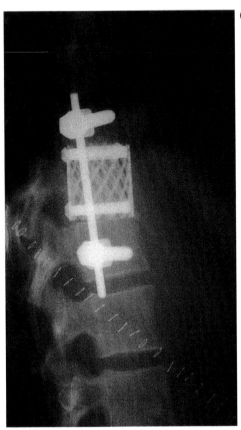

Figure 40.10 (a) MRI showing spine bone metastasis and cord compression at T11 due to vertebral metastasis with soft tissue extension. (b) A matched plain X-ray following surgical decompression and stabilization of the metastasis.

that anticoagulation should be prophylactically prescribed. Logically, the best way of preventing thromboembolism would be with a heparin-like compound rather than with a coumarin. At the moment the evidence is that the low molecular weight heparins are probably more effective than warfarin in the prophylaxis of thromboembolism. There is an additional unexpected benefit to anticoagulation with low molecular weight heparins and this is the modest survival advantage for anticoagulated patients, as demonstrated by randomized clinical trials. In some patients with pelvic tumours and recurrent thromboses, filters may be inserted into the inferior vena cava to reduce the risk of pulmonary embolism (Figures 40.17, 40.18 and 40.19). The benefits of filters are transient. For central venous access catheter-associated thrombosis, removal of the line and anticoagulation should be commenced.

Malignant effusions

Pleural effusions

Although not strictly an emergency, approximately 40% of all pleural effusions are due to malignancy (Table 40.5) and their presence frequently indicates advanced and incurable disease. The pleural space is normally filled with 10–40 mL of hypoproteinaceous plasma that originates from the capillary bed of the parietal pleura and is drained through the parietal pleura lymphatics. A pleural effusion is often the first manifestation of malignancy, and lung cancer and breast cancer account for almost two-thirds of cases. Malignant pleural effusions may be asymptomatic or cause progressive dyspnoea, cough and chest pain which may be pleuritic

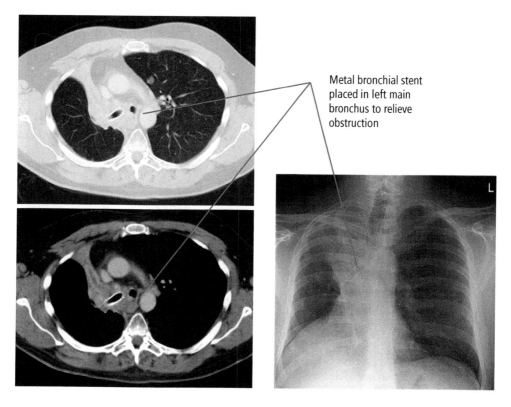

Metal bronchial stent placed in left main bronchus to relieve obstruction

Figure 40.11 Bronchial stent to relieve obstruction.

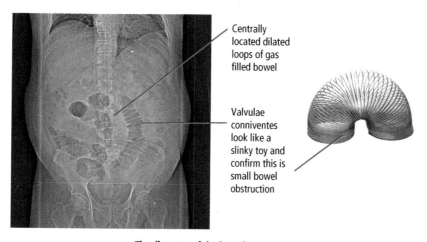

Centrally located dilated loops of gas filled bowel

Valvulae conniventes look like a slinky toy and confirm this is small bowel obstruction

The diameter of the bowel: 3, 6 or 9.

	Abnormal if
Small bowel	>3 cm
Colon	>6 cm
Caecum	>9 cm

Figure 40.12 Small bowel obstruction.

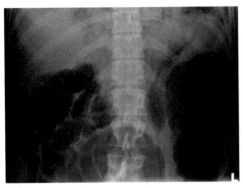
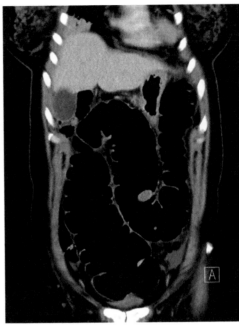

Figure 40.13 Obstructed descending colon. Abdominal X-ray and CT show dilatation of the large bowel (6.5 cm), cecum (9 cm) and distal ileum (2.8 cm) caused by obstructing cancer of the descending colon.

in nature. Malignant pleural effusions are usually exudates and this may be confirmed by a fluid lactate dehydrogenase (LDH) of >200 U/mL, a fluid:serum LDH ratio >0.6, a fluid:serum protein ratio >0.5 and a fluid:serum glucose ratio of <0.5. The fluid may be blood stained and is typically hypercellular, containing lymphocytes, monocytes and reactive mesothelial cells; exfoliated tumour cells may also be present.

The management of malignant effusions should be tailored to the patient's symptoms as only half the patients will be alive at 3 months and over 90% of effusions will recur within 30 days of thoracocentesis. Reaccumulation of pleural effusions may be delayed

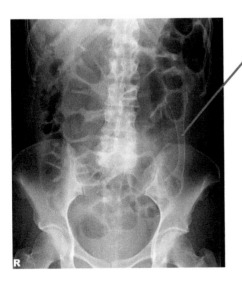

Colonic stent in descending colon has relieved obstruction

Figure 40.14 Colonic stent.

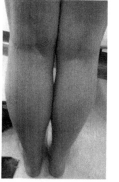
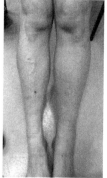

Doppler ultrasound demonstrates central thrombus in left common femoral vein (blue) with a rim of of peripheral blood flow (red)

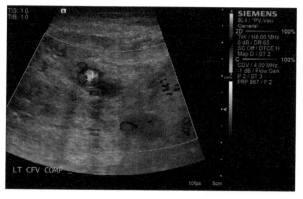

Figure 40.15 Venous thrombosis.

by chemical pleurodesis (usually using talc or tetracycline) or video-assisted thoracic surgery (VATS) with pleurectomy and/or talc insufflation. Pleuroperitoneal shunts or chronic indwelling catheters may be considered for patients who fail pleurodesis, but this is rarely appropriate.

Pericardial effusions

The accumulation of fluid in the pericardial space around the heart may adversely affect cardiac function and like all effusions may be transudate, exudate or haemorrhage. Cardiac tamponade occurs when

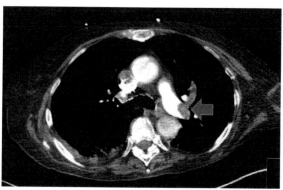

Extensive thrombus in right main pulmonary artery (◀).

Figure 40.16 Pulmonary thrombosis.

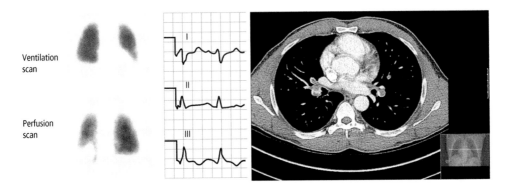

Figure 40.17 V/Q scan, ECG and CT scan features of pulmonary embolism. V/Q scan showing large segmental perfusion defect in the left lower lung and normal ventilation. ECG showing $Q_I S_{III} T_{III}$ pattern (S wave in lead I; Q wave in lead III and inverted T wave in lead III). CT scan shows filling defects occluding the central pulmonary artery and extending into all the lobar branches due to saddle embolus.

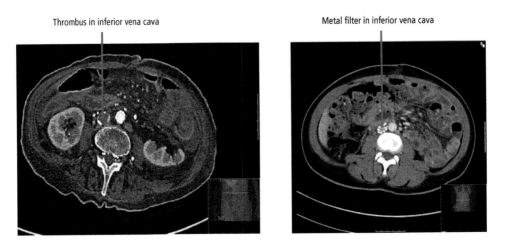

Figure 40.18 CT scan showing an inferior vena cava filter *in situ* in a woman with advanced ovarian cancer and recurrent thromboses.

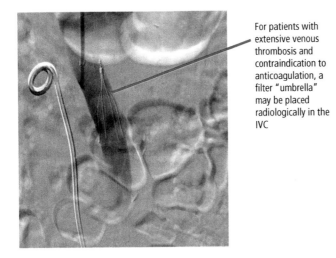

For patients with extensive venous thrombosis and contraindication to anticoagulation, a filter "umbrella" may be placed radiologically in the IVC

Figure 40.19 IVC filter.

Table 40.5 Causes of pleural effusion

Transudate	Cardiac failure
	Nephrotic syndrome
	Cirrhosis
	Protein-losing enteropathy
	Constrictive pericarditis
	Hypothyroidism
	Peritoneal dialysis
	Meig's syndrome (pleural effusion associated with ovarian fibroma)
Exudate Tumour	Primary: lung cancer, mesothelioma
	Secondary: breast or ovary cancer, lymphoma
Infection	Pneumonia
	Tuberculosis
	Subphrenic abscess
Infarction	Pulmonary embolus
Connective tissue disease	Rheumatoid arthritis
	Systemic lupus erythematosus
Others	Pancreatitis (usually left-sided pleural effusion)
	Dressler's syndrome (inflammatory pericarditis and pleurisy following myocardial infarction or heart surgery)
	Yellow nail syndrome (combination of discoloured hypoplastic nails, recurring pleural effusions and lymphedem; aetiology unknown)
	Asbestos exposure

the pressure on the ventricles in diastole prevents them from filling, thus reducing the stroke volume and cardiac output. The classic sign of cardiac tamponade is Beck's triad of hypotension because of decreased stroke volume, jugular–venous distension due to impaired venous return to the heart and muffled heart sounds due to fluid inside the pericardium (Figure 40.20). Tamponade is relived either by direct aspiration or surgically by forming a "pericardial window".

Ascites

The most frequent malignancies causing ascites are primary tumours of the ovaries, pancreas, stomach and colon, breast and lungs (Figures 40.21 and 40.22). The distressing symptoms of ascites include abdominal distension or pain; dyspnoea due to diaphragmatic splinting; oedema of the legs, perineum and lower trunk; and a "squashed stomach syndrome" leading to anorexia. If these symptoms are distressing,

paracentesis is indicated which offers rapid symptom relief but poor long-term control. Whilst anticancer therapy may reduce the subsequent re-accumulation of ascites, if this is not an option or is unsuccessful, diuretics may be helpful. Rarely a peritoneovenous shunt may be surgically placed under general anaesthetic if the ascites cannot be controlled.

Haematological disorders

Hyperviscosity syndrome

Blood hyperviscosity can be caused by too much protein or too many cells in the blood. The clinical features include spontaneous bleeding from mucous membranes, retinopathy, headache, vertigo, coma and seizures. The most frequent causes of excess proteins are monoclonal paraproteinaemias such as Waldrenström's macroglobulinaemia (IgM) and myeloma

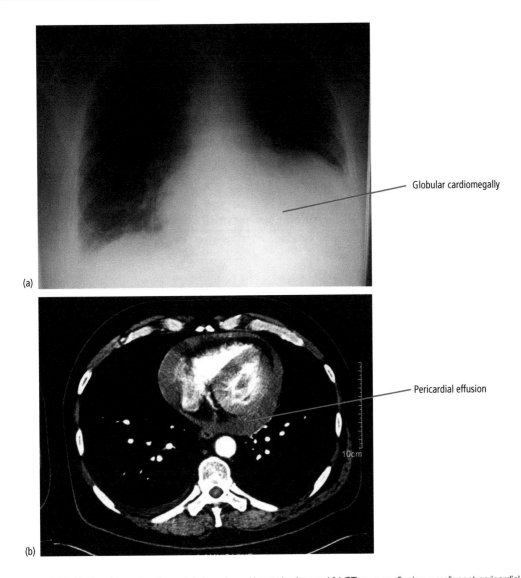

(a)

Globular cardiomegally

(b)

Pericardial effusion

10cm

Figure 40.20 (a) Chest X-ray showing a globular enlarged heart shadow and (b) CT scan confirming a malignant pericardial effusion due to metastatic non-small cell lung cancer. These effusions may present as a medical emergency with cardiac tamponade. The clinical symptoms include dyspnoea and cough and the signs are hypotension, tachycardia, pulsus paradoxus (fall of systolic blood pressure of >10 mmHg on inspiration), quiet muffled heart sounds and a raised jugular–venous pressure (JVP) with Kussmaul's sign (paradoxical rise in JVP on inspiration). The electrocardiograph may show pulsus alternans (alternating QRS voltages). The emergency treatment is pericardiocentesis and subsequent surgical formation of a pericardial window to prevent recurrence may be necessary.

(especially IgA and IgG3 myelomas). Hyperviscosity due to excess cell counts occurs in acute leukaemia blast crises. The retinopathy resembles retinal vein occlusion with dilated retinal veins and retinal haemorrhages. The serum viscosity may be measured (normal range: 0.14–0.18 cPa/s), but treatment of suspected hyperviscosity should be started before the results are available as they often take days to come back. Plasmapheresis should be used to decrease hyperviscosity related to excess proteins, whilst leukapheresis removes excess leukaemic blasts before definitive treatment can begin.

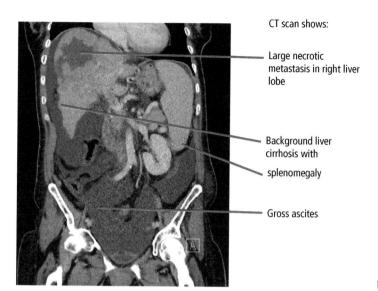

CT scan shows:

Large necrotic metastasis in right liver lobe

Background liver cirrhosis with

splenomegaly

Gross ascites

Figure 40.21 Ascites.

Myelosuppression

Neutropenia

We explain to our patients that chemotherapy puts them at risk of developing bone marrow suppression, as cancer treatments kill "good" as well as "bad" cells. In this case the "good" cells are the haematological progenitor cells and patients are at risk of death if the effects of treatment upon the bone marrow are not recognized. Neutropenic sepsis is very common in cancer treatment and, if undiagnosed, leads to a mortality rate approaching 20–30%. Patients with neutropenic sepsis develop fevers and rigors with associated oral ulceration and candidiasis. It is standard practice for patients with neutropenic sepsis – which is defined by septic symptoms in the presence of a white count that is $<1.0 \times 10^9/L$ – to be admitted to hospital. The patient is resuscitated with intravenous fluids and blood cultures are taken. In the absence of any obvious focus of infection, such as the urinary tract, the advantage of culturing from sites

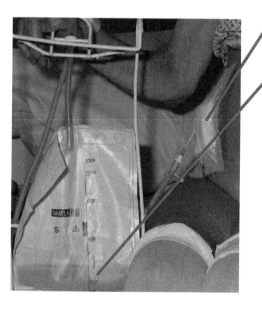

Ascitic drain in place draining milky chylous fluid (a combination of lymph and emulsified fats derived from the small intestine)

Figure 40.22 Ascitic drain.

other than blood is virtually zero. Cultures from other sites merely act to swamp the microbiology lab with unnecessary requests for culture work without yielding any positive advantage. Just 20% of blood cultures from patients with neutropenic sepsis are positive for bacterial organisms. The cause for infection is generally not clear.

Antibiotic policies vary from hospital to hospital, but there is good evidence that treatment with single-agent ceftazidime is as effective as treatment with combination antibiotic regimens. In the United Kingdom patients are generally admitted, though it is interesting to note that this conservative management policy is not strictly necessary. In one randomized study, treatment with oral ciprofloxacin in the community was compared with inpatient treatment with intravenous ceftazidime. The results were absolutely identical in terms of control of fever and patient outcome.

Over the last decade marrow growth factors have become available, and granulocyte colony-stimulating factor (G-CSF), which stimulates the marrow to produce granulocytes, has entered wide use. There is limited evidence that prophylactic use of G-CSF prevents neutropenic sepsis or septic deaths. The evidence for its use in established infection is poor and the consensus view is that G-CSF is of value only in patients with established neutropenic sepsis who have a non-recovering marrow and in whom, additionally, an infective agent has been identified. Nevertheless G-CSF has been adopted as a panacea by oncologists who prescribe it widely as primary and secondary prophylaxis against neutropenia. In contrast G-CSF is of enormous value in transplantation programmes, where the mean period of time to engraftment has been reduced from 28 to 18 days by the use of these agents.

Anaemia

Anaemia is a very common complication of cancer and its treatment. It is estimated that up to 30% of all cancer patients will require a transfusion. In general, anaemia is cumulative and builds up over several cycles of chemotherapy. Recombinant erythropoietin is considered to be a valuable alternative to blood transfusion but is slow acting. The response of patients to erythropoietin is wide ranging and reported at between 20% and 60%. Haemoglobin levels increase after about 6 weeks of treatment with recombinant erythropoietin. The price of this agent used to be considered prohibitive; however, it may become relatively more affordable as the cost of blood continues to increase significantly because of the increased costs of testing blood for infective agents such as Creutzfeldt–Jakob disease (CJD). The pharmaceutical industry markets erythropoietin for its effect upon the asthenia related to cancer treatment; claims are made for a far greater improvement in cancer fatigue than haemoglobin level.

Thrombocytopenia

Thrombocytopenia is not as significant a problem in the treatment of solid tumours as it is in the treatment of haematological malignancies. There is a significant risk of spontaneous major haemorrhage as the platelet count declines below $10–20 \times 10^9$/L and most oncologists advocate prophylactic platelet transfusions at this level or in the presence of bleeding. There are a number of regulatory molecules that stimulate early haematopoietic progenitors and these include the interleukins IL-1, IL-6 and IL-11. IL-1 and IL-6 have poor efficacy and significant toxicity, but IL-11 has been licensed for the prevention of chemotherapy-induced thrombocytopenia. The pharmaceutical industry continues to develop agents for the treatment of thrombocytopenia and the focus recently has been on analogues of thrombopoietin, which appear to have more efficacy and less toxicity than the interleukins.

 KEY POINTS

- Oncological emergencies are common and prompt treatment often results in good outcomes
- Hypercalcaemia presents with diverse clinical manifestations and treatment usually improves these distressing symptoms
- The metabolic chaos of tumour lysis is usually a feature of tumour response to chemotherapy and urgent recognition and treatment is life saving
- Superior vena cava obstruction causes upper body swelling and skin discoloration with venous distension that may be relieved by stenting
- Spinal cord compression causes characteristic pain and neurological signs and rapid treatment by surgical decompression or radiotherapy reduces permanent neurological deficit
- Tumours obstruct tubes including the bowel, urinary tract, bronchi and cerebral ventricular system causing intestinal obstruction,

hydronephrosis, bronchial obstruction and hydrocephalus. Relief is often achieved by radiological or endoscopic stenting

- Cancer-related fluid collections, pleural effusions, pericardial effusions and ascites affect the function of adjacent organs and may be relieved by drains

- Myelosuppression is a common consequence of treatment for cancer and can cause life-threatening neutropenic sepsis and thrombocytopenia that need urgent treatment with intravenous broad-spectrum antibiotics and platelet transfusions, respectively

41

End-of-life care

Learning objectives

✓ Explain the current management of cancer pain

✓ Describe care at the end of life including individualized care plans

✓ Identify those at bereavement risk

Amongst the most important elements of oncological care is recognizing shifting goals as cancer progresses. The balance of benefit and side effects of any intervention should be carefully weighed up. Whilst neurosurgical resection of solitary metastases from melanoma may be appropriate in some circumstances, venipuncture for measuring the serum electrolytes in a dying patient is rarely justifiable. These decisions should involve the patients wherever possible and require skilful use of communication. Throughout the cancer journey patients often enquire about their life expectancy and there is a temptation for clinicians to pluck some figure out of the air. An intelligent doctor will recognize the pitfalls of prognostication when applied to an individual and will appreciate that the median survival (the statistic most relevant in this circumstance) is the time when half the patients will still be alive. Stephen J. Gould, the evolutionary palaeontologist, explained this from a patient's perspective in the essay "The median is not the message" published in the collection *Bully for Brontosaurus* and also published in full online. During the patient's journey with cancer a number of emotions are experienced and these may follow a step-wise succession originally described by the Swiss psychologist Elisabeth Kübler-Ross. In her 1969 book, *On Death and Dying*, she records the stages as denial, anger, bargaining, grieving and finally acceptance.

As the cancer progresses and the patient deteriorates, it is important that reviews are frequent and that problems are anticipated. This close follow-up is often best undertaken in the community by community palliative care services rather than bringing patients up to hospital or GP surgeries for regular appointments, but this approach requires excellent communication between all the health professionals involved. This may be facilitated by patient-held records similar to those used in shared care obstetrics. The anticipation of symptoms, including pain and diminishing mobility, should be addressed in advance so that analgesia is quickly available to patients.

Pain control

Nerve endings, or nociceptors, exist in all tissues and are stimulated by noxious agents including chemical, mechanical and thermal stimuli, giving rise to pain (Table 41.1). These stimuli are relayed by Aβ, Aδ (fast transmitting fibres) and C (slow transmission of sensation) sensory nerve fibres to the dorsal horns of the spinal cord and different qualities of pain may use different sensory fibres.

Analgesic drugs form the mainstay of treating cancer pain and should be chosen based on the severity of the pain rather than the stage of the cancer. Drugs should be administered regularly to prevent pain using a stepwise escalation from non-opioid, to weak opioid and then strong opioid analgesia (Figure 41.1). Adjuvant drugs may be added at any stage of the analgesic ladder as they may have additional analgesic effect in some painful conditions (Figure 41.2). Examples of adjuvant analgesics are corticosteroids,

---

Oncology: Lecture Notes, Third Edition. Mark Bower and Jonathan Waxman.

© 2015 by John Wiley & Sons, Ltd. Published 2015 by John Wiley & Sons, Ltd.

Companion Website: www.lecturenoteseries.com/oncology

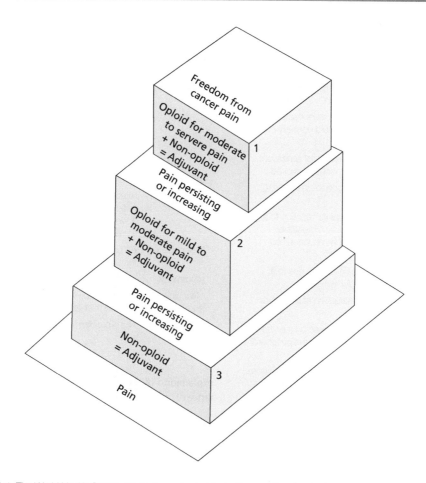

Figure 41.1 The World Health Organization's three step ladder to the use of analgesic drugs.

Other pain ladders

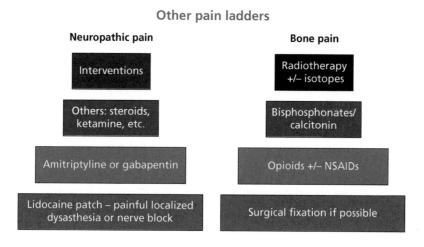

Figure 41.2 The neuropathic and bone pain ladders.

Table 41.1 Definition of pain terms

Term	Definition
Allodynia	Pain due to a stimulus that does not normally cause pain
Analgesia	Absence of pain in response to stimulation that would normally be painful
Dysesthesia	An unpleasant abnormal sensation, whether spontaneous or evoked
Hyperalgesia	Heightened response to a normally painful stimulus
Hyperpathia	An abnormally painful reaction to a stimulus, especially a repetitive stimulus, as well as an increased threshold
Hypoalgesia	Diminished pain in response to a normally painful stimulus
Neuralgia	Pain in the distribution of a nerve or nerves
Neuropathic pain	Pain initiated or caused by a primary lesion or dysfunction in the peripheral nervous system
Nociception	Nervous system activity resulting from potential or actual tissue-damaging stimuli
Paraesthesia	An abnormal sensation, whether spontaneous or evoked

Table 41.2 Side effects of opiates

Side effect	Comments
Constipation	This affects almost all patients and also all patients require prophylaxis with a stimulant laxative (e.g. senna, bisacodyl) and a softener (e.g. docusate sodium) or as a combined preparation (e.g. co-danthramer, co-danthrusate)
Drowsiness	Generally remits after a few days
Nausea	Affects one-third of opioid naïve patients but usually resolves within 1 week. Consider prophylaxis for 1 week.
Hallucinations	An uncommon side effect that often features images in the peripheral vision
Nightmares	Vivid and unpleasant but rare
Myoclonic jerks	Occur usually with excess doses and may be mistaken for fits
Respiratory depression	Not a problem in patients with pain

non-steroidal anti-inflammatory drugs, tricyclic antidepressants, anticonvulsants and some antiarrhythmic drugs. Morphine is the most commonly used strong opioid analgesic and whenever possible should be given by mouth. The dose of morphine needs to be tailored to each patient and be repeated at regular intervals so that the pain does not return between doses. There is no upper dose limit for morphine; however, a number of myths have arisen around opioid prescribing that may deter prescribers as well as patients. Firstly, opioid tolerance is rarely seen in patients with cancer pain and neither psychological dependence nor addiction is a problem in this patient group. The toxicity of opioids may prove to be an obstacle for some patients (Table 41.2). Sedation is common at the start of opioid therapy but resolves in most patients within a few days. Similarly, nausea and vomiting may prove troublesome at the start of regular opioid dosing but usually dissipate within a few days and may be controlled with antiemetics. Constipation develops in almost all patients on opioids and this toxicity persists and necessitates routine prophylactic laxatives for almost everyone receiving opioids. A careful explanation of these issues will result in the acceptance of opioid analgesia by almost all patients.

Care of the dying patient

The continuing attention to the needs and comfort of a dying patient is as important as the care given to any other patient and part of that care includes reducing the distress of relatives. Many issues may be raised by relatives that pose ethical dilemmas and these may make you question the therapy that has been or should be given. Amongst the most frequent scenarios is the role of intravenous hydration, evaluating the balance between painful cannulation and restriction of mobility versus an uncomfortable dry mouth and thirst. To address these questions you should consider whether death from the cancer is now inevitable, whether interventions would relieve symptoms and whether treatment would cause harm. Careful explanation to the relatives is essential; in this circumstance, for example, they need to be reassured that the patient is not dying because of dehydration but rather because of progression of the cancer.

Symptom control in the dying patient often requires a different route of administration as swallowing may be difficult and agitation and restlessness are often prominent features as death approaches. A number of factors may contribute to terminal agitation including physical causes such as pain, sore mouth and full bladder or rectum, along with emotional factors including fear of dying and the distress of relatives. The physical causes should be addressed appropriately and unnecessary medications should be stopped. Often the best method of delivering analgesia, antiemetics and sedation, if appropriate, is via a subcutaneous syringe driver. Similarly, oral secretions accumulating in a patient who is too weak to cough may be distressing to the patient and family alike. Drug treatment for terminal secretions includes hyoscine hydrobromide and glycopyrronium bromide, which is less sedating. It is important to recall that not all patients wish to be sedated and this should be discussed with them and their families.

The last hours and days

For many patients with cancer the last hours and days are heralded by a deterioration to semiconsciousness. At this time patients are usually unable to take oral medication and prescriptions need to be reconsidered. Many medicines may be stopped altogether and alternative routes of administration, including subcutaneous, rectal and transdermal routes, may be employed for other necessary medications including analgesia. Although patients may no longer be receiving medicines by mouth, oral hygiene remains an important part of overall care. It is particularly important to avoid unnecessary unpleasant interventions at this time and to adopt a practical problem-oriented approach to symptom control. A practical guide to the care of the dying patient in a hospital was developed at the Royal Liverpool Hospital in conjunction with Marie Curie Cancer Care to transfer best practice learnt from hospice care. The Liverpool Care of the Dying Pathway (LCP) helps members of the multidisciplinary team in making a decision about which medical interventions should be stopped and which one should be continued (including anticipatory prescribing) and what comfort measures should be started. It also promotes psychological support of the patients, family and carers as well as addressing spiritual needs and bereavement. There has been debate recently about the value of the Liverpool Pathway, with some critics suggesting that it is a one-way road that sanitizes and precipitates the process of dying without allowing thought or revision of decisions. In 2012, half of all NHS trust were to receive financial rewards under the Commissioning

for Quality and Innovation (CQUIN) scheme for hitting targets associated with this pathway. This perhaps inevitably led to a furore about the pathway with media critics accusing clinicians of hastening death with a "sedation and dehydration" tactic. In July 2013 the Department of Health decided to phase out the LCP in favour of more individualized end-of-life care.

When death is inevitable, as it is for all of us, and is approaching rapidly it is the policy in many UK hospitals to discuss resuscitation policies with patients and their relatives. Under these circumstances resuscitation is rarely appropriate and, if deemed futile, the lead clinician may make a "do not attempt resuscitation" (DNAR) decision. These DNAR decisions should be discussed with patients who wish to engage in advanced care planning. However, prolonged discussions about DNAR policies with patients who do not wish to contemplate their future are, in the view of these authors, distressing and irrelevant. The reason for our autocratic view is that cardiac resuscitation cannot return the patient who has died from cancer from his journey across the River Styx, and it causes distress in the relatives and the arrest team.

Bereavement

Bereavement care and support includes recognizing the physical and emotional needs of families and carers and continues after the patient's death. A number of features have been identified that are associated with the risk of severe bereavement reactions (Table 41.3), and the recognition of these risks prior to death can allow planning of care for those left behind after the death. Health professionals are not immune to bereavement, or at least the good ones are not, and our need for support should not be ignored.

Table 41.3 Risk factors for bereavement

Patient	Young
Cancer	Short illness, disfiguring
Death	Sudden, traumatic (haemorrhage)
Relationship to patient	Dependent or hostile
Main carer	Young, other dependents, physical or mental illness, unsupported

The culture of death and dying

Just as different cultures, regardless of the scientific evidence, have developed distinct explanations for the origins of life ranging from Big Bangs and evolution to creationist genesis, similar cultural variations affect attitudes to death. For example, Christians, Jews (Box 41.1) and Sufis believe in resurrection whilst Hindus, Buddhists (Box 41.2) and Sikhs believe in reincarnation. These cultural discrepancies must be recognized and respected, particularly where patients' and carers' views differ.

Box 41.1 Jewish mourners' Kaddish prayer

Glorified and sanctified be God's great name throughout the world which He has created according to His will. May He establish His kingdom in your lifetime and during your days, and within the life of the entire House of Israel, speedily and soon; and say, Amen.

May His great name be blessed forever and to all eternity. Blessed and praised, glorified and exalted, extolled and honoured, adored and lauded be the name of the Holy One, blessed be He, beyond all the blessings and hymns, praises and consolations that are ever spoken in the world; and say, Amen.

May there be abundant peace from heaven, and life, for us and for all Israel; and say, Amen.

He who creates peace in His celestial heights, may He create peace for us and for all Israel; and say, Amen.

With a strong belief in an afterlife, mourning practices in Judaism are extensive, but are not an expression of fear of death. Instead they aim to show respect for the dead and to comfort the living. As an expression of respect, following death the body is never left alone and on hearing of the death, friends and relatives tear a portion of their clothes. Burial is prompt, within 2 days, and is followed by 7 days of mourning (shiva). Mourners sit on low stools or the floor instead of chairs, do not wear leather shoes, do not shave or cut their hair, do not wear cosmetics, do not work and do not do things for comfort or pleasure, such as bathe, have sex or put on fresh clothing. Mourners wear the clothes that they tore at the time of learning of the death and mirrors in the house are covered. The Jewish Kaddish prayer is recited for the first 11 months following a death by identified mourners and on each anniversary of the death (Yahrzeit). It is remarkable that there is no reference to death in the prayer but rather it focuses on the greatness of God and on a call for peace.

Box 41.2 The *Tibetan Book of the Dead* (bardo thodol)

A fundamental tenet of Buddhism is that death is not something that awaits us in some distant future, but something that we bring with us into the world and that accompanies us throughout our lives. Rather than a finality, death offers a unique opportunity for spiritual growth with the ultimate prospect of transformation into an immortal state of benefit to others. Among Tibet's many and varied religious traditions are esoteric teachings that address compassionate death including the *Tibetan Books of the Dead*. These popular texts are manuals of practical instructions for the dying, who are immediately facing death; for those who have died, who are wandering in the intermediate state between lives; and for the living, who are left behind to continue without their loved ones.

Before death, friends and relatives are encouraged to bid farewell without excess drama so that neither regret nor longing is experienced by the dying as their state of mind at death must be positive. This may be facilitated by a spiritual master (lama) whispering guiding instructions from *Liberation Through Hearing during the Intermediate State* commonly known as the *Tibetan Book of the Dead* into the dying person's ear.

Tibetan Buddhism recognizes that spiritual growth may be derived from acknowledging death and proposes detailed meditation strategies that relate to the acceptance of death in order to comprehend the nature of human existence. Four human life cycle stages are recognized: birth, the period between birth and death, death, and the interval between death and rebirth (the bardo). This post-mortem bardo lasts 7 weeks and is followed by rebirth into a worldly state that is influenced by past actions or karma. The cycle of rebirth (samsara) may be broken by enlightenment, culminating in the final liberation of Buddhahood.

🔑 **KEY POINTS**

- Death should not be formalized or sanitized, it should be individualized and end-of-life care should address the needs of the dying and include friends and family in the process
- Anticipating symptoms including pain and diminishing mobility, should be addressed in advance so that analgesia is quickly available to patients
- Logical step ladder approaches to pain should be used
- Bereavement care and support of families and carers should continue after the death

42

Cancer survivorship

Learning objectives

✓ Define cancer survivorship
✓ Recognize the late effects of treatment both physical and psychological that cancer survivors endure

A cancer survivor is thought of as someone who is living with or beyond cancer, but the term is widely interpreted as meaning someone who is alive in remission of their cancer following treatment. In the United Kingdom more than half of all adults diagnosed with cancer will be alive in remission 10 years later (46% of men and 54% of women). The 10-year overall survival following a diagnosis of cancer in adulthood has doubled in the last 40 years and it is estimated that there are over 1.1 million cancer survivors in the United Kingdom who are alive 10 years after their cancer diagnosis (Table 42.1).

These cancer survivors experience a large number of health-related issues both psychological and physical. The psychological issues encountered include the Damacles, Lazarus and guilt complexes discussed in Chapter 4. The physical health concerns encountered by cancer survivors include the late toxicities of treatment and infertility. These late toxicities are determined by the treatments administered as well as the age of the person when he or she receives the treatment. The late effects of treatment on a developing child are substantial. For example, radiotherapy can retard bone and cartilage growth, impair intellectual development and cognitive function and cause endocrine deficiencies of the thyroid gland and hypothalamus. Similarly, chemotherapy at any age may cause organ-specific damage such as pulmonary fibrosis, cardiomyopathy, peripheral neuropathy and nephrotoxicity that may be irreversible. The late toxicities of treatment include second primary cancers and infertility that are of major concerns to cancer survivors (see Chapter 3).

Table 42.1 The 10-year overall survival for common cancers in adults

Male		Female	
Tumour type	10-year overall survival	Tumour type	10-year overall survival
Melanoma	86%	Melanoma	92%
Prostate cancer	84%	Breast cancer	78%
Non-Hodgkin lymphoma	62%	Endometrial cancer	77%
Colorectal cancer	56%	Non-Hodgkin lymphoma	64%
Bladder cancer	54%	Colorectal cancer	57%
Kidney cancer	50%	Kidney cancer	49%
Leukaemia	48%	Ovarian cancer	35%
Brain cancer	13%	Brain cancer	14%
Oesophageal cancer	12%	Lung cancer	7%
Lung cancer	4%	Pancreas cancer	1%

Cancer survivors face health-related discrimination and disadvantages that can seem as unjust as racial or sexual discrimination. Insurance weighting, mortgage loading and work sick leave questioning are everyday experiences of cancer survivors. It should be noted that it is not just the cancer survivor themselves that may experience psychological problems, but also their spouses and families who have higher

Oncology: Lecture Notes, Third Edition. Mark Bower and Jonathan Waxman.
© 2015 by John Wiley & Sons, Ltd. Published 2015 by John Wiley & Sons, Ltd.
Companion Website: www.lecturenoteseries.com/oncology

levels of anxiety many years after the all-clear has sounded.

Most cancer survivors describe the process of living with cancer and enduring successful treatment as a life-changing experience and it is not uncommon for them to use the opportunity to transform themselves, either spiritually or emotionally. Cancer follow-up clinics are full of marathon running, charity donating vegetarians who foster neglected children. So cancer and its treatments can rarely be a force for good in this evil world. Your beloved authors wonder why it is necessary for a person to have cancer to value their days.

Poem written by a doctor just prior to her appointment with a surgeon to discuss treatment for recently diagnosed rectal cancer.

Question mark

Full stop

Semi-colon

New paragraph

Source: Anonymous. In: Powley E & Higson R (eds). (2005). *The Arts in Medical Education: A Practical Guide*, Vol. 1. Reproduced with permission of Radcliffe Publishing.

 KEY POINTS

- More and more people are survivors of cancer who may suffer potential long-term health issues related to treatment
- The authors congratulate you for reading this far and would like to apologize for any mistakes in the text

Index

A

abiraterone 167
ABVD regimen 242
acanthosis nigricans 310
acoustic neurofibromatosis 118
acquired ichthyosis 310
acrokeratosis paraneoplastica 310
actinomycin 173
active specific immunotherapy 88
acupuncture 100
acute lymphoblastic leukaemia (ALL) 229
acute myeloid leukaemia (AML) 227, 229–30
acute promyelocytic leukaemias (APMLs) 229
adrenal cancers
    epidemiology 203
    investigations 203
    medullary tumours 204–5
    presentation 203
    prognosis 204
    treatment 203–4
adrenocorticotrophic hormone (ACTH) 303–4
adriamycin 242
aflatoxins 133
age ranges and cancer 4
age-specific rates 3
age standardized rates 4
alcohol intake 43–4
aldosterone 112
alkylating agents 71–2
allodynia 336
alpha-foetoprotein (AFP) 293
alternative therapies 99–100
alveolar rhabdomyosarcoma 282
amyloidosis (AL) 253
anaemia 78, 332
anal cancer 13
analgesia 336
analgesic drug use 335
anaplastic large cell lymphoma 250
anaplastic lymphoma kinase (ALK) 223
anastrozole 85
androstenedione 112
aneuploid 19
Angelman syndrome 176
angiogenesis 27–8
angiokeratoma corporis diffusum (Fabry's disease) 117
angiosarcoma 132, 282
animal models for human cancers 117
Ann Arbour staging system 53
antimetabolites 71–2
apoptosis 25–6
apple core lesion 145

architecture of cancer 6
ascites 329–31
Aspergillus fumigatus 133
aspirin 144
astrocytomas 119
ataxia telangiectasia 229, 298
atrophy 8–9
    testes 10
axitinib 154

B

Barrett's oesophagus 125
    metaplasia 10
basal cell carcinoma (BCC) 258–9
    five-year survival rates 262
    presentation 259
    treatment 261–2
base excision repair (BER) 32
Bazex syndrome 310
Beau lines 78
Beckwith–Wiedemann syndrome 276
becquerel (Bq) unit 42, 64
benign tumours 11
    connective tissue 14
    epithelial 13
    germ cell 14
    haematological 14
bereavement 337
beta-2-microglobulin 293
bevacizumab 89
    breast cancer 113
    colorectal cancer 148
    kidney cancer 154
bias 93–4
bicalutamide 85
biliary tree cancers
    grading 135
    pathogenesis 132–3
    presentation 134–5
    prevention 134
    prognosis 136
    staging 135
    treatment 135–6
Birbeck granules 277
Birt-Hogg-Dubé syndrome (BHD) 152
bladder cancer
    epidemiology 155
    grading 158
    pathogenesis 155–7
    presentation 157
    staging 158

Oncology: Lecture Notes, Third Edition. Mark Bower and Jonathan Waxman.
© 2015 by John Wiley & Sons, Ltd. Published 2015 by John Wiley & Sons, Ltd.
Companion Website: www.lecturenoteseries.com/oncology

bladder cancer (*Continued*)
  treatment 158–9
  UK registration 157
bleomycin 173
  Hodgkin's lymphoma 242
  side effects 174
bone marrow transplant (BMT) 74
bone metastases 290–91
  differential diagnosis 291
bone sarcomas 281
  clinical features 283–4
  epidemiology 281
  Ewing's sarcomas 287
  investigations 284–7
  osteosarcoma 287
  pathogenesis 281–3
  presentation 283
  prognosis 288
  tumour origins 282
  UK data 283
books about cancer 5
bortezomib 35, 255
Bourneville's disease (tuberous sclerosis) 117–18
Bowen's disease 259
brachytherapy 66–7
  prostate cancer 165–6
brain cancers
  children 119
  gliomas 119
  non-glial brain tumours 119
  prognosis 123
  UK registration 117
brain metastases 290
BRCA gene mutations
  breast cancer 37, 60–1, 108
  ovarian cancer 187–8, 192
  prostate cancer 162
breaking bad news 97–8
breast cancer 12, 107
  carcinoma *in situ* 115
  diagnosis 109–10
  endocrine therapy 85–6
  epidemiology 107–8
  five-year survival 108–11
  gene expression profiles 17
  genes associated with 108
  global incidence 20
  grading 15, 110–11
  immunocytochemical staining 17
  male breast cancer 115
  metastases 113
  Paget's disease of the nipple 115
  presentation 108–9
  prognosis 111
  screening programmes 109
  staging 58, 110–11
  survival rate 57
  treatment 110–15
  UK registration 108
brentuximab 242
Breslow thickness 266–9
bupropion 217
Burkitt lymphoma (BL) 245–50
burn-out in staff 98–9
BVP regimen 174

C

cabozantinib in thyroid cancer 202
cachexia 312–13
café au lait spots 39
calcitonin 293
Campylobacter jejuni 245
cancer 3
  benign 11
  chromosomal abnormalities 18
  diagnosis 7–11
  environmental causes 37–50
  epidemiological perspective 3–4, 16–20
  experimental perspective 5
  genetic causes 35–7
  hallmarks 6–7, 22–30
  histopathological nomenclature 13–14
  histopathological perspective 6
  in situ 11
  invasive 11
  malignant 11
  molecular perspective 6–7
  reading histology reports 7–11
  sociological perspective 4
  staging 53–6, 58–9
  tumour grading 14
  unknown primary identification 14–15
  worldwide contributions 50–51
cancer antigen 125 (CA-125) 293
cancer celebrities 20–21
cancer cells 5
cancer charities 20
cancer hospitals 20
cancer of unknown primary (CUP)
  clinical sites of metastatic spread 289–91
  clinical syndromes 292–3
  epidemiology 289
  histopathological characterization 294
  investigatory approaches 294
  pathogenesis 289
  tumour markers 294
carbohydrate antigen 19-9 (CA19-9) 135–9
carcino embryonic antigen (CEA) 135, 293
carcinoid syndrome 306
carcinoid tumours 206
  comparison by site of origin 207
  investigations 207–8
  presentation 206
  prognosis 209
  treatment 208–9
cardiac tamponade 327–9
care, appropriate 52–3
cell cycle 25
central nervous system (CNS) cancers 116
  aetiology 117–18
  epidemiology 116–17
  investigation 120–22
  pathology 118–19
  presentation 119–20
  prognosis 123
  staging 120–22
  treatment 122–3
cerebral lymphoma, primary 119
cerebroretinal angiomatosis (von Hippel–Lindau syndrome)
    117–18

cervical cancer 178
  CIN 181
  diagnosis 179–80
  epidemiology 178
  grading 180–81
  pathogenesis 178–9
  presentation 179
  prevention 179
  prognosis 181
  screening 179
  staging 180
  terminal care 181–2
  treatment 181
  UK registration 179
cervical glandular intraepithelial neoplasia (CGIN) 181
cervical intraepithelial neoplasia (CIN) 163, 178–81
cervix
  dysplasia 11
  global cancer incidence 20
cetuximab 89
  colorectal cancer 148
chemical carcinogenesis 43
  diet 43–4
  initiation 43
  progression 43
  promotion 43
chemoreceptor trigger zone (CTZ) 74–5
chemotherapy 70–71
  alkylating agents 71–2
  antimetabolites 71–2
  application 73–4
  brain cancers 122
  breast cancer 113
  CNS cancers 122
  complications 242–3
  Hodgkin's lymphoma 242
  intercalating agents 71–2
  kidney cancer 154
  lung cancer 223
  mechanisms of action 71–2
  myeloma 255–7
  non-melanoma skin cancers (NMSCs) 261–2
  pancreatic cancer 139–40
  prostate cancer 167
  soft tissue sarcomas 288
  spindle poisons 71–2
  testicular cancer 173
  topoisomerase inhibitors 72
  tumour resistance 72–3
  tumour sensitivity 73
chemotherapy side effects 74
  alopecia 77–8
  anaphylaxis 75
  carcinogenic side effects 83–4
  cardiological side effects 81
  children 85
  delayed onset, children 85
  delayed onset, idiosyncratic 81–2
  delayed onset, predictable 77–81
  dermatological side effects 81
  early onset 74–7
  extravasation 75–6
  female gonadal toxicity 83
  gastrointestinal tract mucositis 80–81
  gonadal side effects, adults 82–3

gonadal side effects, children 85
  growth disorders in children 85
  hepatic side effects 82
  late onset 82–4
  male gondal toxicity 83
  myelotoxicity 78–80
  nausea and vomiting 74–5
  neurogical side effects 81–2
  onychodystrophy 78
  psychiatric dysfunction 84–5
  pulmonary side effects 82
  teratogenic side effects 83
  tumour lysis 76–7
children
  brain cancers 119
  cancer prevalence 272
  chemotherapy side effects 85
  solid tumours 271–8
chlorambucil 173
cholangiocarcinomas 136
chondrosarcoma 284
choriocarcinoma 176
choroid plexus tumours 119
chromatin modification 34
chromosomal abnormalities in cancer 18
chromosome translocation 84
chronic lymphoblastic leukaemia (CLL) 229, 232, 236–7
chronic myeloid leukaemia (CML) 229, 236–7
cisplatin
  cervical cancer 181
  gastric cancer 131
  side effects 174
  testicular cancer 173
cladribine 277
Clark's levels 266, 269
clinical trials 90
  analysis 92
  bias 93–4
  controls 92
  design 92
  endpoints 92
  ethics 91
  meta-analysis 93
  randomization 92
  result interpretation 93–4
  sample size 92
  screening 91
  side effects 93
  treatments 91–3
cluster designation (CD) 15
CMF treatment programme 113
colon cancer 32
colorectal cancer 24, 143
  diagnosis 145
  dietary intake and risk 144
  epidemiology 143
  grading 145–6
  metastatic disease 148
  pathogenesis 143–5
  presentation 145
  screening 148–50
  staging 145–6
  treatment 146–8
  UK registration 144
combination antiretroviral therapy (cART) 296, 299

common variable immunodeficiency (CVID) 296-7
communication with patients 97-8
comparative genome hybridization (CGH) 113
complementary and alternative medicine (CAM) 99-100
computed tomography (CT) scanning 53-4, 59
  brain cancers 120
connective tissue tumours 14
continuous hyperfractionated accelerated radiotherapy
    (CHART) 64
coping strategies 98
corticosterone 112
corticotrophin-releasing hormone (CRH) 304
cortisol 112
Courvousier's law 138
CpG islands 33
craniopharyngioma 119
Creutzfeldt-Jakob disease (CJD) 332
Cushing's syndrome 210, 303-4, 310
CyberKnife 122
cyclin-dependent kinase (CDK) 23
cyclin-dependent kinase (CDK) inhibitors (CKIs) 23-4
cyclophosphamide 255
  breast cancer 113
  breast cancer, high dose 114-15
cyproterone acetate 85
cytokeratins 18
cytotoxic T-lymphocyte antigen 4 (CTLA-4) 89

D

dacarbazine 242
daily care plan review 94
daratumumab 256-7
dasatinib 89
deep inferior epigastric perforator (DIEP) flap 64
dehydroepiandrosterone (DHEA) 112
deletion 19
deoxycorticosterone 112
deoxycortisol 112
deregulation of cellular metabolism 31
dermatitis herpetiformis 310
dermatomyositis 309-10
Di Bella, Luigi, cure 101
diagnosis of cancer
  benign or malignant 11
  histopathological report 7-11
diet and cancer 43-5
  colorectal cancer 144
diffuse large B-cell lymphoma (DLBL) 245-50
DiGeorge syndrome 298
dihydrofolate reductase (DHFR) 73
dihydrotestosterone 112
dilatation & curettage (D&C) 184
DNA
  chromatin modification 34
  damage recognition 32-3
  epigenetic changes 33
  hereditary repair syndromes 32
  methylation 33
  repair 31-2
  RNA interference 34
docetaxel for breast cancer 113
double minute (DM) chromosomes 275
Down's syndrome 229

ductal carcinoma *in situ* (DCIS) 11-12, 110, 115
Duncan's syndrome 297
duplication 19
Durie and Salmon staging system for myeloma 256
dysesthesia 336
dysplasia 9
  cervix 11

E

Eastern Co-operative Oncology Group (ECOG) functional
    capacity grading 57
Eaton-Lambert syndrome 218
ECF regimen 131
ECX regimen 131
electrocardiology 318
electron beam radiotherapy 66
embryonal rhabdomyosarcoma 282
emergencies in oncology 314
  anaemia 332
  ascites 329, 331
  classification 315
  hypercalcaemia 314-17
  hyperviscosity syndrome 329-30
  neutropenia 331-2
  obstructions 322-3
  pericardial effusions 327-30
  pleural effusions 324-7, 329
  spinal cord compression 320-22
  superior vena cava obstruction (SVCO) 317-21
  thrombocytopenia 332
  thromboses 323-4
  tumour lysis syndrome 317
encephalomyelitis 309
encephalotrigeminal angiomatosis (Sturge-Weber syndrome)
    117
enchondroma 285
end of life care 334
  bereavement 337
  cultural considerations 338
  dying patient care 336-7
  last hours and days 337
  pain control 334-6
endocrine therapy 85
  breast cancer 85, 86, 111-13
  prostate cancer 85-7
endometrial cancer 183
  comparison between type 1 and type 2 subtypes
    184-5
  epidemiological 183
  pathogenesis 183-4
  presentation 184
  prognosis 184-5
  treatment 184-5
  UK registration 184
endoscopic retrograde cholangiopancreatogram (ERCP) 135,
    139
enteropancreatic hormone syndrome 306
environmental causes of cancer 37
  chemical carcinogenesis 43-5
  infections 45-50
  radiation 38-43
EOX regimen 131
ependymoma 119

epidemiology of cancer 3–4
  global 16–20
  UK 16
epidermal growth factor receptor (EGFR/erbB) 23, 113, 138, 140,
    157
epigenetic DNA changes 33
epirubicin
  breast cancer 113
  gastric cancer 131
epithelial tumours 13
Epstein–Barr virus (EBV) 46–8, 238–9, 245, 296
erythema annulare centrifugum 310
erythema gyratum repens 310
erythrocyte sedimentation rate (ESR) 239
erythropoietin (EPO) 79
estradiol/oestradiol 85, 112, 162, 186
estriol 112
estrone 112
ethics 102–3
  clinical trials 91
eumelanin 264
euthanasia 101–2
everolimus for carcinoid tumours 209
evidence-based medicine 93
Ewing's sarcoma 274, 281, 285
  treatment 287
exfoliative dermatitis 310
external beam radiotherapy (EBRT) for prostate cancer
    165
extradural meningioma 119
extragonadal germ cell tumour 119
extranodal marginal zone lymphoma (MALT) 250

F

Fabry's disease (angiokeratoma corporis diffusum)
    117
faecal occult blood (FOB) 143
  screening 149–50
FAM regimen 131
familial adenomatous polyposis (FAP) 60, 144
familial atypical multiple mole-melanoma syndrome (FAMMM)
    264
Fanconi's anaemia 35
Fanconi's syndrome 229
FEC treatment programme 113
α-fetoprotein (ALP) 170
fibroblastic sarcomas 281
fibrosarcoma 282
FIGO classification 189–90
fluorodeoxyglucose-positron emission tomography (FDG-PET)
    imaging 55–6, 59–60
  brain cancers 120
5-fluorouracil (5FU) 261
  breast cancer 113
  gastric cancer 131
flushing 310
flutamide 85
FOLFIRI regimen 148
FOLFOX regimen 148
follicular lymphoma (FL) 245, 250
Frank architecture of cancer 6
functional capacity grading 57
fundamental particles 65

G

G1/S checkpoint 24–5
Gamma Knife 122
gastrectomy 130
gastric cancer
  epidemiology 128
  pathogenesis 128–9
  pathology 129
  presentation 129
  staging 129
  survival 131
  treatment 129–31
  UK registration 129
gastrinomas 138
gastro-oesophageal reflux disease (GORD) 125
gefitinib 89
gender and cancer 4
gene expression profiles 17
gene-directed enzyme prodrug therapy (GDEPT) 140
generalized melanosis 310
genetic causes of cancer
  hereditary 35
  oncogenes 35–6
  tumour suppression genes 36–7
genome instability 28, 31
  chromatin modification 34
  DNA damage recognition 32–3
  DNA methylation 33
  DNA repair 31–2
  epigenetic changes 33
  protein degradation 34–5
  RNA interference 34
germ cell tumours 14
gestational trophoblastic disease (GTD) 175
  epidemiology 175
  pathogenesis 175–6
  presentation 176–7
  prognosis 177
  treatment 177
glial tumours 119
gliomas 24, 119
  gene therapy 122–3
  prognosis 123
  treatment 122
goserelin 85
grading of tumours 14
  breast cancer 15
granulocyte colony-stimulating factor (G-CSF) 79
gray (Gy) unit 42, 64
growth suppressors 23–4
gynaecomastia 308

H

haematological tumours 14
haemopoietic stem cell transplantation 242
haematopoietic growth factors 78–9
hallmarks of cancer 6–7, 22–8
  acquisition 28–30
  emerging 31–5
Hand-Schüller-Christian syndrome 277
Hayflick limit 25
head and neck squamous cancer 24

head cancers 193–6
  anatomy 194
  epidemiology 196
  frequency 196
  pathogenesis 196
  presentation 196–7
  prognosis 196
  treatment 197–8
Helicobacter pylori 49, 128–9, 244–5
hepatitis B virus (HBV) 46–7, 132–3
  vaccination 134
hepatitis C virus (HCV) 49, 132–3
  vaccination 134
hepatobiliary cancer
  epidemiology 132
  grading 135
  pathogenesis 132–4
  presentation 134–5
  prevention 134
  prognosis 136
  staging 135
  treatment 135–6
  UK registration 132
hepatoblastomas 132–4
hepatocellular cancer (HCC) 132–3
herbalism 100
hereditary causes of cancer 35
  predisposition syndromes 37
hereditary DNA repair syndromes 32
hereditary leiomyomatosis renal cell cancer (HLRCC)
  152
hereditary non-polyposis colorectal cancer (HNPCC) 144,
  188
hereditary papillary renal cell cancer (HPRCC) 152
Hirschsprung's disease 213
hirsutism 310
histone acetyltransferase (HAT) 34
histone deacetylases (HDACs) 33–4
histone methyltransferase (HMT) 34
histopathology of cancer 6
  benign or malignant definitions 11
  nomenclature 13–14
  report reading 7–11
HIV patients 296
Hodgkin's lymphoma 238
  chemotherapy complications 242–3
  epidemiology 238
  investigation 239–40
  pathogenesis 238–9
  pathology 240
  presentation 239
  prognosis 242
  staging 240
  treatment and side effects 241–2
  UK data 239
homeopathy 99
Homer's syndrome 219
homogenously staining regions (HSR) 275
hormonal therapy for prostate cancer 166
hormone replacement therapy (HRT) 183–8
human chorionic gonadotropin (HCG) 170, 176–7, 293
human herpesvirus 8 (HHV-8/KSHV) 47–9, 245
human papillomavirus (HPV) 24, 45–6, 47, 178
  vaccination 179
human T-cell leukaemia virus type 1 (HTLV-1) 49

human T-lymphotropic virus, type I (HTLV-1) 245
5-hydroxyindole acetic acid (5HIAA) 207–8
17α hydroxypregnenolone 112
5-hydroxytryptamine (5HT; serotonin) 208
hyper IgE syndrome (HIE) 297
hyper IgM syndrome (HIM) 297
hyperalgesia 336
hypercalcaemia 314–17
  clinical features 315
hyperchromatic nuclei 7
hyperpathia 336
hyperplasia 8–9
  prostate gland 10
hypertrichosis lanuginosa 310
hypertrophic cardiomyopathy (HCM) 10
hypertrophy 8–9
hyperviscosity syndrome 329–30
hypoalgesia 336

I

imatinib 89
immune system avoidance 31
immunodeficiency-related cancers 295
  acquired or secondary immunodeficiency 296
  hereditary or primary immunodeficiency 295–6
  HIV patients 296
  management 299
  tumours in primary immunodeficiency 299
immunological therapy 87
  active specific immunotherapy 88
  non-specific immunotherapy 88–9
  passive specific immunotherapy 87–8
immunotherapy for kidney cancer 154
incidence of cancer 3
  definition 91
infections, carcinogenic
  oncogenic bacteria 49
  oncogenic DNA viruses 45–9
  oncogenic helminths 49–50
  oncogenic RNA viruses 49
inferior gluteal artery perforator (IGAP) flap 64
inflammation 30
insulin-like growth factor (IGF) 138, 140
  gestational trophoblastic disease (GTD) 176
insulinomas 138
intensity modulated radiotherapy (IMRT) 67
  mesothelioma 225
  prostate cancer 165
intercalating agents 71–2
interferon (IFN) 88–9
interleukin-2 (IL-2) 89
intracytoplasmic sperm injection (ICSI) 83
intramedullary ependymoma 119
invasion 9, 28
invasive cancers 11, 16
inversion 19
ionizing radiation
  medical sources 42
  natural sources 40–41
  nuclear warfare 41
  occupational sources 42–3
islet cell tumours 138
isochromosome 19

K

Kaposi's sarcoma (KS) 48, 258, 261
Karnofsky performance status score 57
karyotype nomenclature 19
kidney cancer
　anti-angiogenic therapy 154–5
　diagnosis 152
　epidemiology 151
　familial predisposition 152
　grading 153
　metastatic disease 154
　pathogenesis 151–2
　presentation 152
　prognosis 155
　staging 153
　targeted therapy 155
　treatment 153–4
　UK registration 152
Klinefelter's syndrome 229
Knudson's two hit hypothesis 36, 38

L

laboratory studies of cancer 5
lag time bias 94
Lambert–Eaton myasthenic syndrome 303, 308–9
Langerhans' cell histiocytosis (LCH) 277
　clinical manifestations 277
lapatinib 89
leather bottle stomach 129
leiomyosarcoma 281–2
Letterer–Siwe disease 277
leukaemias 227
　classification 231
　epidemiology 227–9
　investigations 230–31
　myeloid malignancies scheme 228
　pathogenesis 229
　presentation 229–30
　treatment 231–7
　UK data 228
linitis plastica 129
liposarcoma 281–2
Lisch nodules 39
liver cancer
　children 276–7
　epidemiology 132–4
　grading 135
　pathogenesis 132–4
　presentation 134–5
　prevention 134
　prognosis 136
　staging 135
　treatment 135–6
liver flukes 50
liver metastases 291
lobular carcinoma *in situ* (LCIS) 11–12, 110, 115
loop electrosurgical excision procedure (LEEP) 181
Louis–Bar syndrome 298
Luigi Di Bella cure 101
lumpectomy 110–11
lung cancer 214
　epidemiology 214

　global occurrence 216
　grading 220
　pathogenesis 217
　pathology 218–20
　presentation 217–18
　screening 217
　smoking 44
　staging 220
　tobacco smoking 214–17
　treatment 220–23
　UK data 215
lung metastases 291
luteinizing hormone-releasing hormone (LHRH) 83, 85, 192
luteinizing hormone-releasing hormone (LHRH) receptor
　agonists 85, 113
lymphomas
　staging 59
　WHO classification 249
lymphoplasmacytic lymphoma 250
Lynch syndrome 144, 184, 188

M

magnetic resonance imaging (MRI) 54–5
　brain cancers 120
malignant effusions 291
malignant tumours 11
　connective tissue 14
　epithelial 13
　germ cell 14
　haematological 14
mammalian target of rapamycin (mTOR) 155, 209
mammography 109
mantle cell lymphoma (MCL) 245, 250
marginal zone lymphoma (MZ) 245
medical burn-out 98–9
medulloblastoma 119
melanin 264
melanoma
　clinicopathological features 267
　epidemiology 264
　grading 266
　pathogenesis 264
　prognosis 269
　staging 265–6
　suspicious moles 265
　treatment 267–9
　UK data 265
melphalan 255
memingiomas, treatment 123
men
　benign tumours 14
　brain cancer 117
　breast cancer 115
　cancer rates 3–4
　cancer survival 215
　cancer types by age range 4
　chemotherapy side effects 83
　malignant tumours 14
　tobacco smoking 216
menigeal metastases 290
meningioma 119
　imaging 121
　presentation 120

Merkel cell carcinoma 260–61
Merkel cell polyomavirus (MCV) 261
mesothelioma 224
   asbestos types 225
   epidemiology 224
   investigations 225
   pathogenesis 224
   presentation 224
   prognosis 226
   treatment 225–6
   UK data 225
messenger RNA (mRNA) 34
meta-analyses 93
metaplasia 8–9
   Barrett's oesophagus 10
metastases 9, 28, 29–30, 289–91
   breast cancer 113
   central nervous system (CNS) cancers 116–17
   common sites 290
methotrexate for breast cancer 113
methylation of DNA 33
methyl-CpG-binding domain proteins (MBDs) 33
mismatch repair (MMR) 32
mitogen-activated protein kinase (MAPK) 200
mitosis 25
mitotane for adrenal cancers 204
mitotic figure 7
mnemonics 307
Moh's micrographic surgery 261
molecular biology of cancer 6–7
moles, suspicious 265
monoclonal antibodies 87–8
monoclonal gammopathy of undetermined significance
   (MGUS) 252, 255
MOPP regimen 242
mortality from cancer 3
Muir–Torre syndrome 310
multiple endocrine neoplasia (MEN) 201, 212–13
   features 213
mustine 242
mutations 28
myasthenia gravis 309
myelodysplastic syndromes 228
myeloma
   diagnostic criteria 255
   Durie and Salmon staging system 256
   epidemiology 252
   international staging system 256
   investigations 253
   pathogenesis 252–3
   presentation 253
   treatment 253–7
   UK data 253
myeloproliferative neoplasms 227

N

naevi 265–6
neck cancers 193–6
   anatomy 194
   epidemiology 196
   frequency 196
   pathogenesis 196
   presentation 196–7

prognosis 196
   treatment 197–8
necrolytic migratory erythema 310
nesidioblastomas 138
neuralgia 336
neuroblastoma 274–5
neuroectodermal tumours 118–19
neurofibromatosis (von Recklinghausen's disease) 117–18
neuropathic pain 336
neutropenia 79–80, 331–2
Nijmegen syndrome 298
nociception 336
non-glial brain tumours 119
non-Hodgkin's lymphoma (NHL)
   associated infections 245
   epidemiology 244
   grading 249
   pathogenesis 244–5
   staging 246–9
   subtypes 245
   treatment 249–51
   UK data 245
   WHO classification 249
non-homologous end joining (NHEJ) 31
non-islet cell tumour hypoglycaemia 306
non-melanoma skin cancers (NMSCs) 258
   epidemiology 258
   pathogensis 258–9
   presentation 259–61
   prognosis 262
   skin phototypes 262
   treatment 261–2
non-specific immunotherapy 88
   cytotoxic T-lymphocyte antigen 4 (CTLA-4) 89
   interferon (IFN) 88–9
   interleukin-2 (IL-2) 89
   programmed death 1 (PD-1) targeting 89
nuclear:cytoplasmic ratio 7
nucleoli, prominent 7
nucleotide excision repair (NER) 32

O

octreotide 141
   carcinoid tumours 209
odds 4
odds ratio 4
oesophageal cancer 124
   epidemiology 124
   five-year survival rates 127
   grading 126
   pathogenesis 124–5
   presentation 125
   prevention 125
   prognosis 127
   staging 126
   treatment 126–7
   UK registration 125
oesophagectomy 127
oestradiol/estradiol 85, 112, 162, 186
oestrogen receptors (ERs) 111
oligodendroglioma 119
oncogenes 35–6
oncogenic bacteria 49

oncogenic DNA viruses
   Epstein–Barr virus (EBV) 46–8
   hepatitis B virus (HBV) 46
   human herpesvirus 8 (HHV-8/KSHV) 48–9
   human papillomavirus (HPV) 45–6
oncogenic helminths 49–50
oncogenic RNA viruses
   hepatitis C virus (HCV) 49
   human T-cell leukaemia virus type 1 (HTLV-1) 49
oncological mnemonics 307
onco-mice 5–6
oophorectomy 113
opiate side effects 336
opsoclonus–myoclonus syndrome 309
oral cavity anatomy 194
orchidectomy 166–7
Osler–Rendu–Weber syndrome 117
osteosarcoma 274, 281, 285–7
   treatment 287
ovarian cancer 186
   epidemiology 186
   grading 190
   pathogenesis 186–8
   presentation 188–9
   screening 188
   staging 189–90
   treatment 190–92
   UK registration 187
ovarian cyst 192
overdiagnosis bias 94
owl's eyes 239

P

pachydermoperiostosis 310
paclitaxel
   breast cancer 113
   cervical cancer 181
   topotecan 181
paediatric solid tumours
   CNS tumours 272
   complications 278
   epidemiology 271
   five-year survival rates 272
   Langerhans' cell histiocytosis (LCH) 277
   liver tumours 276–7
   lymphomas 272–3
   neuroblastoma 274–5
   pathogenesis 271
   presentation and management 271–2
   retinoblastoma 276
   soft tissue sarcomas and bone tumours 273–4
   Wilm's tumours 275–6
Paget's disease of the nipple 115, 310
pain control 334–6
pain ladders 335
pain terms 336
palliative care 90–95
Pancoast tumour 219
pancreatic cancer 137
   endocrine tumours 141–2
   epidemiology 137
   familial predisposition 138
   grading 139

   pathogenesis 137–8
   presentation 138–9
   prognosis 140–41
   staging 139
   treatment 139–40
   UK registration 138
pancreatic polypeptide (PP) 141
paraesthesia 336
paranasal sinuses anatomy 195
paraneoplastic complications 303
   cachexia 312–13
   dermatological conditions 308–12
   endocrine 303–8
   neurological conditions 308–9
parathyroid cancers
   epidemiology 212
   multiple endocrine neoplasia 212–13
   pathology 212
   presentation 213
   treatment 213
particles, fundamental 65
passive specific immunotherapy 87–8
patched gene (PTC) 157
patients, communicating with 97–8
Patterson–Kelly–Brown syndrome 124
pazopanib 154
peau d'orange 112
pemphigus vulgaris 310
performance status 56–7
pericardial effusions 327–30
periodic anti-Schiff (PAS) test 231
peripheral blood stem cell transplant (PBSCT) 74
peroxisome proliferator-activated receptor (PPAR) gene 200
phaeochromocytoma 306–8
phakomatoses 117
pheomelanin 264
Philadelphia chromosome 229
pituitary adenoma 119
pituitary tumours
   clinical features 211
   epidemiology 210
   pathology 210
   treatment 210–11
placental alkaline phosphatase (PLAP) 293
platelet-derived growth factor (PDGF) 23, 28
   testicular cancer 170
pleomorphic rhabdomyosarcoma 282
pleural effusions 324–7, 329
Plummer–Vinson syndrome 124
poly-ADP ribose polymerase (PARP) inhibitors 113
polycyclic aromatic hydrocarbons (PAHs) 217
polymyositis 309
polyploid 19
positron emission tomography (PET) imaging 54–6
   brain cancers 120
post-transplantation lymphoproliferative diseases (PTLDs) 295–6
Prader-Willi syndrome 176
prednisone 242
pregnenolone 112
prevalence of cancer 3
   definition 91
procarbazine 242
progesterone 112
prognosis 57

programmed death 1 (PD-1) targeting 89
promyelocytic leukaemias (PML) 229
prostate cancer 161
   endocrine therapy 85–7
   epidemiology 161
   grading 163
   pathogenesis 161–2
   presentation 162
   prognosis 167
   screening 167–8
   staging 163, 165
   survival rate 57
   treatment 163–7
   UK registration 162
prostate gland
   global cancer incidence 20
   hyperplasia 10
prostate-specific antigen (PSA) 162–3, 293
prostatic intraepithelial neoplasia (PIN) 163
protein degradation 34–5
protein kinase inhibitors 89–90
proton beam radiotherapy 278
pruritis 310
psychological carcinogenic risk factors 96
psychological distress 96–7
psychosocial problems in cancer survivors 97

Q

quackery 100–101

R

radiation 38–9
   ionizing 40–43
   ultraviolet (UV) 39–40
radio-isotope scanning 56
radio-isotope therapy 66–8
radiology techniques 53
   computed tomography (CT) scanning 53–4
   magnetic resonance imaging (MRI) 54–5
   positron emission tomography (PET) imaging 54–6
   radio-isotope scanning 56
radiotherapy 64
   adverse reactions 69
   brachytherapy 66–7
   breast cancer 111
   cervical cancer 181
   electron beam radiotherapy 66
   fundamental particles 65
   Hodgkin's lymphoma 241–2
   lung cancer 222–3
   measurement of radiation 64–6
   mesothelioma 225
   non-melanoma skin cancers (NMSCs) 261
   radio-isotope therapy 66–8
   soft tissue sarcomas 288
   thyroid cancer 201
   tissue tolerance 69
   toxicity 68–9
   tumour resistance 70
   tumour sensitivity 70
radiotherapy units 42, 64–6

randomized controlled trials (RCTs) 92
Reed–Sternberg (RS) cells 238–9, 241
relative risk 4
replicative immortality 25–7
retinoblastoma 276
retinoblastoma protein (Rb) 23
retinopathy 309
rhabdomyosarcoma 273–4
RNA interference (RNAi) 34
Rous sarcoma virus (RSV) 35
Roux-en-y anastomosis 130

S

salivary glands
   anatomy 195
   tumours 198–9
Schistosoma haematobium 155
schistosomes 49–50
schwannoma 119
screening programmes for breast cancer 109
selective IgA deficiency 297
selective oestrogen receptor modulators (SERMs) 113
senescence 25–7
sensitivity of tests 91
sensory neuropathy 309
serotonin (5-hydroxytryptamine; 5HT) 208
serum protein electrophoresis 254
severe combined immunodeficiency (SCID) syndromes 5,
   298
sex hormone synthesis 112
shark cartilage 101
sievert (Sv) unit 42, 64
sign of Leser–Trelat 310
signal transduction pathways 23
single photon emission computerized tomography (SPECT) for
   brain cancers 120
Sipple's syndrome 213
skin phototypes 262
small lymphocyte lymphoma 245
smoking tobacco 44
   bladder cancer 155
   pancreatic cancer 137
smouldering multiple myeloma (SMM) 255
sociology of cancer 4
sociology of oncology 103
soft tissue sarcomas 281
   clinical features 282
   epidemiology 281
   metastatic disease 288
   pathogenesis 281–3
   presentation 283
   prognosis 288
   treatment 287–8
   UK data 283
sorafenib 89, 154
specificity of tests 91
spinal cord compression 320–22
spinal cord tumours 119
   presentation 120
spindle poisons 71–2
Spiroptera carcinoma 128
squamous cell carcinoma (SCC) 258–9
   five-year survival rates 262

presentation 259–60
treatment 261–2
squamous intraepithelial lesion (SIL) 178
staging cancers 53
    radiology techniques 53–6
    surgery 60–61
    tumours 53, 58–9
standardization 3
standardized ratios 4
Stein–Leventhal syndrome 184
stomach cancer global incidence 20
Sturge–Weber syndrome (encephalotrigeminal angiomatosis)
        117
subacute cerebellar degeneration 309
suberoylanilide hydroxamic acid (SAHA) 34
sunitinib 89, 154
superficial inferior epigastric artery (SIEA) flap 64
superior gluteal artery perforator (SGAP) flap 64
superior vena cava obstruction (SVCO) 317–20
    non-malignant causes 320
    stenting 321
surgery 57–60
    breast cancer 110–11
    colorectal cancer 146–7
    emergencies 62
    gastric cancer 129–30
    kidney cancer 153–4
    lung cancer 220–22
    non-melanoma skin cancers (NMSCs) 261
    oesophagectomy 127
    palliation of cancer 62–3
    pancreatic cancer 139
    prophylaxis 60–1
    reconstruction 63–4
    soft tissue sarcomas 288
    staging 60–61
    treatment for cancer 61–2
survival rates 57
survivorship 339–40
Sweet's syndrome 311
syndrome of inappropriate antidiuresis (SIAD) 304–6
synovial sarcoma 282
systemic nodular panniculitis 311

T

tamoxifen 85, 111
    endometrial cancer 184
targeted therapies for cancer 89–90
taxanes 113
T-cell lymphoma (TCL) 245
T-cell receptor (TCR) genes 15
T-cell receptors 15
teenagers and young adults (TYA)
    cancer frequency and survival 279
    epidemiology of cancers 279
    presentation and management of solid tumours 279–80
telomerase 26–7
telomers 25–7
terminal care for cervical cancer 181–2
testes, atrophy of 10
testicular cancer 169
    epidemiology 169
    grading 172

pathogenesis 169–70
presentation 170
prognosis 174
staging 170–72
treatment 172–4
testicular seminoma 60
testosterone 112
thalidomide 255
thrombocytopenia 80, 332
thrombopoietin (TPO) 79
thyroglobulin 293
thyroid cancer
    epidemiology 200
    five-year survival 201
    investigations 201
    pathogenesis 200–201
    presentation 201
    prognosis 202
    treatment 201–2
thyroid-stimulating hormone (TSH) 176
TIP regimen 174
TNM (Tumour, Nodes, Metastases) classification 53
    bladder cancer 158
    breast cancer 111
    colorectal cancer 146
    gastric cancer 129
    pancreatic cancer 139
    prostate cancer 165
tobacco smoking
    global take-up 216
    lung cancer 214–17
    oesophageal cancer 124
topoisomerase inhibitors 72
totipotential cells 13
Touraine–Solente–Golé syndrome 308
transarterial chemoembolization (TACE) 135
translocations 19
transrectal ultrasonography (TRUS) 163
transurethral resection of bladder tumour (TURBT) 158
transurethral resection of prostate (TURP) 161
transvaginal ultrasound (TVUS) 188
transverse rectus abdominis myocutaneous (TRAM) flap 63
trastuzumab 89
    breast cancer 113
treatment for cancer
    adrenal cancers 203–4
    appropriate care 52–3
    biliary tree cancers 135–6
    bladder cancer 158–9
    brain cancers 122–3
    breast cancer 110–15
    carcinoid tumours 208–9
    cervical cancer 181
    chemotherapy 70–85
    clinical trials 90, 91–4
    CNS cancers 122–3
    colorectal cancer 146–8
    endocrine therapy 85–7
    endometrial cancer 184–5
    Ewing's sarcomas 287
    gastric cancer 129–31
    gestational trophoblastic disease (GTD) 177
    head cancers 197–8
    hepatobiliary cancer 135–6
    Hodgkin's lymphoma 241–2

treatment for cancer (*Continued*)
    immunological therapy 87–9
    kidney cancer 153–4
    leukaemias 231–7
    liver cancer 135–6
    lung cancer 220–23
    melanoma 267–9
    metastatic disease 159
    myeloma 253–7
    neck cancers 197–8
    non-Hodgkin's lymphoma (NHL) 249–51
    non-melanoma skin cancers (NMSCs) 261–2
    oesophageal cancer 126–7
    osteosarcomas 287
    ovarian cancer 190–92
    palliative care 90–95
    pancreatic cancer 139–40
    parathyroid cancers 213
    performance status 56–7
    pituitary tumours 210–11
    prostate cancer 163–7
    radiotherapy 64–70
    soft tissue sarcomas 287–8
    staging 53–6
    surgery 57–64
    targeted therapies 89–90
    testicular cancer 172–4
    thyroid cancer 201–2
treatment for cancer, unconventional 99
    complementary and alternative therapies 99–100
    euthanasia 101–2
    quackery 100–101
tripe palms 311
Trousseau's sign 138
tuberous sclerosis (Bournville's disease) 117–18
tumour grading 14
    breast cancer 15
tumour lysis syndrome 317
tumour protein 53 (TP53) 32
tumour suppression genes 36–7
tumours
    staging 53–6, 58–9

U

ultraviolet (UV) radiation 39–40, 258–9
unknown primary origin cancers (CUPs)
    clinical sites of metastatic spread 289–91
    clinical syndromes 292–3
    epidemiology 289
    histopathological characterization 294

    investigatory approaches 294
    pathogenesis 289
    tumour markers 294
uric acid 76
usefulness of tests 91
uterine cancer 183

V

varenicline 217
vascular endothelial growth factors (VEGFs) 27–8, 32, 138, 140
vasoactive intestinal polypeptide (VIP) 141
video-assisted thoracoscopy (VATS) 225
vinblastine 173
    Hodgkin's lymphoma 242
vincristine 242
VIP regimen 174
von Hippel–Lindau syndrome (cerebroretinal angiomatosis) 35, 117–18, 152
von Recklinghausen's disease (neurofibromatosis) 117–18

W

Weber–Christian disease 311
Werner's syndrome 213
Whipple's procedure 139
wide local excision 110
Wilm's tumours 271, 275–6
Wiskott–Aldrich syndrome 298
women
    benign tumours 14
    brain cancer 117
    cancer rates 3, 5
    cancer survival 215
    cancer types by age range 4
    chemotherapy side effects 83
    malignant tumours 14
    tobacco smoking 216
World Health Organization (WHO) cancer priority ladder 51

X

X-linked agammaglobulinemia (XLA) 297
X-linked lymphoproliferative syndrome (XLPS) 297

Y

young adults *see* teenagers and young adults (TYA)

Printed and bound by CPI Group (UK) Ltd, Croydon, CR0 4YY

09/06/2025

14686001-0001